The ABSITE Review

Fourth Edition

The ABSITE Review

Fourth Edition

Steven M. Fiser, MD

Cardiac Surgery Specialists
Bon Secours Heart and Vascular Institute
Richmond, Virginia

Wolters Kluwer | Lippincott Williams & Wilkins
Health

Philadelphia · Baltimore · New York · London
Buenos Aires · Hong Kong · Sydney · Tokyo

Acquisitions Editor: Keith Donnellan
Product Manager: Brendan Huffman
Production Project Manager: David Orzechowski
Senior Manufacturing Coordinator: Beth Welsh
Marketing Manager: Lisa Lawrence
Senior Design Coordinator: Teresa Mallon
Production Service: Absolute Service, Inc.

Two Commerce Square
2001 Market Street
Philadelphia, PA 19103 USA
LWW.com

Third edition ©2010
Second edition ©2008
First edition ©2004

Printed in China

ABSITE is a trademark of the American Board of Surgery, Inc., which neither sponsors nor endorses this book.

Information contained in this book was obtained from vigorous review of general surgery textbooks and review books, from conferences, and from expert opinions. The ABSITE was not systematically reviewed, nor was it used as an outline for this manual.

Library of Congress Cataloging-in-Publication Data

Fiser, Steven M., 1971-
  The ABSITE review / Steven M. Fiser.—4th ed.
     p. ; cm.
  American Board of Surgery In-Training Examination review
  Includes bibliographical references and index.
  ISBN 978-1-4511-8690-1
  I. Title. II. Title: American Board of Surgery In-Training Examination review.
  [DNLM: 1. Surgical Procedures, Operative—Outlines. 2. Clinical Medicine—Outlines.
WO 18.2]
  RD37.2
  617.0076—dc23

2013008038

Care has been taken to confirm the accuracy of the information presented and to describe generally accepted practices. However, the authors, editors, and publisher are not responsible for errors or omissions or for any consequences from application of the information in this book and make no warranty, expressed or implied, with respect to the currency, completeness, or accuracy of the contents of the publication. Application of the information in a particular situation remains the professional responsibility of the practitioner.

The authors, editors, and publisher have exerted every effort to ensure that drug selection and dosage set forth in this text are in accordance with current recommendations and practice at the time of publication. However, in view of ongoing research, changes in government regulations, and the constant flow of information relating to drug therapy and drug reactions, the reader is urged to check the package insert for each drug for any change in indications and dosage and for added warnings and precautions. This is particularly important when the recommended agent is a new or infrequently employed drug.

Some drugs and medical devices presented in this publication have U.S. Food and Drug Administration (FDA) clearance for limited use in restricted research settings. It is the responsibility of the health care provider to ascertain the FDA status of each drug or device planned for use in their clinical practice.

To purchase additional copies of this book, call our customer service department at (800) 638-3030 or fax orders to (301) 223-2320. International customers should call (301) 223-2300.

Visit Lippincott Williams & Wilkins on the Internet at LWW.com. Lippincott Williams & Wilkins customer service representatives are available from 8:30 am to 6 pm, EST.

CCS0514

CONTENTS

CREDITS

FIGURE CREDITS

Figures on the page numbers listed below are reprinted with permission from: *Greenfield's Surgery: Scientific Principles & Practice, 4e,* Mulholland MW, Lillemoe KD, Doherty GM, Maier RV, Upchurch GR, eds. Philadelphia, PA: Lippincott Williams & Wilkins; 2006.
1, 2, 3, 13 (top), 66 (bottom), 72, 149, 169, 208, 221, 236, 259, 260, 263, 278

Figures on the page numbers listed below are reprinted with permission from: *Greenfield's Surgery: Scientific Principles & Practice, 5e,* Mulholland MW, Lillemoe KD, Doherty GM, Maier RV, Simeone DM, Upchurch GR, eds. Philadelphia, PA: Lippincott Williams & Wilkins; 2011.
5, 13 (bottom), 27, 38, 51, 53, 57, 62, 68, 70, 77, 88, 93, 96, 102, 106, 108, 109, 120, 127, 130, 137, 144, 147, 152, 154, 167, 171, 173, 176, 178, 179, 181, 184, 187, 188, 195, 199, 203, 206, 208, 210, 211, 213, 217, 219, 223, 226, 227, 228, 230, 231, 240, 241, 242, 243, 245, 271, 272, 276

TABLE CREDITS

The table listed below is reprinted and/or modified with permission from: *Greenfield's Surgery: Principles & Practice, 4e.* Mulholland MW, Lillemoe KD, Doherty GM, Maier RV, Upchurch GR, eds. Philadelphia, PA: Lippincott Williams & Wilkins; 2006.

Murphy JT, Gentilello LM. Shock.
79

Tables on the page numbers listed below are reprinted and/or modified with permission from: *Greenfield's Surgery: Scientific Principles & Practice, 5e,* Mulholland MW, Lillemoe KD, Doherty GM, Maier RV, Simeone DM, Upchurch GR, eds. Philadelphia, PA: Lippincott Williams & Wilkins; 2011.

Wait RB, Alouidor R. Fluids, Electrolytes, and Acid-Base Balance.
1

Kheterpal S, Rutter TW, Tremper KK. Anesthesiology and Pain Management.
27, 30 (both tables)

Wait RB, Alouidor R. Fluids, Electrolytes, and Acid-Base Balance.
34

Smith JS Jr, Frankenfield DC. Nutrition and Metabolism.
37

Galiano RD, Mustoe TA. Wound Healing.
53

Chesnut RM. Head Trauma.
59

Nathens AB, Maier RV. Critical Care.
82, 83

Sabel MS, Johnson TM, Bichakjian CK. Cutaneous Neoplams.
94

Miller BS, Gauger PG. Thyroid Gland.
123

PREFACE TO THE FIRST EDITION

Each year, thousands of general surgery residents across the country express anxiety over preparation for the American Board of Surgery In-Training Examination (ABSITE), an exam designed to test residents on their knowledge of the many topics related to general surgery.

This exam is important to the future career of general surgery residents for several reasons. Academic centers and private practices searching for new general surgeons use ABSITE scores as part of the evaluation process. Fellowships in fields such as surgical oncology, trauma, and cardiothoracic surgery use these scores when evaluating potential fellows. Residents with high ABSITE results are looked upon favorably by general surgery program directors, as high scorers enhance program reputation, helping garner applications from the best medical students interested in surgery.

General surgery programs also use the ABSITE scores, with consideration of feedback on clinical performance, when evaluating residents for promotion through residency. Clearly, this examination is important to general surgery residents.

Much of the anxiety over the ABSITE stems from the issue that there are no dedicated outline-format review manuals available to assist in preparation. *The ABSITE Review* was developed to serve as a quick and thorough study guide for the ABSITE, such that it could be used independently of other material and would cover nearly all topics found on the exam. The outline format makes it easy to hit the essential points on each topic quickly and succinctly, without having to wade through the extraneous material found in most textbooks. As opposed to question-and-answer reviews, the format also promotes rapid memorization.

Although specifically designed for general surgery residents taking the ABSITE, the information contained in *The ABSITE Review* is also especially useful for certain other groups:

- General surgery residents preparing for their written American Board of Surgery certification examination
- Surgical residents going into another specialty who want a broad perspective of general surgery and surgical subspecialties (and who may also be required to take the ABSITE)
- Practicing surgeons preparing for their American Board of Surgery recertification examination

PREFACE TO THE FOURTH EDITION

The 4th edition of The ABSITE Review is the most refined to date. It provides a very rapid review of the material found on the ABSITE while still providing sufficient explanations so the reader does not feel lost. Many of the tables and algorithms have been condensed and distilled down to relevant outlines, improving the efficiency of reading time. New sections have been added to reflect recent exams, including outlines on patient safety and surgical quality.

Again, I thank all of the residents who gave me feedback on the books or who I met at surgical meetings saying, "I used your books in residency and they were great." I am glad I could help out.

Thank you again and good luck on the ABSITE.

CELL MEMBRANE
- A **lipid bilayer** that contains protein channels, enzymes, and receptors
- **Cholesterol** increases membrane fluidity
- Cells are negative inside compared to outside; based on Na/K ATPase (3 Na^+ out/2 K^+ in)
- The **Na^+ gradient** that is created is used for **co-transport** of glucose, proteins, and other molecules

Electrolyte Concentrations of Intracellular and Extracellular Fluid Compartments		
	Extracellular Fluid (mEq/L)	**Intracellular Fluid (mEq/L)**
CATIONS		
Na^+	140	12
K^+	4	150
Ca^{2+}	5	10^{-7}
Mg^{2+}	2	7
ANIONS		
Cl^-	103	3
HCO_3^-	24	10
SO_4^{2-}	1	–
HPO_4^{3-}	2	116
Protein	16	40
Organic anions	5	–

Adapted from Wait RB, et al. Fluids and electrolytes and acid–base balance. In: Greenfield LJ, et al., eds. *Surgery: Scientific Principles and Practice*. 3rd ed. Philadelphia, PA: Lippincott Williams & Wilkins; 2001:245.

- **Desmosomes/hemidesmosomes** – adhesion molecules (cell–cell and cell–extracellular matrix, respectively), which anchor cells
- **Tight junctions** – cell–cell occluding junctions; form an impermeable barrier (eg epithelium)
- **Gap junctions** – allow communication between cells (connexin subunits)
- **G proteins** – intramembrane proteins; transduce signal from receptor to response enzyme
- **Ligand-triggered protein kinase** – receptor and response enzyme are a single transmembrane protein

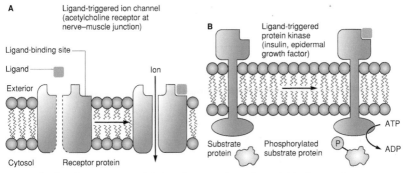

Types of cell surface receptors. *(A)* Ligand-activated ion channel; binding results in a conformational change, opening or activating the channel. *(B)* Ligand-activated protein kinase; binding activates the kinase domain, which phosphorylates substrate proteins. *(continued)*

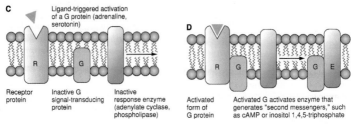

Types of cell surface receptors. (*Continued*)(*C and D*) Ligand activation of a G protein, which then activates an enzyme that generates second, or intracellular, messengers.

- ■ **ABO blood-type antigens** – glycolipids on cell membrane
- ■ **HLA-type antigens** – glycoproteins (Gp) on cell membrane
- ■ **Osmotic equilibrium** – water will move from an area of low solute concentration to an area of high solute concentration and approach osmotic equilibrium

CELL CYCLE
- ■ **G1, S** (protein synthesis, chromosomal duplication), **G2, M** (mitosis, nucleus divides)
- ■ G1 most variable, determines <u>cell cycle length</u>
- ■ **Growth factors** affect cell during G1
- ■ Cells can also go to G0 (quiescent) from G1
- ■ **Mitosis**
  - • **Prophase** – centromere attachment, spindle formation, nucleus disappears
  - • **Metaphase** – chromosome alignment
  - • **Anaphase** – chromosomes pulled apart
  - • **Telophase** – separate nucleus reforms around each set of chromosomes

NUCLEUS, TRANSCRIPTION, AND TRANSLATION
- ■ **Nucleus** – double membrane, outer membrane continuous with rough endoplasmic reticulum
- ■ **Nucleolus** – inside the nucleus, no membrane, **ribosomes** are made here
- ■ **Transcription** – DNA strand is used as a template by **RNA polymerase** for synthesis of an mRNA strand
- ■ **Transcription factors** – bind DNA and help the transcription of genes
  - • **Steroid hormone** – binds receptor in cytoplasm, then enters nucleus and acts as transcription factor
  - • **Thyroid hormone** – binds receptor in nucleus, then acts as a transcription factor
  - • Other transcription factors – AP-1, NF-κB, STAT, NFAT
- ■ **Initiation factors** – bind RNA polymerase and initiate transcription

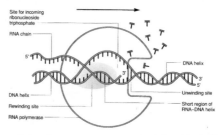

Transcription of DNA. RNA polymerase acts to unwind the DNA helix, catalyzes the formation of a transient RNA–DNA helix, and then releases the RNA as a single-strand copy while the DNA rewinds. In the process, the polymerase moves along the DNA from a start sequence to a stop sequence.

- **DNA polymerase chain reaction** – uses oligonucleotides to amplify specific DNA sequences
- **Purines** – guanine, adenine
- **Pyrimidines** – cytosine, thymidine (only in DNA), uracil (only in RNA)
  - Guanine forms 3 hydrogen bonds with cytosine
  - Adenine forms 2 hydrogen bonds with either thymidine or uracil
- **Translation** – mRNA used as a template by **ribosomes** for the synthesis of **protein**
- **Ribosomes** – have small and large subunits that read mRNA, then bind appropriate tRNAs that have amino acids, and eventually make proteins

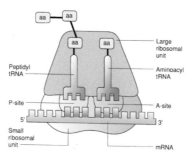

Schematic view of the elongation phase of protein synthesis on a ribosome. As the ribosome moves along the mRNA, incoming aminoacyl–tRNA complexes bind to the A-site on the ribosome, after which a new peptide bond is formed with the nascent polypeptide chain previously attached to the peptide tRNA. The ribosome then moves, ejecting the now-empty tRNA and opening the A-site for the next aminoacyl–tRNA complex.

CELLULAR METABOLISM
- **Glycolysis** – 1 glucose molecule generates 2 ATP and 2 pyruvate molecules
- **Mitochondria** – 2 membranes, Krebs cycle on inner matrix, NADH/FADH$_2$ created
  - **Krebs cycle** – the 2 pyruvate molecules (from the breakdown of 1 glucose) create NADH and FADH$_2$
  - NADH and FADH$_2$ enter the electron transport chain to create ATP
  - Overall, 1 molecule of glucose produces 36 ATP
- **Gluconeogenesis** – mechanism by which **lactic acid** (Cori cycle) and **amino acids** are converted to glucose
  - Used in times of starvation or stress (basically the glycolysis pathway in reverse)
  - **Fat and lipids** are not available for gluconeogenesis because acetyl CoA (breakdown product of fat metabolism) cannot be converted back to pyruvate
- **Cori cycle** – mechanism in which the **liver** converts **muscle lactate** into new **glucose**; pyruvate plays a key role in this process

OTHER CELL ORGANELLES, ENZYMES, AND STRUCTURAL COMPONENTS
- **Rough endoplasmic reticulum** – synthesizes proteins that are exported (increased in pancreatic acinar cells)
- **Smooth endoplasmic reticulum** – lipid/steroid synthesis, detoxifies drugs (increased in liver and adrenal cortex)
- **Golgi apparatus** – modifies proteins with carbohydrates; proteins are then transported to the cellular membrane, secreted, or targeted to lysosomes
- **Lysosomes** – have digestive enzymes that degrade engulfed particles and worn-out organelles
- **Phagosomes** – engulfed large particles; these fuse with lysosomes
- **Endosomes** – engulfed small particles; these fuse with lysosomes

- **Protein kinase C** – activated by **calcium** and **diacylglycerol** (DAG)
  - Phosphorylates other enzymes and proteins
- **Protein kinase A** – activated by **cAMP**
  - Phosphorylates other enzymes and proteins
- **Myosin** – thick filaments, uses ATP to slide along actin to cause **muscle contraction**
- **Actin** – thin filaments, interact with myosin above
- **Intermediate filaments** – keratin (hair/nails), desmin (muscle), vimentin (fibroblasts)
- **Microtubules** – form specialized cellular structures such as cilia, neuronal axons, and mitotic spindles; also involved in the transport of organelles in the cell (form a latticework inside the cell)
  - **Centriole** – a specialized microtubule involved in cell division (forms spindle fibers, which pull chromosome apart)

CHAPTER 2. **HEMATOLOGY**

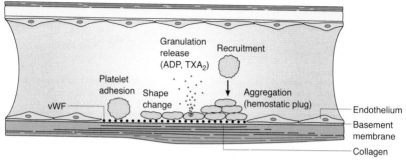

Primary hemostasis is achieved initially with a platelet aggregation as illustrated. Note that platelet adhesion, shape change, granule release followed by recruitment, and the hemostatic plug at the area of subendothelial collagen and collagen exposure are the initial events for thrombus formation.

NORMAL COAGULATION

Three initial responses to vascular injury: vascular vasoconstriction, platelet adhesion, and thrombin generation

<u>Intrinsic pathway</u>: exposed **collagen + prekallikrein + HMW kininogen + factor XII**
↓
activate XI
↓
activate IX, then add VIII
↓
activate X, then add V
↓
convert **prothrombin** (factor II) to **thrombin**
↓
thrombin then converts **fibrinogen** to **fibrin**

<u>Extrinsic pathway</u>:   **tissue factor** (injured cells) + **factor VII**
↓
activate X, then add V
↓
convert **prothrombin** to **thrombin**
↓
thrombin then converts **fibrinogen** to **fibrin**

Prothrombin complex (for intrinsic and extrinsic pathways)
    X, V, Ca, platelet factor 3, and **prothrombin**
    Forms on platelets
    Catalyzes the formation of <u>thrombin</u>

Factor X is the convergence point and is common for both paths
Tissue factor pathway inhibitor – inhibits factor X

Fibrin – links platelets together (binds GpIIb/IIIa molecules) to form <u>platelet plug</u> → hemostasis
XIII – helps crosslink fibrin

Thrombin
    Key to coagulation
    Converts **fibrinogen** to **fibrin** and fibrin split products
    Activates **factors V** and **VIII**
    Activates **platelets**

NORMAL ANTICOAGULATION
Antithrombin III (AT-III)
    Key to anticoagulation
    Binds and inhibits **thrombin**
    Inhibits **factors IX, X, and XI**
    Heparin activates **AT-III** (up to 1000× normal activity)

Protein C – vitamin K–dependent; degrades **factors V and VIII**; degrades **fibrinogen**
Protein S – vitamin K–dependent, <u>protein C cofactor</u>

Fibrinolysis
    Tissue plasminogen activator – released from endothelium and converts plasminogen to plasmin
    Plasmin – degrades **factors V and VIII, fibrinogen**, and **fibrin** → lose platelet plug
    Alpha-2 antiplasmin – natural inhibitor of plasmin, released from endothelium

---

- **Factor VII** – shortest half-life
- **Factors V and VIII** – labile factors, activity lost in stored blood, <u>activity not lost in FFP</u>
- **Factor VIII** – only factor not synthesized in liver (synthesized in **endothelium**)
- **Vitamin K–dependent factors** – II, VII, IX, and X; proteins C and S
- **Vitamin K** – takes <u>6 hours</u> to have effect
- **FFP** – effect is <u>immediate</u> and lasts 6 hours
- **Factor II** – prothrombin
- **Normal half-life** – <u>RBCs</u>: 120 days; <u>platelets</u>: 7 days; <u>PMNs</u>: 1–2 days
- **Prostacyclin** (PGI_2)
  - From **endothelium**
  - <u>Decreases platelet aggregation</u> and promotes <u>vasodilation</u> (antagonistic to TXA_2)
- **Thromboxane** (TXA_2)
  - From **platelets**
  - <u>Increases platelet aggregation</u> and promotes <u>vasoconstriction</u>
  - Triggers release of **calcium** in platelets → exposes **GpIIb/IIIa receptor** and causes platelet-to-platelet binding; platelet-to-collagen binding also occurs (**GpIb receptor**)

COAGULATION FACTORS
- **Cryoprecipitate** – contains highest concentration of **vWF-VIII**; used in <u>von Willebrand's disease</u> and <u>hemophilia A</u> (factor VIII deficiency), also has high levels of fibrinogen
- **FFP** (fresh frozen plasma) – has high levels of all coagulation factors, protein C, protein S, and AT-III
- **DDAVP** and **conjugated estrogens** – cause release of **VIII** and **vWF** from endothelium

COAGULATION MEASUREMENTS
- **PT** – measures II, V, VII, and X; fibrinogen; best for **liver synthetic function**
- **PTT** – measures most factors **except VII and XIII** (*thus does <u>not</u> pick up factor VII deficiency*); also measures fibrinogen
  - Want **PTT 60–90 sec** for routine anticoagulation
- **ACT** = activated clotting time
  - Want **ACT 150–200 sec** for routine anticoagulation, > **460 sec** for cardiopulmonary bypass
- INR > 1.5 – relative contraindication to performing surgical procedures
- INR > 1.3 – relative contraindication to central line placement, percutaneous needle biopsies, and eye surgery

BLEEDING DISORDERS
- **Incomplete hemostasis** – most common cause of surgical bleeding
- **von Willebrand's disease**
  - ***Most common congenital bleeding disorder***
  - Types I and II are autosomal dominant; type III is autosomal recessive

- vWF links **GpIb receptor** on **platelets** to **collagen**
- PT normal; PTT can be normal or abnormal
- Have long **bleeding time** (ristocetin test)
- **Type I** is **most common** (70% of cases) and often has only mild symptoms
- **Type III** causes the **most severe bleeding**
- **Type I** – reduced quantity of vWF
  - Tx: recombinant VIII:vWF, **DDAVP**, cryoprecipitate
- **Type II** – defect in vWF molecule itself, vWF does not work well
  - Tx: recombinant VIII:vWF, **cryoprecipitate**
- **Type III** – complete vWF deficiency (rare)
  - Tx: recombinant VIII:vWF; **cryoprecipitate**; *(DDAVP will <u>not</u> work)*
■ **Hemophilia A** (VIII deficiency)
- Sex-linked recessive
- Need levels 100% pre-op; keep at 80%–100% for 10–14 days after surgery
- **Prolonged PTT** and normal PT
- **Factor VIII** crosses **placenta** → newborns may not bleed at circumcision
- Hemophiliac **joint bleeding** – *do **not** aspirate*
  - Tx: ice, keep joint mobile with range of motion exercises, **factor VIII** concentrate or **cryoprecipitate**
- Hemophiliac **epistaxis**, **intracerebral hemorrhage**, or **hematuria**
  - Tx: **recombinant factor VIII** or **cryoprecipitate**
■ **Hemophilia B** (IX deficiency) – Christmas disease
- Sex-linked recessive
- Need level 100% pre-op; keep at 30%–40% for 2–3 days after surgery
- **Prolonged PTT** and normal PT
- Tx: **recombinant factor IX** or **FFP**
■ **Factor VII deficiency** – **prolonged PT** and normal PTT, bleeding tendency. Tx: **recombinant factor VII** concentrate or **FFP**
■ **Platelet disorders** – cause bruising, epistaxis, mucosal bleeding, petechiae, purpura
- **Acquired thrombocytopenia** – can be caused by H_2 blockers, heparin
- **Glanzmann's thrombocytopenia** – <u>GpIIb/IIIa receptor deficiency</u> on platelets (cannot bind to each other)
  - Fibrin normally links the GpIIb/IIIa receptors together
  - Tx: **platelets**
- **Bernard Soulier** – <u>GpIb receptor deficiency</u> on platelets (cannot bind to collagen)
  - vWF normally links GpIb to collagen
  - Tx: **platelets**
- **Uremia** – inhibits platelet function
  - Tx: **hemodialysis** (1st), DDAVP, platelets
■ **Heparin-induced thrombocytopenia** (HIT)
- Thrombocytopenia due to **antiplatelet antibodies** (IgG PF4 antibody) results in platelet destruction
- Can also cause platelet aggregation and thrombosis (HIT**T**; **T** = thrombosis)
- Forms a **white clot**
- Can occur with low doses of heparin
- Low-molecular-weight heparin has a decreased risk of causing HIT
- Tx: ***stop heparin***; start **argatroban** (direct thrombin inhibitor) to anticoagulate
■ **Disseminated intravascular coagulation** (DIC)
- **Decreased platelets, low fibrinogen, high fibrin split products**, and **high D-dimer**
- Prolonged PT and prolonged PTT
- Often initiated by **tissue factor**
- Tx: need to treat the underlying cause (eg sepsis)
■ **ASA** – stop 7 days before surgery; patients will have prolonged bleeding time
- **Inhibits cyclooxygenase** in platelets and **decreases TXA_2**
- Platelets lack DNA, so they cannot resynthesize cyclooxygenase
■ **Clopidogrel** (Plavix) - stop 7 days before surgery; ADP receptor antagonist; Tx: <u>platelets</u>

- **Coumadin** – stop 7 days before surgery, consider starting heparin while Coumadin wears off
- **Platelets** – want them $> 50,000$ before surgery, $> 20,000$ after surgery
- **Prostate surgery** – can release **urokinase**, activates plasminogen $\rightarrow$ thrombolysis
  - Tx: **ε-aminocaproic acid** (Amicar)
- **H and P** – best way to predict bleeding risk
- **Normal circumcision** – does not rule out bleeding disorders; can still have clotting factors from mother
- **Abnormal bleeding with tooth extraction or tonsillectomy** – picks up 99% patients with bleeding disorder
- **Epistaxis** – common with vWF deficiency and platelet disorders
- **Menorrhagia** – common with bleeding disorders

HYPERCOAGULABILITY DISORDERS

- Present as venous or arterial thrombosis/emboli (eg DVT, PE, stroke)
- **Factor V Leiden mutation** – 30% of spontaneous venous thromboses
  - *Most common congenital hypercoagulability disorder*
  - Causes **resistance to activated protein C**; the defect is on **factor V**
  - Tx: heparin, warfarin
- **Hyperhomocysteinemia** - Tx: **folic acid** and **B$_{12}$**
- **Prothrombin gene defect G20210 A** - Tx: heparin, warfarin
- **Protein C or S deficiency** - Tx: heparin, warfarin
- **Antithrombin III deficiency**
  - *Heparin does <u>not</u> work in these patients*
  - Can develop after previous heparin exposure
  - Tx: recombinant AT-III concentrate or FFP (highest concentration of AT-III) followed by heparin, then warfarin
- **Dysfibrinogenemia, dysplasminogenemia** – Tx: heparin, warfarin
- **Polycythemia vera** – defect in platelet function; can get **thrombosis**
  - Keep Hct < 48 and platelets < 400 before surgery
  - Tx: phlebotomy, ASA
- **Anti-phospholipid antibody syndrome**
  - Not all of these patients have SLE
  - **Procoagulant** (get prolonged PTT but are **hypercoagulable**)
  - Caused by **antibodies** to **cardiolipin** and **lupus anticoagulant** (phospholipids)
  - Dx: **prolonged PTT** (not corrected with FFP), positive Russell viper venom time, false-positive RPR test for syphilis
  - Tx: heparin, warfarin
- **Acquired hypercoagulability** – **tobacco** (most common factor causing acquired hypercoagulability), malignancy, inflammatory states, inflammatory bowel disease, infections, oral contraceptives, pregnancy, rheumatoid arthritis, post-op patients, myeloproliferative disorders
- **Cardiopulmonary bypass** – factor XII (Hageman factor) activated; results in hypercoagulable state
  - Tx: heparin to prevent
- **Warfarin-induced skin necrosis**
  - Occurs when placed on Coumadin without being heparinized first
  - Due to short half-life of proteins C and S, which are first to decrease in levels compared with the procoagulation factors; results in relative hyperthrombotic state
  - *Patients with relative **protein C deficiency** are especially susceptible*
  - Tx: heparin if it occurs; prevent by placing patient on heparin before starting warfarin
- **Key elements in the development of venous thromboses** (Virchow's triad) – stasis, endothelial injury, and hypercoagulability
- **Key element in the development of arterial thrombosis** – endothelial injury

DEEP VENOUS THROMBOSIS (DVT)
■ Stasis, venous injury, and hypercoagulability are risk factors
■ **Post-op DVT Tx:**
  • **1st** – warfarin for 6 months
  • **2nd** – warfarin for 1 year
  • **3rd** or significant PE – warfarin for lifetime
■ **Greenfield filters** – indicated for patients with either:
  • Contraindications to anticoagulation
  • Documented PE while on anticoagulation
  • Free-floating IVC, ilio-femoral, or deep femoral DVT
  • Recent pulmonary embolectomy
■ **Temporary IVC filters** can be inserted in patients at high risk for DVT (eg head injury patients on prolonged bed rest)

PULMONARY EMBOLISM (PE)
■ If the patient is in shock despite massive inotropes and pressors, go to OR; otherwise give heparin (thrombolytics have not shown an improvement in survival) or suction catheter–based intervention
■ Most commonly from the **ilio-femoral** region

HEMATOLOGIC DRUGS
■ **Procoagulant agents** (anti-fibrinolytics)
  • **ε-Aminocaproic acid** (Amicar)
    ∘ Inhibits fibrinolysis by inhibiting **plasmin**
  • Used in DIC, persistent bleeding following cardiopulmonary bypass, ***thrombolytic overdoses***
■ Anticoagulation agents
  • **Warfarin** – prevents vitamin K–dependent decarboxylation of glutamic residues on vitamin K–dependent factors
  • **Sequential compression devices** – improve venous return but also induce fibrinolysis with compression (release of tPA [tissue plasminogen activator] from endothelium)
  • **Heparin**
    ∘ Binds and activates **anti-thrombin III** (1000× more activity)
    ∘ Reversed with **protamine** (binds heparin)
    ∘ Half-life of heparin is 60–90 minutes (want PTT 60–90 seconds)
    ∘ Is cleared by the **reticuloendothelial system**
    ∘ **Long-term heparin** – osteoporosis, alopecia
    ∘ Heparin does not cross placental barrier (can be used in pregnancy) → warfarin does cross the placental barrier (not used in pregnancy)
    ∘ **Protamine** – cross-reacts with NPH insulin or previous protamine exposure; 1% get protamine reaction (hypotension, bradycardia, and decreased heart function)
  • **Low molecular weight heparin** (eg enoxaparin, fondaparinux) – lower risk of HIT compared to unfractionated heparin; binds and activates antithrombin III but increases neutralization of just **Xa** and **thrombin**; *not* reversed with protamine
  • **Argatroban** – reversible direct thrombin inhibitor; metabolized in the **liver**, half-life is 50 minutes, often used in patients w/ **HITT**
  • **Bivalirudin** (Angiomax) – reversible direct thrombin inhibitor, metabolized by **proteinase enzymes** in the blood; half-life is 25 minutes
  • **Hirudin** (Hirulog; from leeches) – irreversible direct thrombin inhibitor; also the most potent direct inhibitor of thrombin; high risk for bleeding complications
  • **Ancrod** – Malayan pit viper venom; stimulates tPA release
■ **Thrombolytics**
  • **Streptokinase** (has high antigenicity), **urokinase**, and **tPA** (tissue plasminogen activator)

- All activate **plasminogen**
- Need to follow **fibrinogen levels** – fibrinogen < 100 associated with increased risk and severity of bleeding
- *Tx for thrombolytic overdose – ε-aminocaproic acid (Amicar)*

Degree	Contraindications
Contraindications to Thrombolytic Use (Urokinase, Streptokinase, tPA)	
Absolute	Active internal bleeding; recent CVA or neurosurgery (< 3 mo); intracranial pathology; recent GI bleeding
Major	Recent (< 10 d) surgery, organ biopsy, or obstetric delivery; left heart thrombus; active peptic ulcer; recent major trauma; uncontrolled hypertension; recent eye surgery
Minor	Minor surgery; recent CPR; atrial fibrillation with mitral valve disease; bacterial endocarditis; hemostatic defects (ie renal or liver disease); diabetic hemorrhagic retinopathy; pregnancy

Modified. Data from NIH Consensus Development Conference. Thrombolytic therapy in treatment. *Ann Intern Med.* 1980;93:141.

CHAPTER 3. BLOOD PRODUCTS

All blood products carry the risk of HIV and hepatitis except **albumin** and **serum globulins** (these are heat treated).

Donated blood is screened for HIV, HepB, HepC, HTLV, syphilis, and West Nile virus.

CMV-negative blood – use in low-birth-weight infants, bone marrow transplant patients, and other transplant patients

Clerical error leading to **ABO incompatibility** is #1 cause of death from transfusion reaction

Type O blood – universal donor, contains no antigens; **Type AB blood** – contains both A and B antigens

Stored blood is low in 2,3-DPG → causes left shift (increased affinity for oxygen)

HEMOLYSIS REACTIONS

- **Acute hemolysis** – from **ABO incompatibility**; antibody mediated
  - Back pain, chills, tachycardia, fever, hemoglobinuria
  - Can lead to ATN, DIC, shock
  - **Haptoglobin < 50** mg/dL (binds Hgb, then gets degraded), **free hemoglobin > 5** g/dL, increase in **unconjugated bilirubin**
  - Tx: fluids, diuretics, HCO_3^-, pressors, histamine blockers (Benadryl)
  - In anesthetized patients, transfusion reactions may present as **diffuse bleeding**
- **Delayed hemolysis** – antibody-mediated against minor antigens
  - Tx: observe if stable
- **Nonimmune hemolysis** – from squeezed blood
  - Tx: fluids and diuretics

OTHER REACTIONS

- **Febrile nonhemolytic transfusion reaction** – *most common transfusion reaction*
  - Usually **recipient antibody** reaction against **donor WBCs**
  - Tx: discontinue transfusion if patient had previous transfusions or if it occurs soon after transfusion has begun
  - Use WBC filters for subsequent transfusions
- **Anaphylaxis** – bronchospasm, hypotension, urticaria
  - Usually **recipient antibodies** against **donor IgA** in an IgA-deficient recipient
  - Tx: fluids, Lasix, pressors, steroids, epinephrine, histamine blockers (Benadryl)
- **Urticaria** – usually nonhemolytic
  - Usually **recipient antibodies** against **donor plasma proteins** or **IgA** in an IgA-deficient patient
  - Tx: histamine blockers (Benadryl), supportive
- **Transfusion-related acute lung injury** (TRALI) – rare
  - Caused by <u>**donor**</u> antibodies to <u>**recipient's**</u> WBCs, clot in pulmonary capillaries

OTHER TRANSFUSION PROBLEMS

- **Cold** – **poor clotting** can be caused by cold products or cold body temperature; patient needs to be warm to clot correctly
- **Dilutional thrombocytopenia** – occurs after 10 units of PRBCs
- **Hypocalcemia** – can cause poor clotting; occurs with massive transfusion; Ca is required for the clotting cascade
- Most common bacterial contaminate – **GNRs** (usually *E. coli*)
- Most common blood product source of contamination – **platelets** (not refrigerated)
- **Chagas' disease** – can be transmitted with blood transfusion

T CELLS (THYMUS) – CELL-MEDIATED IMMUNITY
- **Helper T cells** (CD4)
  - Release **IL-2**, which mainly causes maturation of **cytotoxic T cells**
  - Release **IL-4**, which mainly causes **B-cell** maturation into **plasma cells**
  - Involved in **delayed-type hypersensitivity** (brings in inflammatory cells by chemokine secretion)
- **Suppressor T cells** (CD8) – regulate CD4 and CD8 cells
- **Cytotoxic T cells** (CD8) – recognize and attack non–self-antigens attached to **MHC class I receptors** (eg viral gene products)
- **Intradermal skin test** (ie TB skin test) – used to test cell-mediated immunity
- *Infections associated with defects in cell-mediated immunity – intracellular pathogens (TB, viruses)*

B CELLS (BONE) – ANTIBODY-MEDIATED IMMUNITY (HUMORAL)
- IL-4 from helper T cells stimulates B cells to become plasma cells (antibody secreting)

MHC CLASSES
- **MHC class I** (A, B, and C)
  - **CD8** cell activation
  - Present on **all nucleated cells**
  - Single chain with 5 domains
  - *Target for cytotoxic T cells (binds T cell receptor)*
- **MHC class II** (DR, DP, and DQ)
  - **CD4** cell activation
  - Present on **antigen-presenting cells** (eg monocytes, dendrites)
  - 2 chains with 4 domains each
  - *Activates helper T cells (binds T cell receptor)*
  - *Stimulates antibody formation after interaction with B cell surface IgM*

Viral infection – endogenous viral proteins produced, are bound to class I MHC, go to cell surface, and are recognized by CD8 cytotoxic T cells

Bacterial infection – endocytosis, proteins get bound to class II MHC molecules, go to cell surface, recognized by CD4 helper T cells → B cells which have already bound to the antigen are then activated by the CD4 helper T cells; they then produce the antibody to that antigen and are transformed to plasma cells and memory B cells

NATURAL KILLER CELLS
- Not restricted by MHC, do not require previous exposure, do not require antigen presentation
- Not considered T or B cells
- *Recognize cells that **lack self-MHC***
- Part of the body's natural immunosurveillance for cancer

ANTIBODIES
- **IgM** – initial antibody made after exposure to antigen. It is the largest antibody, having 5 domains (10 binding sites)
- **IgG** – most abundant antibody in body. Responsible for secondary immune response. Can cross the placenta and provides protection in newborn period

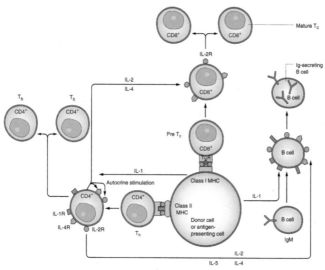

T-cell and B-cell activation. Two signals are required. First, alloantigen binds to antigen-specific receptors—the TCR (T cells) or surface IgM (B cells). The second, or costimulatory, signal is provided by IL-1 released by the antigen-presenting cell. CD4 helper T cells (T_h) release IL-2 and IL-4, which provide help for CD8 T cells (T_c) and for B-cell activation.

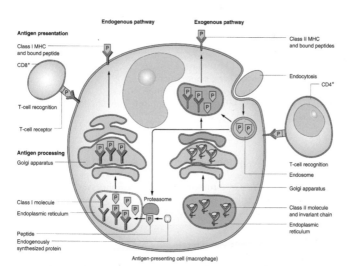

Antigen processing and presentation. <u>Endogenously</u> synthesized or intracellular proteins are degraded into peptides that are transported to the ER. These peptides bind to **class I MHC** molecules and are transported to the surface of the antigen-presenting cell. CD8$^+$ cells recognize the foreign peptide bound to class I MHC by way of the TCR complex. <u>Exogenous</u> antigen is endocytosed and broken down into peptide fragments in endosomes. **Class II MHC** molecules are transported to the endosome, bind the peptide, and are delivered to the surface of the antigen-presenting cell, where they are recognized by CD4$^+$ cells.

- **IgA** – found in secretions, in Peyer's patches in gut, and in breast milk (additional source of immunity in newborn); helps prevent microbial adherence and invasion in gut
- **IgD** – membrane-bound receptor on B cells (serves as an antigen receptor)
- **IgE** – allergic reactions, parasite infections (see table on hypersensitivity reactions, below)
- **IgM** and **IgG** are **opsonins**
- **IgM** and **IgG** fix **complement** (requires 2 IgGs or 1 IgM)
- **Variable region** – antigen recognition
- **Constant region** – recognized by PMNs and macrophages
  - Fc fragment does <u>not</u> carry variable region
- **Polyclonal antibodies** have multiple binding sites to the antigen at multiple epitopes
- **Monoclonal antibodies** have only 1 binding site to 1 epitope

Hypersensitivity Reactions		
Type	Description	Examples
I	**Immediate hypersensitivity reaction** (allergic reaction) **eosinophils** have IgE receptors for the antigen and release major basic protein, which in turns activates **mast cells** and **basophils**, with release histamine, serotonin, and bradykinin	Bee stings, peanuts, hay fever
II	**IgG or IgM reacts with cell-bound antigen**	ABO blood incompatibility, Graves' disease, myasthenia gravis
III	**Immune complex deposition**	Serum sickness, SLE
IV	**Delayed-type hypersensitivity** – antigen stimulation of previously sensitized T cells	TB skin test (PPD), contact dermatitis

- **Basophils** – major source of histamine in blood
- **Mast cells** – major source of histamine in tissue
- **Primary lymphoid organs** – liver, bone, thymus
- **Secondary lymphoid organs** – spleen and lymph nodes
- **Immunologic chimera** – 2 different cell lines in one individual (eg bone marrow transplant patients)

IL-2
- Converts lymphocytes to **lymphokine-activated killer** (LAK) cells by enhancing their immune response to tumor
- Also converts lymphocytes into **tumor-infiltrating lymphocytes** (TILs)
- Has shown some success for melanoma

TETANUS
- **Non–tetanus-prone wounds** – give **tetanus toxoid** only if patient has received < 3 doses or tetanus status is unknown
- **Tetanus-prone wounds** (> 6 hours old; obvious contamination and devitalized tissue; crush, burn, frostbite, or missile injuries) – always give **tetanus toxoid** unless patient has had ≥ 3 doses and it has been < 5 years since last booster
- **Tetanus immune globulin** – give only with tetanus-prone wounds in patients who have not been immunized or if immunization status is unknown

Malnutrition – most common immune deficiency; leads to infection

MICROFLORA
- Stomach – virtually sterile; some GPCs, some yeast
- Proximal small bowel – 10^5 bacteria, mostly GPCs
- Distal small bowel – 10^7 bacteria, GPCs, GPRs, GNRs
- Colon – 10^{11} bacteria, almost all anaerobes, some GNRs, GPCs
- **Anaerobes** (anaerobic bacteria)
  - Most common organisms in the GI tract
  - More common than aerobic bacteria in the colon (1,000:1)
  - *Bacteroides fragilis* – most common anaerobe in the colon
- *Escherichia coli* – most common aerobic bacteria in the colon

FEVER
- MC fever source **within 48 hours**   **Atelectasis**
- MC fever source **48 hours – 5 days**   **Urinary tract infection**
- MC fever source **after 5 days**   **Wound infection**

GRAM-NEGATIVE SEPSIS
- *E. coli* most common
- **Endotoxin** (lipopolysaccharide **lipid A**) is released
- Endotoxin triggers the release of **TNF-α** (from macrophages), activates complement, and activates coagulation cascade
- Early gram-negative sepsis – ↓ insulin, ↑ glucose (impaired utilization)
- Late gram-negative sepsis – ↑ insulin, ↑ glucose secondary to insulin resistance
- **Hyperglycemia** – often occurs just before the patient becomes clinically septic
- **Optimal glucose level in a septic patient** – 100–120 mg/dL

CLOSTRIDIUM DIFFICILE COLITIS
- Dx: *C. difficile* toxin
- Tx: **oral** – vancomycin or Flagyl; **IV** – Flagyl; lactobacillus can also help
- Stop other antibiotics or change them

ABSCESSES
- 90% of abdominal abscesses have anaerobes
- 80% of abdominal abscesses have both anaerobic and aerobic bacteria
- Abscesses are treated by **drainage**
- Usually occur **7–10 days** after operation
- Antibiotics for an abscess are needed in patients with diabetes, cellulitis, clinical signs of sepsis, fever, elevated WBC, or who have bioprosthetic hardware (eg mechanical valves, hip replacements)

WOUND INFECTION (SURGICAL SITE INFECTION)
- **Clean** (hernia): 2%
- **Clean contaminated** (elective colon resection with prepped bowel): 3%–5%
- **Contaminated** (gunshot wound to colon with repair): 5%–10%
- **Gross contamination** (abscess): 30%

- **Prophylactic antibiotics** are given to **prevent surgical site infections** (stop **within 24 hours** of end operation time, except cardiac, which is stopped within 48 hours of end operation time)
- *Staphylococcus aureus* – <u>coagulase-positive</u>
  - **Most common organism overall** in surgical wound infections
- *Staphylococcus epidermidis* – <u>coagulase-negative</u>
- **Exoslime** released by staph species is an **exopolysaccharide matrix**
- *E. coli* – most common **GNR** in surgical wound infections
- *B. fragilis* – most common **anaerobe** in surgical wound infections
  - Recovery from tissue indicates necrosis or abscess (only grows in low redox state)
  - Also implies translocation from the gut
- $\geq 10^5$ **bacteria** needed for wound infection; less bacteria is needed if foreign body present
- **Risk factors for wound infection**: long operations, hematoma or seroma formation, advanced age, chronic disease (eg COPD, renal failure, liver failure, diabetes mellitus), malnutrition, immunosuppressive drugs
- **Surgical infections within 48 hours of procedure**
  - **Injury to bowel** with leak
  - **Invasive soft tissue infection** – *Clostridium perfringens* and beta-hemolytic strep can present within hours postoperatively (produce exotoxins)
- Most common infection in surgery patients – **urinary tract infection**
  - Biggest risk factor – **urinary catheters**; most commonly *E. coli*
- Leading cause of infectious death after surgery – **nosocomial pneumonia**
  - Related to the length of ventilation; aspiration from duodenum thought to have a role
  - Most common organisms in ICU pneumonia – **#1 *S. aureus***, #2 *Pseudomonas*
  - GNRs #1 class of organisms in ICU pneumonia

LINE INFECTIONS
- **#1 *S. epidermidis***, #2 *S. aureus*, #3 yeast
- **Femoral lines** at higher risk for infection compared to subclavian and intrajugular lines
- 50% line salvage rate with antibiotics; much less likely with yeast line infections
- **Central line cultures**: > 15 colony forming units = line infection → need new site
- **Site shows signs of infection** → move to new site
- If worried about line infection, best to pull out the central line and place peripheral IVs if central line not needed

NECROTIZING SOFT TISSUE INFECTIONS
- Beta-hemolytic *Streptococcus* (group A), *C. perfringens*, or mixed organisms
- Usually occur in patients who are immunocompromised (diabetes mellitus) or who have poor blood supply
- Can present very quickly after surgical procedures (within hours)
- Pain out of proportion to skin findings, WBCs > 20, thin gray drainage, can have skin blistering/necrosis, induration and edema, crepitus or soft tissue gas on x-ray, can be septic
- **Necrotizing fasciitis** – usually **beta-hemolytic group A strep**; can be poly-organismal
  - Overlying skin may be pale red and progress to purple with blister or bullae development
  - Overlying skin can look normal in the early stages
  - Thin, gray, foul-smelling drainage; crepitus
  - Beta-hemolytic group A strep has **exotoxin**
  - Tx: **early debridement**, high-dose penicillin; may want broad spectrum if thought to be poly-organismal

- **C. perfringens infections**
  - **Necrotic tissue** decreases oxidation-redux potential, setting up environment for C. perfringens
  - C. perfringens has **alpha toxin**
  - Pain out of proportion to exam; may not show skin signs with deep infection
  - Gram stain shows GPRs without WBCs
  - **Myonecrosis** and **gas gangrene** – common presentations
  - Can occur with farming injuries
  - Tx: **early debridement**, high-dose penicillin
- **Fournier's gangrene**
  - Severe infection in perineal and scrotal region
  - Risk factors – diabetes mellitus and immunocompromised state
  - Caused by mixed organisms (GPCs, GNRs, anaerobes)
  - Tx: **early debridement**; try to preserve testicles if possible; antibiotics
- **Mixed organism infection** can also cause necrotizing soft tissue infections

FUNGAL INFECTION

- Need fungal coverage for positive blood cultures, 2 sites other than blood, 1 site with severe symptoms, endophthalmitis, or patients on prolonged bacterial antibiotics with failure to improve
- **Actinomyces** (not a true fungus) – pulmonary symptoms most common; can cause tortuous abscesses in cervical, thoracic, and abdominal areas
  - Tx: **drainage** and **penicillin G**
- **Nocardia** (not a true fungus) – pulmonary and CNS symptoms most common
  - Tx: **drainage** and **sulfonamides** (Bactrim)
- **Candida** – common inhabitant of the respiratory tract
  - Tx: **fluconazole** (some *Candida* resistant), **anidulafungin** for severe infections
- **Aspergillosis**
  - Tx: **voriconazole** for severe infections
- **Histoplasmosis** – pulmonary symptoms usual; Mississippi and Ohio River valleys
  - Tx: **liposomal amphotericin** for severe infections
- **Cryptococcus** – CNS symptoms most common; usually in AIDS patients
  - Tx: **liposomal amphotericin** for severe infections
- **Coccidioidomycosis** – pulmonary symptoms; Southwest
  - Tx: **liposomal amphotericin** for severe infections

SPONTANEOUS BACTERIAL PERITONITIS (SBP; PRIMARY)

- **Low protein** (< 1 g/dL) in peritoneal fluid – risk factor
- **Monobacterial** (50% *E. coli*, 30% *Streptococcus*, 10% *Klebsiella*)
- Secondary to decreased host defenses (intrahepatic shunting, impaired bactericidal activity in ascites); <u>not</u> due to transmucosal migration
- Fluid cultures are negative in many cases
- **PMNs > 500 cells/cc** diagnostic
- Tx: **ceftriaxone** or other 3rd-generation cephalosporin
- Need to rule out intra-abdominal source (eg bowel perforation) if not getting better on antibiotics or if cultures are polymicrobial
- Liver transplantation not an option with active infection
- **Fluoroquinolones** good for **prophylaxis** (norfloxacin)

SECONDARY BACTERIAL PERITONITIS

- Intra-abdominal source (implies perforated viscus)
- Polymicrobial – *B. fragilis*, *E. coli*, *Enterococcus* most common organisms
- Tx: usually need laparotomy to find source

HIV
- **Exposure risk**
  - HIV blood transfusion 70%
  - Infant from positive mother 30%
  - Needle stick from positive patient 0.3%
  - Mucous membrane exposure 0.1%
  - Seroconversion occurs in 6–12 weeks
  - **AZT** (zidovudine, reverse transcriptase inhibitor) and **ritonavir** (protease inhibitor) can help decrease seroconversion after exposure
  - Antivirals should be given within 1–2 hours of exposure
- **Opportunistic infections** – most common cause for laparotomy in HIV patients (CMV infection most common)
  - Neoplastic disease – 2nd most common reason for laparotomy
- **CMV colitis** – most common intestinal manifestation of AIDS (can present with pain, bleeding, or perforation)
- **Kaposi's sarcoma** – MC neoplasm in AIDS patients (although surgery rarely needed)
- **Lymphoma in HIV patients** – <u>stomach</u> most common followed by rectum
  - Mostly non-Hodgkin's (B cell)
  - Tx: chemotherapy usual; may need surgery with significant bleeding or perforation
- **GI bleeds – lower GI bleeds** are more common than upper GI bleeds in HIV patients
  - **Upper GI bleeds** – <u>Kaposi's sarcoma</u>, lymphoma
  - **Lower GI bleeds** – <u>CMV</u>, bacterial, HSV
- **CD4 counts**: 800–1,200 normal; 300–400 symptomatic disease; < 200 opportunistic infections

HEPATITIS C
- Now rarely transmitted with blood transfusion (0.0001%/unit)
- 1%–2% of population infected
- Fulminant hepatic failure <u>rare</u>
- <u>Chronic infection</u> in 60%; <u>cirrhosis</u> in 15%; <u>hepatocellular carcinoma</u> in 1%–5%
- Interferon may help prevent development of cirrhosis

OTHER INFECTIONS
- **Brown recluse spider bites** – Tx: **dapsone** initially; may need resection of area and skin graft for large ulcers later
- **Acute septic arthritis** – *Gonococcus*, staph, *H. influenzae*, strep
  - Tx: **drainage**, 3rd-generation cephalosporin and vancomycin until cultures show organism
- **Diabetic foot infections** – mixed staph, strep, GNRs, and anaerobes
  - Tx: broad-spectrum antibiotics (Unasyn)
- **Cat/dog/human bites** – polymicrobial
  - *Eikenella* found only in human bites; can cause permanent joint injury
  - *Pasteurella multocida* found in cat and dog bites
  - Tx: broad-spectrum antibiotics (Augmentin)
- **Impetigo, erysipelas, cellulitis**, and **folliculitis** – staph and strep most common
- **Furuncle** – boil; usually *S. epidermidis* or *S. aureus*. Tx: drainage ± antibiotics
- **Carbuncle** – a multiloculated furuncle
- **Peritoneal dialysis catheter infections**
  - *S. aureus* and *S. epidermidis* most common
  - Fungal infections hard to treat
  - Tx: intraperitoneal vancomycin and gentamicin; increased dwell time and intraperitoneal heparin may help
  - Removal of catheter for peritonitis that lasts for 4–5 days

- Fecal peritonitis requires laparotomy to find perforation
- Some say need removal of peritoneal dialysis catheter for all fungal, tuberculous, and *Pseudomonas* infections

■ **Sinusitis**
  - **Risk factors** – nasoenteric tubes, intubation, patients with severe facial fractures
  - Usually polymicrobial
  - CT head shows air–fluid levels in the sinus
  - Tx: broad-spectrum antibiotics; rare to have to tap sinus percutaneously for systemic illness

■ Use **clippers** preoperatively instead of razors to decrease chance of wound infection

■ **Antiseptic** – kills and inhibits organisms on body
■ **Disinfectant** – kills and inhibits organisms on inanimate objects
■ **Sterilization** – all organisms killed
■ **Common antiseptics in surgery**
  • **Iodophors** (Betadine) – good for GPCs and GNRs; poor for fungi
  • **Chlorhexidine gluconate** (Hibiclens) – good for GPCs, GNRs, and fungi

MECHANISM OF ACTION
■ **Inhibitors** of **cell wall synthesis** – penicillins, cephalosporins, carbapenems, monobactams, vancomycin
■ **Inhibitors** of the **30s ribosome and protein synthesis** – tetracycline, aminoglycosides (tobramycin, gentamicin), linezolid
■ **Inhibitors** of the **50s ribosome and protein synthesis** – erythromycin, clindamycin, Synercid
■ **Inhibitor** of **DNA helicase** (DNA gyrase) – quinolones
■ **Inhibitor** of **RNA polymerase** – rifampin
■ **Produces oxygen radicals** that **breakup DNA** – metronidazole (Flagyl)
■ **Sulfonamides** – PABA analogue, inhibits purine synthesis
■ **Trimethoprim** – inhibits dihydrofolate reductase, which inhibits purine synthesis
■ **Bacteriostatic antibiotics** – tetracycline, clindamycin, erythromycin (all have reversible ribosomal binding), Bactrim
■ **Aminoglycosides** – have irreversible binding to ribosome and are considered **bactericidal**

MECHANISM OF ANTIBIOTIC RESISTANCE
■ **PCN resistance** – due to plasmids for beta-lactamase
■ **Transfer of plasmids** – most common method of antibiotic resistance
■ **Methicillin-resistant *S. aureus*** (MRSA) – resistance caused by a **mutation of cell wall-binding protein**
■ **Vancomycin-resistant *Enterococcus*** (VRE) – resistance caused by a **mutation in cell wall–binding protein**
■ **Gentamicin resistance** – resistance due to modifying enzymes leading to a **decrease in active transport of gentamicin** into the bacteria

APPROPRIATE DRUG LEVELS
■ **Vancomycin** – peak 20–40 μg/mL; trough 5–10 μg/mL
■ **Gentamicin** – peak 6–10 μg/mL; trough < 1 μg/mL
■ **Peak too high** → decrease amount of each dose
■ **Trough too high** → decrease frequency of doses (increase time interval between doses)

SPECIFIC ANTIBIOTICS
■ **Penicillin**
  • **GPCs** – streptococci, syphilis, *Neisseria meningitides* (GPR), *Clostridium perfringens* (GPR), beta-hemolytic *Streptococcus*, anthrax
  • Not effective against *Staphylococcus* or *Enterococcus*
■ **Oxacillin** and **nafcillin**
  • **Anti-staph** penicillins (staph only)

- **Ampicillin** and **amoxicillin**
  - Same as penicillin but also picks up <u>enterococci</u>
- **Unasyn** (ampicillin/sulbactam) and **Augmentin** (amoxicillin/clavulanic acid)
  - Broad spectrum – pick up **GPCs** (staph and strep), **GNRs**, ± anaerobic coverage
  - Effective for enterococci; <u>not</u> effective for *Pseudomonas, Acinetobacter,* or *Serratia*
  - **Sulbactam** and **clavulanic acid** are beta-lactamase inhibitors
- **Ticarcillin** and **piperacillin** (antipseudomonal penicillins)
  - **GNRs** – enterics, *Pseudomonas, Acinetobacter,* and *Serratia*
  - Side effects: **inhibits platelets**; high salt load
- **Timentin** (ticarcillin/clavulanic acid) and **Zosyn** (piperacillin/sulbactam)
  - Broad spectrum – pick up **GPCs** (staph and strep), **GNRs**, and **anaerobes**
  - Effective for enterococci; effective for *Pseudomonas, Acinetobacter,* and *Serratia*
  - Side effects: **inhibits platelets**; high salt load
  - **Zosyn** has **QID dosing**
- **First-generation cephalosporins** (cefazolin, cephalexin)
  - **GPCs** – staph and strep
  - <u>Not</u> effective for *Enterococcus*; does not penetrate CNS
  - Ancef (cefazolin) has the longest half-life → best for prophylaxis
- **Second-generation cephalosporins** (cefoxitin, cefotetan, cefuroxime)
  - **GPCs, GNRs,** ± anaerobic coverage; lose some staph activity
  - <u>Not</u> effective for *Enterococcus, Pseudomonas, Acinetobacter,* or *Serratia*
  - Effective only for community-acquired GNRs
  - Cefotetan has longest half-life → best for prophylaxis
- **Third-generation cephalosporins** (ceftriaxone, ceftazidime, cefepime, cefotaxime)
  - **GNRs** mostly, ± anaerobic coverage
  - <u>Not</u> effective for *Enterococcus*; effective for *Pseudomonas, Acinetobacter,* and *Serratia*
  - Side effects: **cholestatic jaundice**, sludging in gallbladder (ceftriaxone)
- **Monobactam** (aztreonam)
  - **GNRs**; picks up *Pseudomonas, Acinetobacter,* and *Serratia*
- **Carbapenems** (meropenem, imipenem) – is given with cilastatin
  - Broad spectrum – **GPCs, GNRs,** and **anaerobes**
  - <u>Not</u> effective for **MEP**: MRSA, *Enterococcus,* and *Proteus*
  - **Cilastatin** – prevents renal hydrolysis of the drug and increases half-life
  - Side effects: **seizures**
- **Bactrim** (Trimethoprim/sulfamethoxazole)
  - **GNRs,** ± GPCs
  - <u>Not</u> effective for *Enterococcus, Pseudomonas, Acinetobacter,* and *Serratia*
  - Side effects (numerous): teratogenic, allergic reactions, renal damage, Stevens–Johnson syndrome (erythema multiforme), hemolysis in G6PD-deficient patients
- **Quinolones** (ciprofloxacin, levofloxacin, norfloxacin)
  - Some **GPCs**, mostly **GNRs**
  - <u>Not</u> effective for *Enterococcus*; picks up *Pseudomonas, Acinetobacter,* and *Serratia*
  - 40% of MRSA sensitive; same efficacy PO and IV
  - **Ciprofloxacin** has **BID dosing**; **levofloxacin** has **QD** dosing
- **Aminoglycosides** (gentamicin, tobramycin)
  - **GNRs**
  - Good for *Pseudomonas, Acinetobacter,* and *Serratia*; not effective for anaerobes (need O_2)
  - Resistance due to **modifying enzymes** leading to **decreased active transport**
  - Synergistic with ampicillin for *Enterococcus*
  - Beta-lactams (ampicillin, amoxicillin) facilitate aminoglycoside penetration
  - Side effects: reversible **nephrotoxicity**, irreversible **ototoxicity**

- **Erythromycin** (macrolides)
  - **GPCs;** best for community-acquired pneumonia and atypical pneumonias
  - Side effects: **nausea** (PO), **cholestasis** (IV)
  - Also binds motilin receptor and is **prokinetic** for bowel
- **Vancomycin** (glycopeptides)
  - **GPCs,** *Enterococcus, Clostridium difficile* (with PO intake), MRSA
  - Binds cell wall proteins
  - Resistance develops from a **change in cell wall–binding protein**
  - Side effects: HTN, **Redman syndrome** (histamine release), nephrotoxicity, ototoxicity
- **Synercid** (streptogramin – quinupristin-dalfopristin)
  - **GPCs;** includes MRSA, VRE
- **Linezolid** (oxazolidinones)
  - **GPCs;** includes MRSA, VRE
- **Tetracycline**
  - **GPCs, GNRs, syphilis**
  - Side effects: tooth discoloration in children
- **Clindamycin**
  - **Anaerobes,** some GPCs
  - Good for aspiration pneumonia
  - Can be used to treat *C. perfringens*
  - Side effects: pseudomembranous colitis
- **Metronidazole** (Flagyl)
  - **Anaerobes**
  - Side effects: disulfiram-like reaction, **peripheral neuropathy** (long-term use)
- **Antifungal drugs**
  - **Amphotericin** – binds **sterols** in wall and alters membrane permeability
    - Side effects: **nephrotoxic**, fever, hypokalemia, hypotension, anemia
    - Liposomal type has fewer side effects
  - **Voriconazole** and **itraconazole** – inhibit **ergosterol** synthesis (needed for cell membrane)
  - **Anidulafungin** (Eraxis) – inhibits synthesis of **cell wall glucan**
  - **Prolonged broad-spectrum antibiotics** ± fever → **itraconazole**
  - **Invasive aspergillosis** → **voriconazole**
  - **Candidemia** → **anidulafungin**
  - **Fungal sepsis** other than candida and aspergillus → **liposomal amphotericin**
- **Antituberculosis drugs**
  - **Isoniazid** – inhibits mycolic acids (give with pyridoxine)
    - Side effects: hepatotoxicity, **B$_6$ deficiency**
  - **Rifampin** – inhibits RNA polymerase
    - Side effects: hepatotoxicity; GI symptoms; high rate of resistance
  - **Pyrazinamide**
    - Side effect: hepatotoxicity
  - **Ethambutol**
    - Side effect: **retrobulbar neuritis**
- **Antiviral drugs**
  - **Acyclovir** – inhibits viral DNA polymerase; used for **HSV** infections, EBV
  - **Ganciclovir** – inhibits viral DNA polymerase; used for **CMV** infections
    - Side effects: decreased bone marrow, CNS toxicity
- Broad-spectrum antibiotics can lead to **superinfection**
- **Effective for *Enterococcus*** – vancomycin, Timentin/Zosyn, ampicillin/amoxicillin, or gentamicin with ampicillin

- **Effective for *Pseudomonas*, *Acinetobacter*, and *Serratia*** – ticarcillin/piperacillin, Timentin/Zosyn, third-generation cephalosporins, aminoglycosides (gentamicin and tobramycin), meropenem/imipenem, or fluoroquinolones
- **Double cover *Pseudomonas***
- **Perioperative antibiotics**
  - Used to **prevent surgical site infections**
  - Need to be given **within 1 hour** before incision

- **Sublingual** and **rectal drugs** – do not pass through liver first (no first-pass metabolism)
- **Skin absorption** – based on lipid solubility through the epidermis
- **CSF absorption** – restricted to nonionized, lipid-soluble drugs
- **Albumin** – largely responsible for binding drugs (PCNs and warfarin 90% bound)
- **Sulfonamides** – will displace unconjugated bilirubin from albumin in newborns (avoid in newborns)
- **Tetracycline** and **heavy metals** – stored in bone
- **0 order kinetics** – constant amount of drug is eliminated regardless of dose
- **1st order kinetics** – drug eliminated proportional to dose
- **Takes 5 half-lives** for a drug to reach steady state
- **Volume of distribution** = amount of drug in the body divided by amount of drug in plasma or blood
  - Drugs with a high volume of distribution have higher concentrations in the **extravascular compartment** (eg fat tissue) compared with intravascular concentrations
- **Bioavailability** – fraction of unchanged drug reaching the systemic circulation
  - Assumed to be 100% for intravenous drugs, less for other routes (ie oral)
- **ED$_{50}$** – drug level at which <u>desired effect</u> occurs in 50% of patients
- **LD$_{50}$** – drug level at which <u>death</u> occurs in 50% of patients
- **Hyperactive** – effect at an unusually low dose
- **Tachyphylaxis** – tolerance after only a few doses
- **Potency** – dose required for effect
- **Efficacy** – ability to achieve result without untoward effect
- **Drug metabolism** (hepatocyte smooth endoplasmic reticulum, P-450 system)
  - **Phase I** – demethylation, oxidation, reduction, hydrolysis reactions (mixed function oxidases, requires NADPH/oxygen)
  - **Phase II** – glucuronic acid (**#1**) and sulfates attached (forms **water-soluble metabolite**); usually inactive and ready for excretion. Biliary excreted drugs may become deconjugated in intestines with reabsorption, some in active form (termed entero-hepatic recirculation; eg cyclosporine)
  - **Inhibitors of P-450** – cimetidine, isoniazid, ketoconazole, erythromycin, Cipro, Flagyl, allopurinol, verapamil, amiodarone, MAOIs, disulfiram
  - **Inducers of P-450** – cruciform vegetables, ETOH, insecticides, cigarette smoke, phenobarbital (barbiturates), Dilantin, theophylline, warfarin
- **Kidney** – most important organ for eliminating most drugs (glomerular filtration and tubular secretion)
- **Polar drugs** (ionized) – <u>water</u> soluble; more likely to be eliminated in unaltered form
- **Nonpolar drugs** (non-ionized) – <u>fat</u> soluble; more likely metabolized before excretion

- **Gout** – caused by **uric acid** buildup; end product of purine metabolism
  - **Colchicine** – anti-inflammatory; binds **tubulin** and inhibits migration of WBCs
  - **Indomethacin** – NSAID; inhibits prostaglandin synthesis (reversible cyclooxygenase inhibitor)
  - **Allopurinol** – xanthine oxidase inhibitor, blocks uric acid formation from xanthine
  - **Probenecid** – increases renal secretion of uric acid

- ■ **Lipid-lowering agents**
  - **Cholestyramine** – binds bile acids in gut, forcing body to resynthesize bile acids from cholesterol, thereby lowering body cholesterol; can bind vitamin K and cause bleeding tendency
  - **HMG-CoA reductase inhibitors** (statin drugs) – can cause liver dysfunction, rhabdomyolysis
  - **Niacin** (inhibits cholesterol synthesis) – can cause flushing. Tx: **ASA**
- ■ **GI drugs**
  - **Promethazine** (Phenergan, antiemetic) – **inhibits dopamine receptors**; S/E - **tardive dyskinesia** (Tx: **diphenhydramine** [Benadryl])
  - **Metoclopramide** (Reglan, prokinetic) – **inhibits dopamine receptors**; can be used to increase gastric and gut motility
  - **Ondansetron** (Zofran, antiemetic) – central-acting **serotonin receptor inhibitor**
  - **Omeprazole** – proton pump inhibitor; **blocks H/K ATPase** in stomach parietal cells
  - **Cimetidine/ranitidine** – histamine H_2 **receptor blockers**; decrease acid in stomach
  - **Octreotide** – long-acting **somatostatin analogue**; decreases gut secretions
- ■ **Cardiac drugs**
  - **Digoxin**
    - **Inhibits Na/K ATPase** and increases myocardial **calcium**
    - **Slows atrial-ventricular conduction**
    - Also acts as an **inotrope**
    - Decreases **blood flow** to intestines – has been implicated in causing **mesenteric ischemia**
    - **Hypokalemia** increases sensitivity of heart to digitalis; can precipitate arrhythmias or AV block
    - Is **not** cleared with dialysis
    - Other side effects: visual changes (yellow hue), fatigue, arrhythmias
  - **Amiodarone** – good for acute atrial and ventricular arrhythmias
    - S/Es: **pulmonary fibrosis** w/ prolonged use; can also cause **hypo-** and **hyperthyroidism**
  - **Magnesium** – used to treat torsades de pointes (ventricular tachycardia)
  - **Adenosine** – causes transient interruption of the AV node
  - **ACE inhibitors** (angiotensin-converting enzyme inhibitors) – captopril
    - Best single agent shown to improve survival in patients with <u>CHF</u>
    - Can prevent CHF after myocardial infarction
    - Can prevent progression of renal dysfunction in patients with hypertension and DM
    - Can precipitate renal failure in patients with renal artery stenosis
  - **Beta-blockers** – may prolong life in patients with severe LV failure
    - Reduce risk of **MI** and **atrial fibrillation** postoperatively
    - Best single agent shown to improve survival after <u>myocardial infarction</u>
  - **Atropine** – acetylcholine antagonist; increases heart rate
- ■ **Metyrapone** and **aminoglutethimide** – inhibit adrenal steroid synthesis
  - Used in patients with adrenocortical CA
- ■ **Leuprolide** – analogue of GnRH and LHRH
  - Inhibits release of LH and FSH from pituitary when given continuously (paradoxic effect); used in patients with metastatic prostate CA
- ■ **NSAIDs** – inhibit prostaglandin synthesis and lead to ↓ mucus and HCO_3^- secretion and ↑ acid production (mechanism of ulcer formation in patients on NSAIDs)
- ■ **Misoprostol** – a PGE_1 derivative; a **protective prostaglandin** used to prevent peptic ulcer disease; consider use in patients on chronic NSAIDs
- ■ **Haldol** – antipsychotic, inhibits dopamine receptors; can cause extrapyramidal manifestations (Tx: Benadryl)

- **ASA poisoning** – tinnitus, headaches, nausea, and vomiting
  - 1st – respiratory alkalosis
  - 2nd – metabolic acidosis
- **Gadolinium** – MC side effect: nausea
- **Iodine contrast**
  - MC side effect – **nausea**
  - MC side effect requiring medical Tx – **dyspnea**
- **Tylenol overdose** – Tx: *N*-acetylcysteine

CHAPTER 8. ANESTHESIA

Standard Airway Examination for Nonanesthesiologists

Exam Element	Concerning Findings
Body mass index (kg/m^2)	Body mass index ≥ 31
Mouth opening	Interincisor or intergingival distance > 3 cm
Mallampati classification	Class III or IV
Mandibular protrusion	Inability to protrude lower incisors to meet or extend past upper incisors
Neck anatomy	Radiation changes, or thick obese neck
Cervical spine mobility	Limited extension or possibly unstable cervical spine
Beard	Presence of full beard

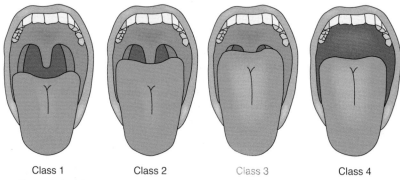

Class 1   Class 2   Class 3   Class 4

Mallampati classification of the airway examination

INHALATIONAL INDUCTION AGENTS

- **MAC** – minimum alveolar concentration = smallest concentration of inhalational agent at which 50% of patients will not move with incision
  - Small MAC → more lipid soluble = more potent
  - Speed of induction is inversely proportional to solubility
  - Nitrous oxide is fastest but has high MAC (low potency)
- Inhalational agents cause unconsciousness, amnesia, and some analgesia (pain relief)
- Blunt hypoxic drive
- Most have some **myocardial depression**, ↑ cerebral blood flow, and ↓ renal blood flow
- **Nitrous oxide** (NO_2) – fast, minimal myocardial depression; tremors at induction
- **Halothane** – slow onset/offset, highest degree of cardiac depression and arrhythmias; <u>least pungent</u>, which is good for children
  - Halothane hepatitis – fever, eosinophilia, jaundice, ↑ LFTs
- **Sevoflurane** – fast, less laryngospasm and less pungent; <u>good for mask induction</u>
- **Isoflurane** – good for <u>neurosurgery</u> (lowers brain O_2 consumption; no increase in ICP)
- **Enflurane** – can cause <u>seizures</u>

INTRAVENOUS INDUCTION AGENTS
- **Sodium thiopental** (barbiturate) – fast acting
  - Side effects: ↓ cerebral blood flow and metabolic rate, ↓ blood pressure
- **Propofol** – very rapid distribution and on/off; amnesia; sedative
  - Side effects: hypotension, respiratory depression
  - **Not an analgesic**
  - Do not use in patients with egg allergy
  - Metabolized in liver and by plasma cholinesterases
- **Ketamine** – dissociation of thalamic/limbic systems; places patient in a cataleptic state (amnesia, analgesia)
  - No respiratory depression
  - Side effects: **hallucinations**, catecholamine release (↑ CO_2, tachycardia), ↑ airway secretions, and ↑ cerebral blood flow
  - **Contraindicated in patients with head injury**
  - Good for **children**
- **Etomidate** – fewer hemodynamic changes; fast acting
  - Continuous infusions can lead to adrenocortical suppression
- **Rapid sequence intubation** – can be indicated for recent oral intake, GERD, delayed gastric emptying, pregnancy, bowel obstruction (pre-oxygenate, etomidate, succinylcholine typical sequence)

MUSCLE RELAXANTS (PARALYTICS)
- **Diaphragm** – last muscle to go down and 1st muscle to recover from paralytics
- **Neck muscles and face** – 1st to go down and last to recover from paralytics
- **Depolarizing agents** – only one is **succinylcholine**; depolarizes neuromuscular junction
- **Succinylcholine** – fast, short acting; causes fasciculations, ↑ ICP; many side effects →
  - **Malignant hyperthermia**
    - Caused by a defect in calcium metabolism
    - Calcium released from sarcoplasmic reticulum causes **muscle excitation – contraction syndrome**
    - Side effects: 1st sign is ↑ **end-tidal CO_2**, then fever, tachycardia, rigidity, acidosis, hyperkalemia
    - Tx: **dantrolene** (10 mg/kg) inhibits Ca release and decouples excitation complex; cooling blankets, HCO_3, glucose, supportive care
  - **Hyperkalemia** – depolarization releases K
    - **Do not use** in patients with severe burns, neurologic injury, neuromuscular disorders, spinal cord injury, massive trauma, or acute renal failure
  - **Open-angle glaucoma** can become closed-angle glaucoma
  - **Atypical pseudocholinesterases** – cause prolonged paralysis (Asians)
- Nondepolarizing agents
  - Inhibit neuromuscular junction by competing with acetylcholine
  - Can get prolongation of these agents with myasthenia gravis
  - **Cis-atracurium** – undergoes **Hoffman degradation**
    - Can be used in **liver** and **renal failure**
    - Histamine release
  - **Rocuronium** – fast, intermediate duration; hepatic metabolism
  - **Pancuronium** – slow acting, long-lasting; renal metabolism
    - Most common side effect – *tachycardia*
  - **Reversing drugs for nondepolarizing agents**
    - **Neostigmine** – blocks **acetylcholinesterase**, increasing acetylcholine
    - **Edrophonium** – blocks **acetylcholinesterase**, increasing acetylcholine
    - **Atropine** or **glycopyrrolate** should be given with <u>neostigmine or edrophonium</u> to counteract effects of generalized acetylcholine overdose

LOCAL ANESTHETICS
- Work by **increasing action potential threshold**, preventing Na influx
- Can use 0.5 cc/kg of 1% lidocaine
- **Infected tissues** are hard to anesthetize secondary to **acidosis**
- **Length of action** – bupivacaine > lidocaine > procaine
- Side effects: tremors, seizures, tinnitus, arrhythmias (CNS symptoms occur before cardiac)
- **Epinephrine** allows higher doses to be used, stays locally
  - **No epinephrine** with arrhythmias, unstable angina, uncontrolled hypertension, poor collaterals (penis and ear), uteroplacental insufficiency
- **Amides** (all have an "i" in first part of the name) – lidocaine, bupivacaine, mepivacaine; rarely cause allergic reactions
- **Esters** – tetracaine, procaine, cocaine; ↑ allergic reactions due to PABA analogue

NARCOTICS (OPIOIDS)
- Morphine, fentanyl, Demerol, codeine
- Act on **mu-opioid receptors**
- Profound analgesia, respiratory depression (↓ CO_2 drive), no cardiac effects, blunt sympathetic response
- Metabolized by the liver and excreted via kidney
- Overdose of narcotics – Tx: **Narcan** (works for all)
- Avoid use of narcotics in patients on **MAOIs** → can cause **hyperpyrexic coma**
- **Morphine** – analgesia, euphoria, respiratory depression, miosis, <u>constipation, histamine release</u> (causes hypotension), ↓ cough
- **Demerol** – analgesia, euphoria, respiratory depression, miosis, <u>tremors, fasciculations, convulsions</u>
  - **No histamine release**
  - Can cause **seizures** (buildup of **normeperidine** analogues) – <u>*avoid* in patients with **renal failure**</u> and be careful with total amount given for other patients
- **Methadone** – simulates morphine, less euphoria
- **Fentanyl** – fast acting; 80× strength of **morphine** (does not cross-react in patients with morphine allergy); no histamine release
- **Sufentanil** and **remifentanil** – <u>very</u> fast-acting narcotics with short half-lives
- Most potent narcotic – *sufentanil*

BENZODIAZEPINES
- Anticonvulsant, amnesic, anxiolytic, **respiratory depression**; <u>not</u> analgesic; liver metabolism
- **Versed** (midazolam) – short acting; contraindicated in pregnancy, crosses placenta
- **Valium** (diazepam) – intermediate acting
- **Ativan** (lorazepam) – long acting
- Overdose of these drugs – Tx: **flumazenil** (competitive inhibitor; may cause seizures and arrhythmias; contraindicated in patients with elevated ICP or status epilepticus)

EPIDURAL AND SPINAL ANESTHESIA
- **Epidural anesthesia** – allows analgesia by **sympathetic denervation**; vasodilation
  - **Morphine** in epidural can cause **respiratory depression**
  - **Lidocaine** in epidural can cause **decreased heart rate** and **blood pressure**
  - Dilute concentrations allow sparing of motor function
  - Tx for **acute hypotension** and **bradycardia**: turn epidural down; fluids, phenylephrine, atropine
  - T-5 epidural can affect cardiac accelerator nerves
  - Epidural contraindicated with <u>hypertrophic cardiomyopathy</u> or <u>cyanotic heart disease</u> → **sympathetic denervation** causes decreased afterload, which worsens these conditions

- **Spinal anesthesia** – injection into subarachnoid space, spread determined by baricity and patient position
  - Neurologic blockade is above motor blockade
  - Spinal contraindicated with hypertrophic cardiomyopathy, cyanotic heart disease
- **Caudal block** – through sacrum, good for pediatric hernias and perianal surgery
- **Epidural and spinal complications** – hypotension, headache, urinary retention (need urinary catheter in these patients), abscess/hematoma formation, respiratory depression (with high spinal)
- **Spinal headaches** – caused by CSF leak after spinal/epidural; headache gets worse sitting up; Tx: rest, fluids, caffeine, analgesics; **blood patch** to site if it persists > 24 hours.

PERIOPERATIVE COMPLICATIONS

- Pre-op **renal failure** (#1) and **CHF** – associated with most postop hospital **mortality**
- **Postop MI** – may have no pain or EKG changes; can have hypotension, arrhythmias, ↑ filling pressures, oliguria, bradycardia
- **Patients who need cardiology workup pre-op** – angina, previous MI, shortness of breath, CHF, walks < 2 blocks due to shortness of breath or chest pain, FEV_1 < 70% predicted, severe valvular disease, PVCs > 5/min, high grade heart block, age > 70, DM, renal insufficiency, patients undergoing major vascular surgery (peripheral and aortic)

ASA Physical Status (PS) Classes

Class	Description
1	Healthy
2	Mild disease without limitation (controlled hypertension, obesity, diabetes mellitus, significant smoking history, older age)
3	Severe disease (angina, previous MI, poorly controlled hypertension, diabetes mellitus with complications, moderate COPD)
4	Severe constant threat to life (unstable angina, CHF, renal failure, liver failure, severe COPD)
5	Moribund (ruptured AAA, saddle pulmonary embolus)
6	Donor
E	Emergency

- Most **aortic, major vascular,** and **peripheral vascular surgeries** are considered high risk
- **Carotid endarterectomy** (CEA) is considered <u>moderate</u> risk surgery
- **Biggest risk factors for postop MI**: age > 70, DM, previous MI, CHF, unstable angina

Cardiac Risk[a] Stratification for Noncardiac Surgical Procedures

High (cardiac risk > 5%) – emergent operations (especially in elderly); aortic, peripheral, and other major vascular surgery (*except* CEA); long procedure with large fluid shifts
Intermediate (cardiac risk < 5%) – CEA; head and neck surgery; intraperitoneal and intrathoracic surgery; orthopedic surgery; prostate surgery
Low[b] (cardiac risk < 1%) – endoscopic procedures; superficial procedures; cataract surgery; breast surgery

[a]Combined incidence of cardiac death and nonfatal myocardial infarction.
[b]Do not generally require further preoperative cardiac testing.

- Best determinant of esophageal vs. tracheal intubation – **end-tidal CO$_2$** (ETCO$_2$)
- Intubated patient undergoing surgery with **sudden transient <u>rise</u> in ETCO$_2$**
  - Dx: most likely **hypoventilation**
  - Tx: ↑ tidal volume or ↑ respiratory rate
- Intubated patient with **sudden <u>drop</u> in ETCO$_2$** – likely became **disconnected from the vent**; could also be due to pulmonary embolism (patient would have hypotension)
- **Endotracheal tube** – should be placed 2 cm above the carina
- **MC PACU complication** – *nausea and vomiting*
- **Higher volume hospitals** are associated with lower mortality for <u>abdominal aortic aneurysm repair</u> and for <u>pancreatic resection</u>

TOTAL BODY WATER

- Roughly ⅔ of the total body weight is water (men); **infants** have a little more body water, **women** have a little less
- ⅔ of water weight is intracellular (mostly muscle)
- ⅓ of water weight is extracellular
  - ⅔ of extracellular water is interstitial
  - ⅓ of extracellular water is in plasma
- **Proteins** – determine <u>plasma/interstitial</u> compartment osmotic pressures
- **Na** – determines <u>intracellular/extracellular</u> osmotic pressure
- **Volume overload** – most common cause is iatrogenic; first sign is **weight gain**
- **Cellular catabolism** – can release a significant amount of H_2O
- **0.9% normal saline**: Na 154 and Cl 154; **3% normal saline**: Na 513 and Cl 513
- **Lactated Ringer's** (LR; ionic composition of plasma): Na 130, K 4, Ca 2.7, Cl 109, bicarb 28
- **Plasma osmolarity**: $(2 \times Na) + (glucose/18) + (BUN/2.8)$
  - Normal: 280–295
- **Water** shifts from areas of low solute concentration (low osmolarity) to areas of high solute concentration (high osmolarity) to achieve osmotic equilibration

ESTIMATES OF VOLUME REPLACEMENT

- 4 cc/kg/h for 1st 10 kg
- 2 cc/kg/h for 2nd 10 kg
- 1 cc/kg/h for each kg after that
- Best indicator of adequate volume replacement is **urine output**
- During open abdominal operations, fluid loss is **0.5–1.0 L/h** unless there are measurable blood losses
- Usually do not have to replace blood lost unless it is **> 500 cc**
- **Insensible fluid losses** – 10 cc/kg/day; 75% skin, 25% respiratory, pure water
- **Replacement fluids** after **major adult gastrointestinal surgery**
  - During operation and 1st 24 hours, use **LR**
  - After 24 hours, switch to **D5 ½ NS with 20 mEq K⁺**
    - 5% dextrose will stimulate **insulin release**, resulting in amino acid uptake and protein synthesis (also prevents protein catabolism)
    - D5 ½ NS @ 125/h provides 150 g glucose per day (525 kcal/day)

GI FLUID SECRETION

- Stomach   1–2 L/day
- Biliary system   500–1,000 mL/day
- Pancreas   500–1,000 mL/day
- Duodenum   500–1,000 mL/day
- **Normal K⁺ requirement**: 0.5–1.0 mEq/kg/day
- **Normal Na⁺ requirement**: 1–2 mEq/kg/day

GI ELECTROLYTE LOSSES

- Sweat – hypotonic (Na concentration 35–65)
- Saliva – K⁺ *(highest concentration of K⁺ in body)*
- Stomach – H⁺ and Cl⁻
- Pancreas – HCO_3^-
- Bile – HCO_3^-

- Small intestine – HCO_3^-, K^+
- Large intestine – K^+
- **Gastric losses** – replacement is D5 ½ NS with 20 mg K^+
- **Pancreatic/biliary/small intestine losses** – replacement is LR with HCO_3^-
- **Large intestine losses** (diarrhea) – replacement is LR with K^+
- **GI losses** – should generally be replaced **cc/cc**
- **Dehydration** (eg marathon runner) – replacement with **normal saline**
- **Urine output** – should be kept at least 0.5 cc/kg/h; should not be replaced, usually a sign of normal postoperative diuresis

POTASSIUM (NORMAL 3.5–5.0)
- **Hyperkalemia** – peaked T waves on EKG; often occurs with <u>renal failure</u>; Tx →
  - **Calcium gluconate** (membrane stabilizer for heart)
  - **Sodium bicarbonate** (causes alkalosis, K enters cell in exchange for H)
  - **10 U insulin** and **1 ampule of 50% dextrose** (K driven into cells with glucose)
  - **Kayexalate**
  - **Dialysis** if refractory
- **Hypokalemia** – T waves disappear (usually occurs in setting of <u>overdiuresis</u>)
  - May need to replace Mg^+ before you can correct K^+

SODIUM (NORMAL 135–145)
- **Hypernatremia** – usually from **dehydration**; restlessness, irritability, seizures
  - Correct with **D5 water** <u>slowly</u> to avoid brain swelling
- **Hyponatremia** – usually from **fluid overload**; headaches, nausea, vomiting, seizures
  - **Water restriction** is first-line treatment for hyponatremia, then **diuresis**
  - Correct Na slowly to avoid **central pontine myelinosis** (no more than 1 mEq/h)
  - **Hyperglycemia** can cause **pseudohyponatremia** – for each 100 increment of glucose over normal, add 2 points to the Na value
  - **SIADH** (syndrome of inappropriate antidiuretic hormone) causes hyponatremia

CALCIUM (NORMAL 8.5–10.0; NORMAL IONIZED CA 4.4–5.5)
- **Hypercalcemia** (Ca usually > 13 or ionized > 6-7 for symptoms) - causes lethargic state
  - **Breast cancer** most common malignant cause
  - **Hyperparathyroidism** most common benign cause
  - <u>No</u> lactated Ringer's (contains Ca^{2+})
  - <u>No</u> thiazide diuretics (these retain Ca^{2+})
  - Tx: **normal saline** at 200-300 cc/h and **Lasix**
  - For **malignant disease** → mithramycin, calcitonin, alendronic acid, dialysis
- **Hypocalcemia** (Ca usually < 8 or ionized Ca < 4 for symptoms) - hyperreflexia, Chvostek's sign (tapping on face produces twitching), perioral tingling and numbness, Trousseau's sign (carpopedal spasm), prolonged QT interval; can occur after **parathyroidectomy**
  - May need to replace Mg^+ before you can correct Ca
  - **Protein adjustment for calcium** – for every 1g decrease in protein, add 0.8 to Ca

MAGNESIUM (NORMAL 2.0–2.7)
- **Hypermagnesemia** – causes lethargic state; usually in **renal failure** patients taking magnesium containing products
  - Tx: calcium
- **Hypomagnesemia** – usually occurs with **massive diuresis, chronic TPN** without mineral replacement or **ETOH abuse**; signs similar to hypocalcemia

METABOLIC ACIDOSIS

- **Anion gap = Na – (HCO_3 + Cl)**; Normal is < 10–15
- **High anion gap acidosis – "MUDPILES"** = **m**ethanol, **u**remia, **d**iabetic ketoacidosis, **p**ar-aldehydes, **i**soniazid, **l**actic acidosis, **e**thylene glycol, **s**alicylates
- **Normal anion gap acidosis** – usually loss of Na/HCO_3^- (ileostomies, small bowel fistulas)
- Tx: underlying cause; keep pH > 7.20 with bicarbonate; severely ↓ pH can affect myocardial contractility

METABOLIC ALKALOSIS

- Usually a contraction alkalosis
- **Nasogastric suction** – results in **hypochloremic, hypokalemic, metabolic alkalosis,** and **paradoxical aciduria** →
  - Loss of Cl^- and H ion from stomach secondary to nasogastric tube (hypochloremia and alkalosis)
  - Loss of water causes kidney to reabsorb Na in exchange for K^+ (Na/K ATPase), thus losing K^+ (hypokalemia)
  - Na^+/H^- exchanger activated in an effort to reabsorb water along with K^+/H^- exchanger in an effort to reabsorb K^+ → results in paradoxical aciduria
  - Tx: **normal saline** (need to correct the Cl- deficit)

Acid–Base Balance			
Condition	pH (7.4)	CO_2 (40)	HCO_3 (24)
Respiratory acidosis	↓	↑	↑
Respiratory alkalosis	↑	↓	↓
Metabolic acidosis	↓	↓	↓
Metabolic alkalosis	↑	↑	↑

- **Respiratory compensation** (CO_2 regulation) for acidosis/alkalosis takes **minutes**
- **Renal compensation** (HCO_3^- regulation) for acidosis/alkalosis takes **hours to days**

ACUTE RENAL FAILURE

- **FeNa** = (urine Na/Cr)/(plasma Na/Cr) – fractional excretion of Na; *best test for azotemia*
- **Prerenal** – FeNa < 1%, urine Na < 20, BUN/Cr ratio > 20, urine osmolality > 500 mOsm
  - 70% of renal mass must be damaged before ↑ Cr and BUN
- **Contrast dyes** – prehydration best prevents renal damage; HCO_3^- and N-acetylcysteine
- **Myoglobin** – converted to ferrihemate in acidic environment, which is toxic to renal cells; Tx: alkalinize urine

TUMOR LYSIS SYNDROME

- Release of purines and pyrimidines leads to ↑ PO_4 and **uric acid**, ↓ Ca
- Can result in ↑ BUN and Cr (from renal damage), EKG changes
- Tx: **hydration** *(best)*, rasburicase (converts uric acid in inactive metabolite allantoin), allopurinol (↓ uric acid production), diuretics, alkalinization of urine

VITAMIN D (CHOLECALCIFEROL)

- Made in skin (UV sunlight converts 7-dehydrocholesterol to cholecalciferol)
- Goes to **liver** for **(25-OH)**, then **kidney** for **(1-OH)**. This creates the active form of vitamin D

- **Active form of vitamin D** – increases **calcium-binding protein**, leading to increased intestinal Ca absorption

CHRONIC RENAL FAILURE
- ↓ **Active vitamin D** (↓ 1-OH hydroxylation) → ↓ Ca reabsorption from gut (↓ Ca-binding protein)
- **Anemia** – from low erythropoietin

Transferrin – transporter of iron
Ferritin – storage form of iron

- **Caloric need** – approximately 20–25 calories/kg/day
- **Calories**:

Fat	9 calories/g
Protein	4 calories/g
Oral carbohydrates	4 calories/g
Dextrose	3.4 calories/g

- **Nutritional requirements for average healthy adult male**
  - **20% protein** calories (**1 g protein/kg/day**; 20% should be essential amino acids)
  - **30% fat** calories – important for essential fatty acids
  - **50% carbohydrate** calories
- **Trauma**, **surgery**, or **sepsis** stress can increase kcal requirement 20%–40%
- **Pregnancy** increases kcal requirement 300 kcal/day
- **Lactation** increases kcal requirement 500 kcal/day
- **Protein requirement** also increases with above
- **Burns**
  - Calories: 25 kcal/kg/day + (30 kcal/day × % burn)
  - Protein: 1–1.5 g/kg/day + (3 g × % burn)
- Much of **energy expenditure** is used for **heat production**
- **Fever** increases **basal metabolic rate** (10% for each degree above 38.0°C)
- If overweight and trying to calculate caloric need, use equation: weight = [(actual weight − ideal body weight) × 0.25] + IBW
- **Harris–Benedict equation** calculates basal energy expenditure based on **weight**, **height**, **age**, and **gender**
- **Central line TPN** – glucose based; maximum glucose administration – 3 g/kg/h
- **Peripheral line parenteral nutrition** (PPN) – fat based
- **Short-chain fatty acids** (eg butyric acid) – fuel for **colonocytes**
- **Glutamine** – fuel for **small bowel enterocytes**
  - Most common amino acid in **bloodstream** and **tissue**
  - Releases NH_4 in kidney, thus helping with **nitrogen excretion**
  - Can be used for **gluconeogenesis**
- **Primary fuel for most neoplastic cells** – glutamine

PREOPERATIVE NUTRITIONAL ASSESSMENT
- **Approximate half-lives**
  - Albumin – 18 days
  - Transferrin – 10 days
  - Prealbumin – 2 days
- Normal **protein** level: 6.0–8.5
- Normal **albumin** level: 3.5–5.5
- **Acute** indicators of nutritional status – retinal binding protein, prealbumin, transferrin
- **Ideal body weight** (IBW)
  - Men = 106 lb + 6 lb for each inch over 5 ft
  - Women = 100 lb + 5 lb for each inch over 5 ft
- **Preoperative signs of poor nutritional status**
  - Acute weight loss > 10% in 6 months
  - Weight < 85% of IBW
  - Albumin < 3.0
- **Low albumin** (< 3.0) – strong risk factor for **morbidity** and **mortality** after surgery

RESPIRATORY QUOTIENT (RQ)
- Ratio of CO_2 produced to O_2 consumed – is a measurement of energy expenditure
- **RQ > 1** = lipogenesis (overfeeding)
  - Tx: ↓ carbohydrates and caloric intake
  - High carbohydrate intake can lead to CO_2 buildup and ventilator problems
- **RQ < 0.7** = ketosis and fat oxidation (starving)
  - Tx: ↑ carbohydrates and caloric intake
- Pure **fat utilization** – RQ = 0.7
- Pure **protein utilization** – RQ = 0.8
- Pure **carbohydrate utilization** – RQ = 1.0

POSTOPERATIVE PHASES
- **Diuresis phase** – postoperative days 2–5
- **Catabolic phase** – postoperative days 0–3 (negative nitrogen balance)
- **Anabolic phase** – postoperative days 3–6 (positive nitrogen balance)

STARVATION OR MAJOR STRESS (SURGERY, TRAUMA, SYSTEMIC ILLNESS)

Metabolic Differences Between the Responses to Simple Starvation and to Injury		
	Starvation	Injury
Basal metabolic rate	−	+ +
Presence of mediators (eg TNF-alpha, IL-1)	−	+ + +
Major fuel oxidized	Fat	Mixed (fat, protein)
Ketone body production	+ + +	±
Gluconeogenesis	+	+ + +
Protein metabolism	+	+ + +
Negative nitrogen balance	+	+ + +
Hepatic ureagenesis	+	+ + +
Muscle proteolysis	+	+ + +
Hepatic protein synthesis	+	+ + +

- The magnitude of metabolic response is proportional to the degree of injury
- **Glycogen stores**
  - Depleted after 24–36 hours of starvation (⅔ in skeletal muscle, ⅓ in liver) → body then switches to **fat**
  - Skeletal muscle lacks **glucose-6-phosphatase** (found only in **liver**)
  - Glucose-6-phosphate stays in muscle after breakdown from glycogen and is utilized
- **Gluconeogenesis precursors** – amino acids (especially **alanine**), lactate, pyruvate, glycerol
  - **Alanine** is the simplest amino acid precursor for gluconeogenesis
    - Is the **primary substrate** for gluconeogenesis
  - **Alanine** and **phenylalanine** – only amino acids to increase during times of stress
  - **Late starvation** – gluconeogenesis occurs in <u>kidney</u>
- **Starvation**
  - Protein-conserving mechanisms **do not occur after trauma** (or surgery) secondary to catecholamines and cortisol
  - Protein-conserving mechanisms do occur with **starvation**
  - **Fat** (ketones) is the main source of energy in **starvation** and in **trauma**; however, with trauma the energy source is more mixed (fat and protein)
  - Most patients can tolerate a 15% weight loss without major complications
  - Patients can tolerate about **7 days** without eating; if longer than that, place a **Dobbhoff tube** or start TPN

- Try to feed gut to avoid **bacterial translocation** (bacterial overgrowth, increased permeability due to starved enterocytes, bacteremia) and **TPN complications**
- **PEG tube** – consider when regular feeding not possible (eg CVA) or predicted to not occur for > 4 weeks
- **Brain** – utilizes <u>ketones</u> with progressive starvation (normally uses **glucose**)
- **Peripheral nerves, adrenal medulla, red blood cells**, and **white blood cells** are all **obligate glucose users**
- **Refeeding syndrome**
  - Occurs when feeding after prolonged starvation/malnutrition
  - Results in decreased **K**, **Mg**, and **PO$_4$**; causes cardiac dysfunction, profound weakness, encephalopathy
  - Prevent this by starting to re-feed at a **low rate** (10–15 kcal/kg/day)
- **Cachexia** – anorexia, weight loss, wasting
  - Thought to be mediated by **TNF-α**
  - Glycogen breakdown, lipolysis, protein catabolism
- **Kwashiorkor** – protein deficiency
- **Marasmus** – starvation

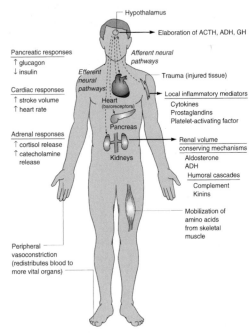

Homeostatic adjustments initiated after injury

NITROGEN BALANCE

- **6.25 g of protein** contains **1 g of nitrogen**
- N balance = (N in – N out) = ([protein/6.25] – [24-hour urine N + 4 g])
  - **Positive N balance** – more protein ingested than excreted (anabolism)
  - **Negative N balance** – more protein excreted than taken in (catabolism)
- Total protein synthesis for a healthy, normal 70-kg male is **250 g/day**

■ **Liver**
  • Responsible for amino acid production and breakdown
  • **Urea production** is used to get rid of **ammonia** from amino acid breakdown
  • Majority of protein breakdown from skeletal muscle is **glutamine** and **alanine**

FAT DIGESTION

■ **Triacylglycerides** (TAGs), **cholesterol**, and **lipids**
  • Broken down by pancreatic lipase, cholesterol esterase, and phospholipase to micelles and free fatty acids
  • **Micelles** – aggregates of bile salts, **long-chain free fatty acids**, and monoacylglycerides
    • Enter enterocyte by fusing with membrane
    • **Bile salts** – increase absorption area for fats, helping form **micelles**
    • **Cholesterol** – used to synthesize bile salts
    • **Fat-soluble vitamins** (A, D, E, K) – absorbed in micelles
  • **Medium-** and **short-chain fatty acids** – enter enterocyte by simple diffusion
■ **Micelles and other fatty acids enter enterocytes**
  • **Chylomicrons** are formed (90% TAGs, 10% phospholipids/proteins/cholesterol) which enter **lymphatics** (thoracic duct)
  • **Long-chain fatty acids** – enter **lymphatics** along with chylomicrons
  • **Medium-** and **short-chain fatty acids** – enter **portal system** (same as amino acids and carbohydrates)
■ **Lipoprotein lipase** – on endothelium in liver and adipose tissue; clears <u>chylomicrons and TAGs</u> from the blood, breaking them down to <u>fatty acids</u> and <u>glycerol</u>
■ **Free fatty acid–binding protein** – on endothelium in the liver and adipose tissue; binds short- and medium-chain fatty acids
■ **Saturated fatty acids** – used for **fuel** by **cardiac** and **skeletal muscles**
  • **Fatty acids** (ketones – acetoacetate, beta-hydroxybutyrate) – preferred source of energy for **colonocytes**, **liver**, **heart**, and **skeletal muscle**
■ **Unsaturated fatty acids** – used as **structural components** for cells
■ **Hormone-sensitive lipase** (HSL) – in fat cells; breaks down **TAGs** (storage form of **fat**) to **fatty acids** and **glycerol**, which are released into the bloodstream (HSL is sensitive to growth hormone, catecholamines, glucocorticoids)
■ <u>**Essential**</u> **fatty acids** – linolenic, linoleic
  • Needed for prostaglandin synthesis (long-chain fatty acids)
  • Important for immune cells

CARBOHYDRATE DIGESTION

■ Begins with **salivary amylase**, then pancreatic amylase and disaccharidases
■ **Glucose** and **galactose** – absorbed by secondary active transport; released into portal vein
■ **Fructose** – facilitated diffusion; released into portal vein
■ **Sucrose** = fructose + glucose
■ **Lactose** = galactose + glucose
■ **Maltose** = glucose + glucose

PROTEIN DIGESTION

■ Begins with **stomach pepsin**, then trypsin, chymotrypsin, and carboxypeptidase
■ **Trypsinogen** released from pancreas and activated by **enterokinase**, which is released from the duodenum
  • Other pancreatic protein enzymes are then activated by trypsin
  • Trypsin can then also autoactivate other trypsinogen molecules
■ **Protein** broken down to amino acids, dipeptides, and tripeptides by proteases
■ Absorbed by secondary active transport; released as free amino acids into portal vein

- Limit protein intake in patients with **liver failure** and **renal failure** to **avoid ammonia buildup** and possible worsening encephalopathy
- **Branched-chain** amino acids – leucine, isoleucine, valine ("LIV")
  - Metabolized in **muscle**
  - Possibly important in patients with liver failure
  - Are **essential amino acids**
- **Essential** amino acids – leucine, isoleucine, valine, arginine, histidine, lysine, methionine, phenylalanine, threonine, and tryptophan

CENTRAL VENOUS TPN (GENERAL COMPOSITION)

- **10% amino acid solution**
- **50% dextrose solution**
- **Electrolytes** (Na, Cl, K, Ca, Mg, PO4, acetate)
- **Mineral** and **vitamins**
- **Lipids** – given separately from TPN
  - 10% lipid solution contains 1.1 kcal/cc; 20% lipid solution contains 2 kcal/cc

Mineral and Vitamin Deficiencies

Deficiency	Effect
Chromium	Hyperglycemia, encephalopathy, neuropathy
Selenium	Cardiomyopathy, weakness
Copper	Pancytopenia
Zinc	Poor wound healing
Phosphate	Weakness (failure to wean off ventilator), encephalopathy, decreased phagocytosis
Thiamine (B_1)	Wernicke's encephalopathy, cardiomyopathy
Pyridoxine (B_6)	Sideroblastic anemia, glossitis, peripheral neuropathy
Cobalamin (B_{12})	Megaloblastic anemia, peripheral neuropathy, beefy tongue
Folate	Megaloblastic anemia, glossitis
Niacin	Pellagra (diarrhea, dermatitis, dementia)
Essential fatty acids	Dermatitis, hair loss, thrombocytopenia
Vitamin A	Night blindness
Vitamin K	Coagulopathy
Vitamin D	Rickets, osteomalacia, osteoporosis
Vitamin E	Neuropathy

CORI CYCLE

- Glucose is utilized and converted to **lactate** in muscle
- Lactate then goes to the **liver** and is converted back to **pyruvate** and eventually **glucose** via gluconeogenesis
- Glucose is then transported back to muscle

- Cancer **#2 cause of death in the United States**
- **MC CA in women** – breast CA
- **MC cause of CA-related death in women** – lung CA
- **MC CA in men** – prostate CA
- **MC cause of CA-related death in men** – lung CA
- **PET** (positron emission tomography) – used to identify **metastases**; detects **fluorodeoxyglucose** molecules
- **Cytotoxic T cells** need MHC complex to attack tumor
- **Natural killer cells** can independently attack tumor cells
- Tumor antigens are random unless viral-induced tumor
- **Hyperplasia** – increased number of cells
- **Metaplasia** – replacement of one tissue with another (GERD squamous epithelium in esophagus changed to columnar gastric tissue; eg Barrett's esophagus)
- **Dysplasia** – altered size, shape, and organization (eg Barrett's dysplasia)

TUMOR MARKERS
- CEA – colon CA
- AFP – liver CA
- CA 19-9 – pancreatic CA
- CA 125 – ovarian CA
- Beta-HCG – testicular CA, choriocarcinoma
- PSA – prostate CA (thought to be the tumor marker with the **highest sensitivity**, although specificity is low)
- NSE – small cell lung CA, neuroblastoma
- BRCA I and II – breast CA
- Chromogranin A – carcinoid tumor
- Ret oncogene – thyroid medullary CA
- **Half-lives** – CEA: 18 days; PSA: 18 days; AFP: 5 days

ONCOGENESIS
- **Cancer transformation**:
  1) Heritable alteration in genome *and;*
  2) Loss of growth regulation
- **Latency period** – time between exposure and formation of clinically detectable tumor
  - **Initiation** – carcinogen acts with DNA
  - **Promotion** of cancer cells then occurs
  - **Progression** of cancer cells to clinically detectable tumor
- Neoplasms can arise from **carcinogenesis** (eg smoking), **viruses** (eg EBV), or **immunodeficiency** (eg HIV)
- **Retroviruses** contain **oncogenes**
  - Epstein-Barr virus – associated with Burkitt's lymphoma (8:14 translocation) and nasopharyngeal CA (c-myc)
- **Proto-oncogenes** are **human genes** with **malignant potential**

Malignancy	Associated Infectious Agent
Cervical cancer	Human papillomavirus
Gastric cancer	*Helicobacter pylori*
Hepatocellular carcinoma	Hepatitis B and hepatitis C viruses
Nasopharyngeal carcinoma	EBV
Burkitt's lymphoma	EBV
Various lymphomas	HIV

EBV, Epstein-Barr virus; HIV, human immunodeficiency virus.
Modified from O'Connell C, Dickey VL. *Blueprints: Hematology and Oncology*. Philadelphia, PA: Lippincott Williams & Wilkins; 2005, with permission.

RADIATION THERAPY (XRT)

■ **M phase** – most vulnerable stage of cell cycle for XRT
■ Most damage done by formation of **oxygen radicals** → maximal effect with **high oxygen levels**
■ Main target is **DNA** – oxygen radicals and XRT itself damage DNA and other molecules
■ **Higher-energy radiation** has **skin-preserving effect** (maximal ionizing potential not reached until deeper structures)
■ **Fractionate XRT doses**
  • Allows **repair** of normal cells
  • Allows **re-oxygenation** of tumor
  • Allows **redistribution** of tumor cells in cell cycle
■ Very radiosensitive tumors – **seminomas**, **lymphomas**
■ Very radioresistant tumors – **epithelial**, **sarcomas**
■ **Large tumors** – less responsive to XRT due to <u>lack of oxygen in the tumor</u>
■ **Brachytherapy** – source of radiation in or next to tumor (Au-198, I-128); delivers high, concentrated doses of radiation

CHEMOTHERAPY AGENTS

■ **Cell cycle–specific agents** (5FU, methotrexate) – exhibit plateau in cell-killing ability
■ **Cell cycle–nonspecific agents** – linear response to cell killing
■ **Tamoxifen** (blocks estrogen receptor) – decreases short-term (5-year) risk of breast CA 45% (1% risk of blood clots, 0.1% risk of endometrial CA)
■ **Taxol** promotes microtubule formation and stabilization that cannot be broken down; cells are ruptured
■ **Bleomycin** and **busulfan** – can cause pulmonary fibrosis
■ **Cisplatin** (platinum alkylating agent) – nephrotoxic, neurotoxic, ototoxic
■ **Carboplatin** (platinum alkylating agent) – **bone** (myelo) suppression
■ **Vincristine** (microtubule inhibitor) – peripheral neuropathy, neurotoxic
■ **Vinblastine** (microtubule inhibitor) – **bone** (myelo) suppression
■ **Alkylating agents** – transfer alkyl groups; form covalent bonds to DNA
  • **Cyclophosphamide** – **acrolein** is the active metabolite
    ◦ Side effects: gonadal dysfunction, SIADH, hemorrhagic cystitis
    ◦ **Mesna** can help with hemorrhagic cystitis
■ **Levamisole** – **anthelminthic drug** thought to stimulate immune system against cancer
■ **Methotrexate** – inhibits <u>dihydrofolate reductase</u> (DHFR), which inhibits purine and DNA synthesis
  • Side effects: renal toxicity, radiation recall
  • **Leucovorin rescue** (folinic acid) – reverses effects of methotrexate by re-supplying folate

- **5-Fluorouracil (5FU)** – inhibits <u>thymidylate synthetase</u>, which inhibits purine and DNA synthesis
  - **Leucovorin** (folinic acid) – increases toxicity of 5FU
- **Doxorubicin** – DNA intercalator, O_2 radical formation
  - **Heart toxicity** secondary to **O_2 radicals** at total doses > 500 mg/m^2
- **Etoposide** (VP-16) – inhibits topoisomerase (which normally unwinds DNA)
- **Least myelosuppression** – bleomycin, vincristine, busulfan, cisplatin
- **GCSF** (granulocyte colony–stimulating factor) - used for **neutrophil recovery** after chemo; side effects - **Sweet's syndrome** (acute febrile neutropenic dermatitis)

MISCELLANEOUS

- **Resection of a normal organ to prevent cancer**
  - Breast – BRCA I or II with strong family history
  - Thyroid – RET proto-oncogene with family history thyroid CA
- **Tumor suppressor genes**
  - **Retinoblastoma** (Rb1) – chromosome 13; involved in **cell cycle** regulation
  - **p53** – chromosome 17; involved in **cell cycle** (normal gene induces cell cycle arrest and **apoptosis**; abnormal gene allows unrestrained cell growth)
  - **APC** – chromosome 5; involved with **cell cycle** regulation and movement
  - **DCC** – chromosome 18; involved in **cell adhesion**
  - **bcl** – involved in **apoptosis** (programmed cell death)
  - **BRCA**
- **Proto-oncogenes**
  - **ras** proto-oncogene – G protein defect
  - **src** proto-oncogene – tyrosine kinase defect
  - **sis** proto-oncogene – platelet-derived growth factor receptor defect
  - **erb B** proto-oncogene – epidermal growth factor receptor defect
  - **myc** (c-myc, n-myc, l-myc) proto-oncogenes – transcription factors
- **Li–Fraumeni syndrome** – defect in **p53 gene** → patients get childhood sarcomas, breast CA, brain tumors, leukemia, adrenal CA
- **Colon CA**
  - Genes involved in development include **APC, p53, DCC,** and **K-ras**
  - **APC** thought to be the **initial step** in the evolution of colorectal CA
  - **Colon CA usually does not go to bone**
- **Carcinogens**
  - **Coal tar** – larynx, skin, bronchial CA
  - **Beta-naphthylamine** – urinary tract CA (bladder CA)
  - **Benzene** – leukemia
  - **Asbestos** – mesothelioma
- **Cancer spread**
  - Suspicious supraclavicular nodes – neck, breast, lung, stomach (Virchow's node), pancreas
  - Suspicious axillary node – **lymphoma** (#1), breast, melanoma
  - Suspicious periumbilical node – pancreas (Sister Mary Joseph's node)
  - Ovarian metastases – stomach (Krukenberg tumor), colon
  - Bone metastases – **breast** (#1), prostate
  - Skin metastases – breast, melanoma
  - Small bowel metastases – **melanoma** (#1)
- **Clinical trials**
  - Phase I – is it safe and at what dose?
  - Phase II – is it effective?
  - Phase III – is it better than existing therapy?
  - Phase IV – implementation and marketing

- **Types of therapy**
  - **Induction** – sole treatment; used for advanced disease or when no other Tx exists
  - **Primary** (neoadjuvant) – chemo given 1st (usually), followed by another (secondary) therapy
  - **Adjuvant** – combined with another modality; given after other therapy is used
  - **Salvage** – for tumors that fail to respond to initial chemotherapy
- **Lymph nodes** have poor barrier function → better to view them as signs of **probable metastasis**
- **En bloc multiorgan resection** can be attempted for some tumors (colon into uterus, adrenal into liver, gastric into spleen); aggressive local invasiveness is different from metastatic disease
- **Palliative surgery** – tumors of hollow viscus causing obstruction or bleeding (colon CA), breast CA with skin or chest wall involvement
- **Sentinel lymph node biopsy** – <u>no role in patients with clinically palpable nodes</u>; you need to go after and sample these nodes
- **Colon metastases to the liver** – 35% 5-year survival rate if successfully resected
- **Prognostic indicators for survival after resection of hepatic colorectal metastases** – disease-free interval > 12 months, tumor number < 3, CEA < 200, size < 5 cm, negative nodes
- **Most successfully cured metastases with surgery** – colon CA in liver, sarcoma to the lung, <u>but</u> survival still low overall for these
- **Ovarian CA** – one of the few tumors for which **surgical debulking** improves chemotherapy (not seen in other tumors)
- **Curable solid tumors with chemotherapy only** – Hodgkin's and non-Hodgkin's lymphoma
- **T-cell lymphomas** – HTLV-1 (skin lesions), mycosis fungoides (Sézary cells)
- **HIV-related malignancies** – Kaposi's sarcoma, non-Hodgkin's lymphoma
- **V-EGF** (vascular epidermal growth factor) – causes angiogenesis; involved in tumor metastasis

CHAPTER 12. TRANSPLANTATION

TRANSPLANT IMMUNOLOGY
- **HLA-A, -B,** and **-DR** – most important in recipient/donor matching
  - **HLA-DR** – most important overall (HLA = human leukocyte antigen)
- **ABO blood compatibility** – generally required for all transplants (except liver)
- **Cross-match** – detects **preformed recipient antibodies** to the donor organ by mixing recipient serum with donor lymphocytes → if these antibodies are present, it is termed a **positive cross-match** and **hyperacute rejection** would likely occur with TXP
- **Panel reactive antibody** (PRA)
  - Technique identical to cross-match; detects preformed recipient antibodies using a panel of HLA typing cells
  - Get a percentage of cells that the recipient serum reacts with → a **high PRA** (> 50%) is often a contraindication to TXP (increased risk of hyper-acute rejection)
  - Transfusions, pregnancy, previous transplant, and autoimmune diseases can all increase PRA
- **Mild rejection** – pulse steroids
- **Severe rejection** – steroid and antibody therapy (ATG or daclizumab)
- **Skin cancer** – #1 malignancy following any transplant (squamous cell CA #1)
- **Post-transplant lympho-proliferative disorder** (PTLD) – next most common malignancy following transplant (**Epstein-Barr virus** related)
  - Tx: withdrawal of immunosuppression; may need chemotherapy and XRT for aggressive tumor

DRUGS
- **Mycophenolate** (MMF, CellCept)
  - Inhibits de novo purine synthesis, which **inhibits growth of T cells**
  - Side effects: myelosuppression
  - Need to keep WBCs > 3
  - Used as maintenance therapy to prevent rejection
  - Azathioprine (Imuran) has similar action
- **Steroids** – inhibit **inflammatory cells** (macrophages) and **genes for cytokine synthesis** (IL-1, IL-6); used for induction after TXP, maintenance, and acute rejection episodes
- **Cyclosporin** (CSA)
  - Binds **cyclophilin protein** and **inhibits genes for cytokine synthesis** (IL-2, IL-4, etc.); used for maintenance therapy
  - Side effects: nephrotoxicity, hepatotoxicity, tremors, seizures, hemolytic-uremic syndrome
  - Need to keep trough 200–300
  - Undergoes **hepatic metabolism** and **biliary excretion** (reabsorbed in the gut, get entero-hepatic recirculation)
- **FK-506** (Prograf, tacrolimus)
  - Binds **FK-binding protein**; actions similar to CSA but more potent
  - Side effects: nephrotoxicity, more GI symptoms and mood changes than CSA, much less entero-hepatic recirculation compared to CSA
  - Less rejection episodes in Kidney TXP's w/ FK-506 compared to CSA
  - Need to keep trough 10–15
- **Sirolimus** (Rapamycin)
  - Binds FK-binding protein like FK-506 but **inhibits mammalian target of rapamycin (mTOR)**; result is that it **inhibits T and B cell response to IL-2**
  - Used as maintenance therapy
- **Anti-thymocyte globulin** (ATG)
  - Equine (ATGAM) or rabbit (Thymoglobulin) **polyclonal antibodies** against T cell antigens (CD2, CD3, CD4)

- Used for induction and acute rejection episodes
- Is **cytolytic** (complement dependent)
- Need to keep WBCs > 3
- Side effects: **cytokine release syndrome** (fever, chills, pulmonary edema, shock) – steroids and Benadryl given before drug to try to prevent this
- **Zenapax** (daclizumab) – human monoclonal antibody against **IL-2 receptors**
  - Used for induction and acute rejection episodes
  - Is <u>not</u> cytolytic

TYPES OF REJECTION
- **Hyperacute rejection** (occurs within minutes to hours)
  - Caused by **preformed antibodies** that should have been picked up by the cross-match
  - Activates the **complement** cascade and thrombosis of vessels occurs
  - Tx: **emergent re-transplant** (or just removal of organ if kidney)
- **Accelerated rejection** (occurs < 1 week)
  - Caused by sensitized **T cells** to donor antigens
  - Tx: ↑ immunosuppression, pulse steroids, and possibly antibody Tx
- **Acute rejection** (occurs 1 week to 1 month)
  - Caused by **T cells** (cytotoxic and helper T cells)
  - Tx: ↑ immunosuppression, pulse steroids, and possibly antibody Tx
- **Chronic rejection** (months to years)
  - Partially a type IV hypersensitivity reaction (sensitized **T cells**)
  - **Antibody formation** also plays a role
  - Leads to graft fibrosis
  - Tx: ↑ immunosuppression – no really effective treatment

KIDNEY TRANSPLANTATION
- Can store kidney for 48 hours
- Need ABO type compatibility and cross-match
- **UTI** – can still use kidney
- **Acute ↑ in creatinine** (1.0–3.0) – can still use kidney
- Mortality primarily from **stroke** and **MI**
- Attach to **iliac vessels**
- **Complications**
  - **Urine leaks** (#1) – Tx: drainage and stenting best
  - **Renal artery stenosis** – diagnose with ultrasound
    - Tx: PTA with stent
  - **Lymphocele** – most common cause of external ureter compression
    - Tx: 1st try **percutaneous drainage**; if that fails, then need **peritoneal window** (make hole in peritoneum, lymphatic fluid drains into peritoneum and is re-absorbed – 95% successful)
  - **Postop oliguria** – usually due to **ATN** (pathology shows hydrophobic changes)
  - **Postop diuresis** – usually due to **urea** and **glucose**
  - **New proteinuria** – suggestive of **renal vein thrombosis**
  - **Postop diabetes** – side effect of CSA, FK, steroids
  - **Viral infections** – **CMV** – Tx: ganciclovir; **HSV** – Tx: acyclovir
  - **Acute rejection** – usually occurs in 1st 6 months; pathology shows tubulitis (vasculitis with more severe form)
  - **Kidney rejection workup** – usually for ↑ in Cr or poor urine output
    - **Ultrasound with duplex** (to rule out vascular problem and ureteral obstruction) and **biopsy**
    - Empiric **decrease in CSA** or **FK** (these can be nephrotoxic)
    - Empiric **pulse steroids**
  - **Chronic rejection** – usually do not see until after 1 year; no good treatment
  - **5-year graft survival overall** – 70% (cadaveric 65%, living donors 75%)

■ **Living kidney donors**
- Most common complication – wound infection (1%)
- Most common cause of death – fatal PE
- The remaining kidney hypertrophies

LIVER TRANSPLANTATION

■ Can store for 24 hours
■ Contraindications to liver TXP – **current ETOH abuse**, **acute ulcerative colitis**
■ Chronic **hepatitis C** – most common reason for liver TXP in adults
■ **MELD score** uses **creatinine**, **INR**, and **bilirubin** to predict if patients with cirrhosis will benefit more from liver TXP than from medical therapy (MELD > 15 benefits from liver TXP)
■ Criteria for **urgent TXP** – fulminant hepatic failure (**encephalopathy** – stupor, coma)
■ Patients with hepatitis B antigenemia can be treated with **HBIG** (hepatitis B immunoglobulin) and **lamivudine** (protease inhibitor) after liver TXP to help prevent reinfection
■ **Hepatitis B** – reinfection rate is reduced to 20% with the use of HBIG and lamivudine
■ **Hepatitis C** – disease most likely to recur in the new liver allograft; reinfects essentially all grafts
■ **Hepatocellular CA** – if no vascular invasion or metastases can still consider TXP
■ **Portal vein thrombosis** – not a contraindication to TXP
■ **ETOH** – 20% will start drinking again (recidivism)
■ **Macrosteatosis** – extracellular fat globules in the liver allograft
- Risk-factor for **primary non-function -** if 50% of cross-section is macrosteatatic in potential donor liver, there is a 50% chance of primary non-function
■ Duct-to-duct anastomosis is performed
- Hepaticojejunostomy in kids
■ Right subhepatic, right, and left subdiaphragmatic drains are placed
■ **Biliary system** (ducts, etc.) depends on **hepatic artery** blood supply
■ Most common arterial anomaly – **right hepatic coming off SMA**
■ **Complications**
- **Bile leak** (#1) – Tx: place **drain**, then **ERCP with stent** across leak
- **Primary nonfunction**
  - **1st 24 hours** – total bilirubin > 10, bile output < 20 cc/12 h, elevated PT and PTT; **After 96 hours** – mental status changes, ↑ LFTs, renal failure, respiratory failure
  - Usually requires **re-transplantation**
- <u>Early</u> hepatic artery thrombosis
  - **MC early vascular Cx**
  - ↑ LFTs, ↓ bile output, **fulminant hepatic failure**
  - Tx: MC will need **emergent re-transplantation** for ensuing fulminant hepatic failure (can try to stent or revise anastomosis)
- <u>Late</u> hepatic artery thrombosis
  - Results in biliary strictures and abscesses (<u>not</u> fulminant hepatic failure)
- **Abscesses** – most commonly from **late** (chronic) **hepatic artery thrombosis**
- **IVC stenosis / thrombosis** (rare) – edema, ascites, renal insufficiency; Tx: thrombolytics, IVC stent
- **Portal vein thrombosis** (rare): <u>early</u> – abdominal pain; <u>late</u> – UGI bleeding, ascites, may be asymptomatic; Tx - if <u>early</u>, **re-op thrombectomy** and **revise anastomosis**
- **Cholangitis** – get **PMNs** around portal triad (<u>not</u> mixed infiltrate)
- **Acute rejection** – T cell mediated against blood vessels
  - Clinical – fever, jaundice, ↓ bile output
  - Labs – leukocytosis, eosinophilia, ↑ LFTs, ↑ total bilirubin, and ↑ PT
  - Pathology – shows **portal triad lymphocytosis**, **endotheliitis** (mixed infiltrate), and **bile duct injury**
  - Usually occurs in 1st 2 months

- **Chronic rejection** – <u>unusual</u> after liver TXP; get disappearing bile ducts (antibody and cellular attack on bile ducts); gradually get bile duct obstruction with ↑ in alkaline phosphatase, portal fibrosis
- **Retransplantation rate** – 20%
- **5-year survival rate** – 70%

PANCREAS TRANSPLANTATION
- Need both **donor celiac artery** and **SMA** for arterial supply
- Need **donor portal vein** for venous drainage
- Attach to iliac vessels
- Most use **enteric drainage** for pancreatic duct. Take second portion of duodenum from donor along with ampulla of Vater and pancreas, then perform anastomosis of donor duodenum to recipient bowel
- **Successful pancreas/kidney TXP** results in stabilization of retinopathy, ↓ neuropathy, ↑ nerve conduction velocity, ↓ autonomic dysfunction (gastroparesis), ↓ orthostatic hypotension
  - <u>No</u> reversal of vascular disease
- **Complications**
  - **Venous thrombosis** (#1) – hard to treat
  - **Rejection** – hard to diagnose if patient does not also have a kidney transplant
    - Can see ↑ glucose or amylase; fever, leukocytosis

HEART TRANSPLANTATION
- Can store for 6 hours
- Need ABO compatibility and crossmatch
- For patients with life expectancy < 1 year
- Persistent **pulmonary hypertension** after heart transplantation
  - Associated with <u>early mortality</u> after heart TXP
  - Tx: inhaled nitric oxide, ECMO if severe
- **Acute rejection** – shows <u>perivascular lymphocytic infiltrate</u> with varying grades of <u>myocyte inflammation and necrosis</u>
- *Chronic allograft vasculopathy* (progressive diffuse coronary atherosclerosis) – MCC of late death and death overall following heart TXP

LUNG TRANSPLANTATION
- Can store for 6 hours
- Need ABO compatibility and crossmatch
- For patients with life expectancy < 1 year
- #1 cause of <u>early mortality</u> – **reperfusion injury** (Tx: similar to ARDS)
- Indication for double-lung TXP – **cystic fibrosis**
- Exclusion criteria for using lungs – aspiration, moderate to large contusion, infiltrate, purulent sputum, $PO_2 < 350$ on 100% FiO_2 and PEEP 5
- **Acute rejection** – perivascular lymphocytosis
- **Chronic rejection** – *bronchiolitis obliterans*; MCC of late death and death overall following lung TXP

OPPORTUNISTIC INFECTIONS
- **Viral** – CMV, HSV, VZV
- **Protozoan** – *Pneumocystis jiroveci* pneumonia (reason for **Bactrim** prophylaxis)
- **Fungal** – *Aspergillus, Candida, Cryptococcus*

Hierarchy for Permission for Organ Donation from Next of Kin – 1) Spouse, 2) adult son or daughter, 3) either parent, 4) adult brother or sister, 5) guardian, 6) any other person authorized to dispose of the body

INFLAMMATION PHASES

- **Injury** – leads to exposed <u>collagen</u>, <u>platelet-activating factor</u> release, and <u>tissue factor</u> release from endothelium
- **Platelets bind collagen** – release growth factors (platelet-derived growth factor [<u>PDGF</u>]); leads to PMN and macrophage recruitment
- **Macrophages** – *dominant role in wound healing*; release important **growth factors** (PDGF) and **cytokines** (IL-1 and TNF-α)

GROWTH AND ACTIVATING FACTORS

- **PDGF**
  - Chemotactic and activates **inflammatory cells** (PMNs and macrophages)
  - Chemotactic and activates **fibroblasts** → collagen and ECM proteins
  - **Angiogenesis**
  - **Epithelialization**
  - Chemotactic for smooth muscle cells
  - Has been shown to accelerate wound healing
- **EGF** (epidermal growth factor)
  - Chemotactic and activates **fibroblasts**
  - **Angiogenesis**
  - **Epithelialization**
- **FGF** (fibroblastic growth factor)
  - Chemotactic and activates **fibroblasts** → collagen and ECM proteins
  - **Angiogenesis**
  - **Epithelialization**
- **PAF** (platelet-activating factor) – is not stored, generated by **phospholipase** in endothelium; is a **phospholipid**
  - Chemotactic for inflammatory cells; ↑ adhesion molecules
- **Chemotactic factors**
  - For inflammatory cells – PDGF, IL-8, LTB-4, C5a and C3a, PAF
  - For fibroblasts – PDGF, EGF, FGF
- **Angiogenesis factors** – PDGF, EGF, FGF, IL-8, hypoxia
- **Epithelialization factors** – PDGF, EGF, FGF
- **PMNs** – last 1–2 days in tissues (7 days in blood)
- **Platelets** – last 7–10 days
- **Lymphocytes** – involved in chronic inflammation (T cells) and antibody production (B cells)
- **TXA$_2$** and **PGI$_2$** – see Chapter 2 (Hematology)

TYPE I HYPERSENSITIVITY REACTIONS

- **Eosinophils**
  - Have IgE receptors that bind to allergen
  - Release **major basic protein**, which stimulates basophils and mast cells to release **histamine**
  - Eosinophils are increased in <u>parasitic infections</u>
- **Basophils**
  - Main source of <u>histamine</u> in **blood**; not found in tissue
- **Mast cells** – primary cell in **type I hypersensitivity reactions**
  - Main source of <u>histamine</u> in **tissues**
- **Histamine** – vasodilation, tissue edema, postcapillary leakage
  - Primary effector in **type I hypersensitivity reactions** (<u>allergic reactions</u>)

- **Bradykinin** – peripheral vasodilation, increased permeability, pain, pulmonary vasoconstriction
  - **Angiotensin-converting enzyme** (ACE) – inactivates bradykinin; located in **lung**

NITRIC OXIDE (NO)
- Has **arginine** precursor (substrate for nitric oxide synthase)
- NO activates **guanylate cyclase** and increases **cGMP**, resulting in vascular smooth muscle **dilation**
- Is also called endothelium-derived relaxing factor
- **Endothelin** – causes vascular smooth muscle **constriction** (opposite effect of nitric oxide)

IMPORTANT CYTOKINES
- Main initial cytokine response to injury and infection is release of **TNF-α** and **IL-1**
- **Tumor necrosis factor-alpha** (TNF-α)
  - **Macrophages** – largest producers of TNF
  - Increases adhesion molecules
  - Overall, a procoagulant
  - Causes cachexia in patients with cancer
  - Activates neutrophils and macrophages → more cytokine production, cell recruitment
  - High concentrations of TNF-α can cause circulatory collapse and multisystem organ failure
- **IL-1**
  - Main source also macrophages; effects similar to TNF-α and synergizes TNF-α
  - Responsible for **fever** (PGE$_2$ mediated in hypothalamus)
    - Raises thermal set point, causing fever
    - **NSAIDs** decrease fever by reducing PGE$_2$ synthesis
  - **Alveolar macrophages** – cause fever with **atelectasis** by releasing **IL-1**
- **IL-6** – increases **hepatic acute phase proteins** (C-reactive protein, amyloid A)

INTERFERONS
- Released by **lymphocytes** in response to <u>viral infection</u> or other stimulants
- Activate macrophages, natural killer cells, and cytotoxic T cells
- **Inhibit viral replication**

HEPATIC ACUTE PHASE RESPONSE PROTEINS
- **IL-6** – most potent stimulus
- *Increased* – **C-reactive protein** (an opsonin, activates complement), **amyloid A** and P, fibrinogen, haptoglobin, ceruloplasmin, alpha-1 antitrypsin, and C3 (complement)
- *Decreased* – albumin, **pre-albumin**, and **transferrin**

CELL ADHESION MOLECULES
- **Selectins** – <u>L-selectins</u>, located on leukocytes, bind to <u>E- (endothelial)</u> and <u>P- (platelets) selectins</u>; **rolling adhesion**
- **Beta-2 integrins** (CD 11/18 molecules) – on leukocytes; bind ICAMs, etc., **anchoring adhesion**
- **ICAM, VCAM, PECAM, ELAM** – on endothelial cells, bind beta-2 integrin molecules located on leukocytes and platelets. These are also involved in **transendothelial migration**

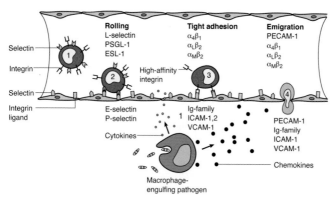

Leukocyte recruitment. (1) Circulating leukocytes express integrins in a low-affinity conformation. (2) Exposure to activated endothelium leads to rolling, which is mediated by L-selectin and P-selectin on the neutrophil and E-selectin on the endothelium. (3) Leukocyte exposure to cytokines released by macrophages phagocytosing pathogens induces a high-affinity integrin conformation. Tight leukocyte—endothelial adhesion involves integrin engagement with counter-ligand expressed on the endothelium. (4) Subsequent exposure to chemokines leads to diapedesis, which is further mediated by the family of β_1- and β_2-integrins.

COMPLEMENT
- **Classic pathway** (IgG or IgM) – antigen–antibody complex activates
  - Factors **C1**, **C2**, and **C4** – found only in the classic pathway
- **Alternative pathway** – endotoxin, bacteria, other stimuli activate
  - Factors **B**, **D**, and **P** (properdin) – found only in the alternate pathway
- **C3** – common to and is the convergence point for both pathways
- **Mg** – required for both pathways
- **Anaphylatoxins** – C3a, C4a, C5a; ↑ vascular permeability, bronchoconstriction; activate mast cells and basophils
- **Membrane attack complex** – C5b-9b; causes **cell lysis** (usually bacteria) by creating a hole in the cell membrane
- **Opsonization** (targets antigen for immune response) – **C3b** and C4b
- **Chemotaxis** for inflammatory cells – **C3a** and C5a

PROSTAGLANDINS
- Produced from arachidonic precursors
- **PGI$_2$** and **PGE$_2$** – vasodilation, bronchodilation, ↑ permeability; inhibit platelets
- **NSAIDs** – inhibit cyclooxygenase (reversible)
- **Aspirin** – inhibits cyclooxygenase (irreversible), inhibits platelet adhesion by decreasing TXA$_2$
- **Steroids** – inhibit phospholipase, which converts phospholipids to arachidonic acid → inhibits inflammation

LEUKOTRIENES
- Produced from arachidonic precursors
- **LTC$_4$, LTD$_4$, LTE$_4$** – slow-reacting substances of anaphylaxis; bronchoconstriction, vasoconstriction followed by increased permeability (wheal and flare)
- **LTB$_4$** – chemotactic for inflammatory cells

CATECHOLAMINES
- Peak **24–48 hours** after injury
- Norepinephrine released from sympathetic postganglionic neurons
- Epinephrine and norepinephrine released from adrenal medulla (neural response to injury)

MISCELLANEOUS
- **Neuroendocrine response to injury** – afferent nerves from site of injury stimulate CRF, ACTH, ADH, growth hormone, epinephrine, and norepinephrine release
- **Thyroid hormone** – does *not* play a major role in injury or inflammation
- **CXC chemokines** – chemotaxis, angiogenesis, wound healing
  - **IL-8** and **platelet factor 4** are CXC chemokines
  - C = cysteine; X = another amino acid
- **Oxidants** generated in inflammation (oxidants/main producer oxidase):
  Superoxide anion radical (O_2^-)   NADPH oxidase
  Hydrogen peroxide (H_2O_2)   xanthine oxidase
- **Cellular defenses** against oxidative species (oxidants/defense):
  Superoxide anion radical   *Superoxide dismutase*
  Converts to hydrogen peroxide
  Hydrogen peroxide   *Glutathione* **peroxidase**, **catalase**
- **Reperfusion injury** – **PMNs** are the primary mediator
- **Chronic granulomatous disease** – NADPH-oxidase system enzyme defect in PMNs
  - Results in ↓ superoxide radical (O_2^-) formation

WOUND HEALING

■ **Inflammation** (days 1–10) – PMNs, macrophages; **epithelialization** (1–2 mm/day)
■ **Proliferation** (5 days–3 weeks) – fibroblasts, **collagen deposition**, neovascularization, **granulation tissue** formation; type III collagen replaced with type I
■ **Remodeling** (3 weeks–1 year) – decreased vascularity
 • Net amount of collagen does not change with remodeling, although significant production and degradation occur
 • Collagen **cross-linking** occurs
■ **Peripheral nerves** regenerate at **1 mm/day**
■ **Order of cell arrival in wound**
 • **Platelets**
 • **PMNs**
 • **Macrophages**
 • **Lymphocytes** (recent research shows arrival before fibroblasts)
 • **Fibroblasts**

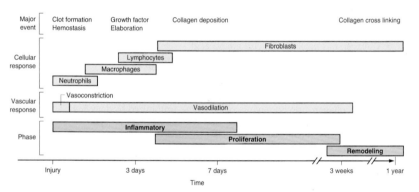

Timeline of phases of wound healing with dominant cell types and major physiologic events.

■ *Macrophages are essential for wound healing (release of growth factors, cytokines, etc.)*
■ **Fibronectin** – chemotactic for macrophages; anchors fibroblasts
■ **Fibroblasts** – replace fibronectin-fibrin with **collagen**
■ **Predominant cell type by day**
 • **Days 0–2** – PMNs
 • **Days 3–4** – macrophages
 • **Days 5 and on** – fibroblasts
■ **Platelet plug** – platelets and fibrin
■ **Provisional matrix** – platelets, fibrin, and fibronectin
■ **Accelerated wound healing** – reopening a wound results in quicker healing the 2nd time (as healing cells are already present there)
■ **Epithelial integrity** – most important factor in healing **open wounds** (secondary intention)
 • Migration from **hair follicles** (#1 site), wound edges, and sweat glands
 • Dependent on **granulation tissue** in wound
 • Unepithelialized wounds leak serum and protein, promote bacteria

- **Tensile strength** – most important factor in healing **closed incisions** (primary intention)
  - Depends on collagen deposition and cross-linking of collagen
- **Submucosa** – strength layer of bowel
  - Weakest time point for small bowel anastomosis – 3–5 days
- **Myofibroblasts** (smooth muscle cell–fibroblast; communicate by **gap junctions**)
  - Involved in **wound contraction** and healing by **secondary intention**
  - Perineum has better wound contraction than leg

Collagen

Type	Description
I	Most common type of collagen: **skin**, **bone**, and **tendons** Primary collagen in a **healed wound**
II	Cartilage
III	Increased in **healing wound**, also in **blood vessels** and **skin**
IV	**Basement membranes**
V	Widespread, particularly found in the **cornea**

- **Alpha-ketoglutarate**, **vitamin C**, **oxygen**, and **iron** are required for hydroxylation (prolyl hydroxylase) and subsequent **cross-linking of proline residues** in collagen
  - Collagen has proline every 3rd amino acid
  - Proline cross-linking improves **wound tensile strength**
- **Scurvy** – vitamin C deficiency
- **Tensile strength never equal to pre-wound** (80%)
  - **Type III collagen** – predominant collagen type synthesized for days 1–2
  - **Type I collagen** – predominant collagen type synthesized by days 3–4
  - Type III replaced by type I collagen by 3 weeks
    - **At 8 weeks**, wound reaches maximum tensile strength, which is 80% of its original strength
    - Maximum collagen accumulation at 2–3 weeks → after that the amount of collagen stays the same, but continued cross-linking improves strength
    - **d-Penicillamine** – inhibits collagen cross-linking
- **Essentials for wound healing**
  - **Moist** environment (avoid desiccation)
  - **Oxygen delivery** – optimize fluids, no smoking, pain control, arterial revascularization, supplemental oxygen
    - Want transcutaneous oxygen measurement (TCOM) > 25 mm Hg
  - **Avoid edema** – leg elevation
  - **Remove necrotic tissue**
- **Impediments to wound healing**
  - **Bacteria** > $10^5/cm^2$ – ↓ oxygen content, collagen lysis, prolonged inflammation
  - **Devitalized tissue** and **foreign bodies** – retards granulation tissue formation and wound healing
  - **Cytotoxic drugs** – 5FU, methotrexate, cyclosporine, FK-506, etc. can impair wound healing in 1st 14 days after injury
  - **Diabetes** – can contribute to poor wound healing by impeding the early-phase inflammation response (hyperglycemia causes poor leukocyte chemotaxis)
  - **Albumin** < 3.0 – risk factor for poor wound healing
  - **Steroids** – prevent wound healing by inhibiting macrophages, PMNs, and collagen synthesis by fibroblasts; ↓ wound tensile strength as well
    - **Vitamin A** (25,000 IU qd) – counteracts effects of steroids on wound healing

- **Wound ischemia** (hypoxia) – can be caused by fibrosis, pressure (sacral decubitus ulcer, pressure sores), poor arterial inflow (atherosclerosis), poor venous outflow (venous stasis), smoking, radiation, edema, vasculitis
- **Diseases associated with abnormal wound healing**
  - **Osteogenesis imperfecta** – type I collagen defect
  - **Ehlers–Danlos syndrome** – 10 types identified, all collagen disorders
  - **Marfan's syndrome** – fibrillin defect (connective tissue protein)
  - **Epidermolysis bullosa** – excessive fibroblasts. Tx: phenytoin
  - **Scurvy** – Vitamin C deficiency
  - **Pyoderma gangrenosum**
- **Diabetic foot ulcers** – usually at **Charcot's joint** (2nd MTP joint); secondary to **neuropathy** (can't feel feet, pressure from walking leads to ischemia); also on **toes**
- **Leg ulcers** - 90% due to **venous insufficiency**; Tx - Unna boot (elastic wrap)
- **Scars** – contain a lot of proteoglycans, **hyaluronic acid**, and water
  - **Scar revisions** – wait for 1 year to allow maturation; may improve with age
  - **Infants** heal with **little or no scarring**
- **Cartilage** – contains no blood vessels (get nutrients and oxygen by **diffusion**)
- **Denervation** – has no effect on wound healing
- **Chemotherapy** – has no effect on wound healing after 14 days
- **Keloids** – autosomal dominant; dark skinned
  - **Collagen <u>goes beyond</u> original scar**
  - Tx: **intra-lesion steroid injection**; silicone, pressure garments, XRT
- **Hypertrophic scar tissue** – dark skinned; flexor surfaces of upper torso
  - **Collagen <u>stays within confines</u> of original scar**
  - Often occurs in burns or wounds that take a long time to heal
  - Tx: **steroid injection**, silicone, pressure garments

PLATELET GRANULES
- **Alpha granules**
  - **Platelet factor 4** – aggregation
  - **Beta-thrombomodulin** – binds thrombin
  - **Platelet-derived growth factor** (PDGF) – chemoattractant
  - Transforming growth factor beta (TGF-beta) – modulates above responses
- **Dense granules** – contain **adenosine, serotonin**, and **calcium**
- Platelet aggregation factors – **TXA_2, thrombin, platelet factor 4**

- **1st peak** for trauma deaths (0–30 minutes) – deaths due to lacerations of heart, aorta, brain, brainstem, or spinal cord; cannot really save these patients; death is too quick
- **2nd peak** for trauma deaths (30 minutes–4 hours) – deaths due to head injury (#1) and hemorrhage (#2); these patients can be saved with rapid assessment (golden hour)
- **3rd peak** for trauma deaths (days to weeks) – deaths due to multisystem organ failure and sepsis
- **Blunt injury** – 80% of all trauma; <u>liver</u> most commonly injured (some texts say spleen)
    - Kinetic energy $= \frac{1}{2} MV^2$, where M $=$ mass, V $=$ velocity
    - **Falls** – age and body orientation biggest predictors of survival. LD_{50} is 4 stories
- **Penetrating injury** – <u>small bowel</u> most commonly injured (some texts say liver)
- **Hemorrhage** – most common cause of death in 1st hour
    - **Blood pressure** is usually OK until 30% of total blood volume is lost
    - Resuscitate with **2 L Lactated Ringers**, then switch to **blood**
- **Head injury** – most common cause of death after reaching the ER alive
- **Infection** – most common cause of death in the long term
- **Tongue** – most common cause of upper airway obstruction $\rightarrow$ perform jaw thrust
- **Seat belts** – small bowel perforations, lumbar spine fractures, sternal fractures
- **Saphenous vein** at ankle – best site for cutdown for venous access
- **Diagnostic peritoneal lavage** (DPL)
    - Used in hypotensive patients with blunt trauma
    - Positive if > 10 cc blood, > 100,000 RBCs/cc, food particles, bile, bacteria, > 500 WBC/cc
    - Need laparotomy if DPL is positive
    - DPL needs to be supraumbilical if pelvic fracture present
    - **DPL misses** – retroperitoneal bleeds, contained hematomas
- **FAST scan** (focused abdominal sonography for trauma)
    - Ultrasound scan used in lieu of DPL
    - Checks for blood in perihepatic fossa, perisplenic fossa, pelvis, and pericardium
    - Examiner dependent
    - Obesity can obstruct view
    - May not detect free fluid < 50–80 mL
    - Need laparotomy if FAST scan is positive
    - **FAST scan misses** – retroperitoneal bleeding, hollow viscous injury
- In hypotensive patients with a **negative FAST scan** (or negative DPL) you need to find the source of bleeding (**pelvic fracture**, **chest**, or **extremity**)
- **Need a CT scan following blunt trauma in patients** with abdominal pain, need for general anesthesia, closed head injury, intoxicants on board, paraplegia, distracting injury, or hematuria
    - Patients requiring DPL that turned out negative will need an abdominal CT scan
    - **CT scan misses** – hollow viscous injury, diaphragm injury
- **Need laparotomy** with peritonitis, evisceration, positive DPL, uncontrolled visceral hemorrhage, free air, diaphragm injury, intraperitoneal bladder injury, contrast extravasation from hollow viscus, specific renal, pancreas, and biliary tract injuries

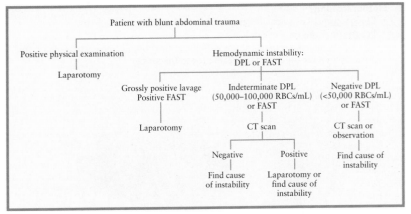

Diagnosis of blunt abdominal trauma.

- **Penetrating abdominal injury** (eg GSW) – generally need laparotomy
- **Possible penetrating abdominal injuries** (knife or low-velocity injuries) – local exploration and observation if fascia not violated

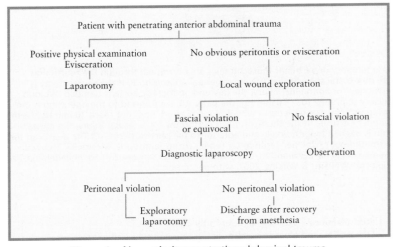

Diagnosis of **low-velocity** penetrating abdominal trauma.

- **Abdominal compartment syndrome**
  - Occurs after massive fluid resuscitation, trauma, or abdominal surgery
  - **Bladder pressure** > 25–30 suggests compartment syndrome
  - **IVC compression** is the final common pathway for **decreased cardiac output**
  - Low cardiac output causes **visceral** and **renal malperfusion** (↓ urine output)
  - Upward displacement of diaphragm affects ventilation
  - Tx: decompressive laparotomy
- **Pneumatic antishock garment** – controversial; use in patients with SBP < 50 and no thoracic injury. Release compartments one at a time after reaching ER

- **ER thoracotomy**
  - Blunt trauma – use only if pressure/pulse lost **in ER**
  - Penetrating trauma – use only if pressure/pulse lost **on way to ER** or **in ER**
  - Thoracotomy – open pericardium anterior to the phrenic nerve, cross-clamp the aorta, watch for the esophagus (anterior to the aorta)

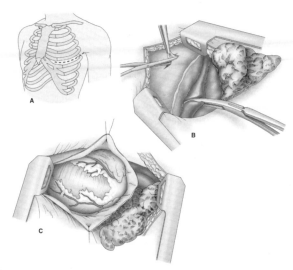

(A) Emergency department thoracotomies are performed through the fourth and fifth intercostal spaces using the anterolateral approach. *(B)* If the thoracotomy is performed for abdominal injury, the descending thoracic aorta is clamped. If blood pressure improved to > 70 mm Hg, the patient is transported to the operating room for laparotomy. For patients in whom blood pressure does not reach 70 mm Hg, further treatment is futile. If the thoracotomy is performed for a cardiac injury, the pericardium is opened longitudinally and anterior to the phrenic nerve. *(C)* The heart can then be rotated out of the pericardium for repair. (From Johnson JL, Moore EE. Thoracic trauma. In: Fischer JE, Bland KI, et al, eds. *Mastery of Surgery.* 5th ed. Philadelphia, PA: Lippincott Williams & Wilkins; 2007, with permission.)

- **Catecholamines** – peak 24–48 hours after injury
- **ADH, ACTH,** and **glucagon** – also ↑ after trauma (fight or flight response)

BLOOD TRANSFUSION

- Type O blood (universal donor) – contains no A or B antigens; males can receive Rh-positive blood; females who are prepubescent or of childbearing age should receive Rh-negative blood
- Type-specific blood (nonscreened, non–cross-matched) – can be administered relatively safely, but there may be effects from antibodies to HLA minor antigens in the donated blood

HEAD INJURY
- ■ **Glasgow Coma Scale (GCS)**
  - • **Motor**
    - • **6** – follows commands
    - • **5** – localizes pain
    - • **4** – withdraws from pain
    - • **3** – flexion with pain (decorticate)
    - • **2** – extension with pain (decerebrate)
    - • **1** – no response
  - • **Verbal**
    - • **5** – oriented
    - • **4** – confused
    - • **3** – inappropriate words
    - • **2** – incomprehensible sounds
    - • **1** – no response
  - • **Eye opening**
    - • **4** – spontaneous opening
    - • **3** – opens to command
    - • **2** – opens to pain
    - • **1** – no response
- ■ **GCS score** – ≤ **14**: head CT; ≤ **10**: intubation; ≤ **8**: ICP monitor

---

Indications for Head CT

- ■ Suspected skull penetration by a foreign body
- ■ Discharge of cerebrospinal fluid (CSF), blood, or both from the nose
- ■ Hemotympanum or discharge of blood or CSF from the ear
- ■ Head injury with alcohol or drug intoxication
- ■ Altered state of consciousness at the time of examination
- ■ Focal neurologic signs or symptoms
- ■ Any situation precluding proper surveillance
- ■ Head injury plus additional trauma
- ■ Protracted unconsciousness

- ■ **Epidural hematoma** – most commonly due to arterial bleeding from the **middle meningeal artery**
  - • Head CT – shows lenticular (lens-shaped) deformity
  - • Patients often have loss of consciousness (LOC) → then lucid interval → then sudden deterioration (vomiting, restlessness, LOC)
  - • Operate for significant neurologic degeneration or significant mass effect (shift > 5 mm)
- ■ **Subdural hematoma** – most commonly from tearing of **venous plexus** (bridging veins) that cross between the dura and arachnoid
  - • **Head CT** – shows crescent-shaped deformity
  - • Operate for significant neurologic degeneration or mass effect (> 1 cm)
  - • **Chronic subdural hematomas** – usually in elderly after minor fall
- ■ **Intracerebral hematoma** – usually frontal or temporal
  - • Can cause significant mass effect requiring operation
- ■ **Cerebral contusions** – can be coup or contrecoup
- ■ **Traumatic intraventricular hemorrhage** – need **ventriculostomy** if causing hydrocephalus
- ■ **Diffuse axonal injury** – shows up better on MRI than CT scan
  - • Tx: supportive; may need craniectomy if ICP elevated
  - • Very poor prognosis

- **Cerebral perfusion pressure** (CPP = MAP − ICP)
  - **CPP** = mean arterial pressure (MAP) *minus* intracranial pressure (ICP)
  - **Signs of elevated ICP** − ↓ ventricular size, loss of sulci, loss of cisterns
  - **ICP monitors** − indicated for GCS ≤ 8, suspected ↑ ICP, or patient with moderate to severe head injury and inability to follow clinical exam (eg is intubated)
  - **Supportive treatment for elevated ICP**
    - Normal ICP is 10; > 20 needs treatment
    - Want CPP > 60
      - **Sedation** and **paralysis**
      - **Raise head of bed**
      - **Relative hyperventilation** for modest cerebral vasoconstriction (CO_2 30–35); do not want to over-hyperventilate and cause cerebral ischemia from too much vasoconstriction
      - Keep **Na 140–150, serum Osm 295–310** − may need to use <u>hypertonic saline</u> at times (draws fluid out of brain)
      - **Mannitol** − load 1 g/kg, give 0.25 mg/kg q4h after that (draws fluid from brain)
      - **Barbiturate coma** − consider if above not working
      - **Ventriculostomy w/ CSF drainage** (keep ICP < 20)
      - **Craniotomy decompression** − if not able to get ICP down medically (can also perform Burr hole)
      - **Fosphenytoin** or **Keppra** − can be given prophylactically to prevent seizures with moderate to severe head injury
      - **Peak ICP** − occurs **48–72 hours** after injury
      - **Dilated pupil** − **temporal pressure** on the same side (CN III, oculomotor, compression)
- **Basal skull fractures**
  - **Raccoon eyes** (peri-orbital ecchymosis) − anterior fossa fracture
  - **Battle's sign** (mastoid ecchymosis) − middle fossa fracture; can injure **facial nerve** (CN VII)
    - If acute facial nerve injury, need exploration and repair
    - If delayed, likely secondary to edema and exploration not needed
  - Can also have hemotympanum and CSF rhinorrhea/otorrhea with basal skull fractures
- **Temporal skull fractures** − can injure CN VII and VIII (vestibulocochlear nerve)
  - Most common site of **facial nerve injury** − *geniculate ganglion*
  - Temporal skull fractures most commonly associated with lateral skull or orbital blows
- **Most skull fractures do <u>not</u> require surgical treatment**
  - Operate if **significantly depressed** (> 1 cm), **contaminated**, or **persistent CSF leak** not responding to conservative therapy
- **CSF leaks** after skull fracture − treat expectantly; can use **lumbar CSF drainage** if persistent
- **Coagulopathy** with **traumatic brain injury** − due to release of **tissue factor**

SPINE TRAUMA
- **Cervical spine**
  - **C-1 burst** (Jefferson fracture) − caused by axial loading
    - Tx: rigid collar
  - **C-2 hangman's fracture** − caused by distraction and extension
    - Tx: traction and halo
  - **C-2 odontoid fracture**
    - Type I − above base, stable
    - Type II − at base, unstable (will need fusion or halo)
    - Type III − extends into vertebral body (will need fusion or halo)
  - **Facet** fractures or dislocations − can cause cord injury; usually associated with hyperextension and rotation with ligamentous disruption

- **Thoracolumbar spine**
  - 3 columns of the thoracolumbar spine:
    - <u>Anterior</u> – anterior longitudinal ligament and anterior ½ of the vertebral body
    - <u>Middle</u> – posterior ½ of the vertebral body and posterior longitudinal ligament
    - <u>Posterior</u> – facet joints, lamina, spinous processes, interspinous ligament
  - If more than 1 column is disrupted, the spine is considered unstable
    - **Compression** (wedge) **fractures** usually involve the anterior column only and are considered stable
    - **Burst fractures** are considered unstable (> 1 column) and require spinal fusion
  - **Upright fall** – at risk for calcaneus, lumbar, and wrist/forearm fractures
- Need **MRI** for neurologic deficits without bony injury to check for ligamentous injury
- **Indications for emergent surgical spine decompression**
  - Fracture or dislocation not reducible with distraction
  - Open fractures
  - Soft tissue or bony compression of the cord
  - Progressive neurologic dysfunction

MAXILLOFACIAL TRAUMA
- Fracture of **temporal bone** is the most common cause of <u>facial nerve injury</u>
- Try to preserve skin and not trim edges with facial lacerations

Le Fort Classification of Facial Fractures		
Type	Description	Treatment
I	Maxillary fracture straight across (–)	Reduction, stabilization, intramaxillary fixation (IMF) ± circumzygomatic and orbital rim suspension wires
II	Lateral to nasal bone, underneath eyes, diagonal toward maxilla (/ \)	Same as Le Fort I
III	Lateral orbital walls (- -)	Suspension wiring to stable frontal bone; may need external fixation

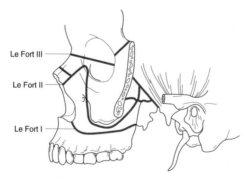

Le Fort classification system of maxillofacial fractures.

- **Nasoethmoidal orbital fractures** – 70% have a CSF leak
  - Conservative therapy for up to 2 weeks
  - Can try epidural catheter to ↓ CSF pressure and help it close CSF leak
  - May need surgical closure of dura to stop leak
- **Nosebleeds**
  - **Anterior** – packing
  - **Posterior** – can be hard to deal with; try balloon tamponade 1st
    - May need angioembolization of **internal maxillary artery** or ethmoidal artery

- **Orbital blowout fractures** – patients with impaired upward gaze or diplopia with upward vision need repair; perform restoration of orbital floor with bone fragments or bone graft
- **Mandibular injury** – malocclusion #1 indicator of injury
  - Diagnosis – fine-cut facial CT scans with reconstruction to assess injury
  - Most repaired with IMF (metal arch bars to upper and lower dental arches, 6–8 weeks) or open reduction and internal fixation (ORIF)
- **Tripod fracture** (zygomatic bone) – ORIF for cosmesis
- Patients w/ maxillofacial fractures are at high risk for **cervical spine injuries**

NECK TRAUMA
- **Asymptomatic blunt** – neck CT scan
- **Asymptomatic penetrating** – controversial; most common method below

Neck Zones	
Zone	**Method**
I	Clavicle to cricoid cartilage; need angiography, bronchoscopy, esophagoscopy, and barium swallow; a pericardial window may be indicated. May need **median sternotomy** to reach these lesions
II	Cricoid to angle of mandible. **Need neck exploration in OR**
III	Angle of mandible to the base of skull. Need angiography and laryngoscopy. May need jaw subluxation/digastric and sternocleidomastoid muscle release/ mastoid sinus resection to reach vascular injuries in this location

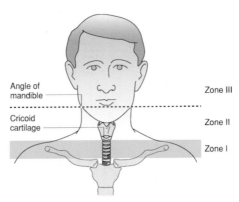

Angle of mandible — Zone III
Cricoid cartilage — Zone II
Zone I

Zones of the neck. Zones I is the cricoid cartilage to the top of the clavicles. The important implication of a zone I injury is the greater potential for intrathoracic great vessel injury.

- **Symptomatic blunt** or **penetrating neck trauma** – shock, bleeding, expanding hematoma, losing or lost airway, subcutaneous air, stridor, dysphagia, hemoptysis, neurologic deficit → *all need neck exploration*
- **Esophageal injury**
  - *Hardest neck injury to find*
  - **Esophagoscopy** and **esophagogram** – best combined modality (find essentially 95% of injuries when using both methods)
  - **Contained injuries** – can be observed

- **Noncontained injuries**:
  - If **small** injury and **minimal contamination** → <u>primary closure</u>
  - If **extensive** injury or **contamination** →
    Neck esophageal injuries – just place drains (will heal)
    Chest esophageal injuries – chest tubes to drain injury and place spit fistula in neck (will eventually need esophagectomy)
- Always drain esophageal and hypopharyngeal repairs – 20% leak rate
- Approach to esophageal injuries
  - Neck – **left side**
  - Upper ⅔ of thoracic esophagus – **right thoracotomy**
  - Lower ⅓ of thoracic esophagus – **left thoracotomy**
- **Laryngeal fracture** and **tracheal injuries**
  - These are **airway emergencies**
  - Symptoms: **crepitus, stridor, respiratory compromise**
  - Need to **secure airway emergently in ER** (cricothyroidotomy usual)
  - Tx: primary repair, can use strap muscle for airway support; tracheostomy necessary for most to allow edema to subside and to check for stricture (need to convert cricothyroidotomy to tracheostomy)
- **Thyroid gland injuries** – control bleeding and drain (<u>not</u> thyroidectomy)
- **Recurrent laryngeal nerve injury** – can try to repair or can reimplant in <u>cricoarytenoid muscle</u> (Sx - hoarseness)
- **Shotgun injures to neck** – need angiogram and neck CT; esophagus/trachea evaluation
- **Vertebral artery bleeds** – can embolize or ligate without sequela in majority
- **Common carotid bleeds** – ligation will cause stroke in 20%

CHEST TRAUMA
- **Chest tube**
  - > 1,500 cc after initial insertion, > 250 cc/h for 3 hours, > 2,500 cc/24 h, or bleeding with instability → all relative indications for **thoracotomy in OR**
  - Need to drain all of the blood (in < 48 hours) to prevent fibrothorax, pulmonary entrapment, infected hemothorax
  - **Unresolved hemothorax** after 2 well-placed chest tubes → thoracoscopic drainage
- **Sucking chest wound** (open pneumothorax)
  - Needs to be at least ⅔ the diameter of the trachea to be significant
  - Cover wound with dressing that has tape on three sides → prevents development of <u>tension pneumothorax</u> while allowing lung to expand with inspiration
- **Tracheobronchial injury**
  - Patient may have worse oxygenation after chest tube placement
  - One of the very few indications in which clamping the chest tube may be indicated
  - Bronchus injuries are more common on the **right**
  - May need to **mainstem intubate** patient on unaffected side
  - Dx: bronchoscopy
  - Tx: repair if <u>large air leak and respiratory compromise</u> or after <u>2 weeks of persistent air leak</u>
  - **Right thoracotomy** for <u>right mainstem, trachea, and proximal left mainstem injuries</u> (avoids the aorta)
  - **Left thoracotomy** for <u>distal left mainstem injuries</u>
- **Esophageal injury** – see section "Neck Trauma"
- **Diaphragm**
  - Injuries are more likely to be found on **left** and to result from **blunt trauma**
  - CXR – see **air–fluid level** in chest from <u>stomach herniation</u> through hole (diagnosis can be made essentially with CXR)
  - **Transabdominal** approach if **< 1 week**
  - **Chest** approach if **> 1 week** (need to take down adhesions in the chest)
  - May need mesh

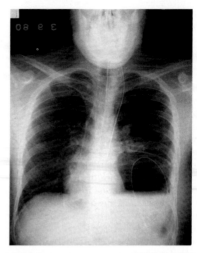

Chest roentgenogram demonstrating a nasogastric tube within the left chest (From Thal ER, Friese RS. Traumatic rupture of the diaphragm. In: Fischer JE, Bland KI, et al, eds. *Mastery of Surgery.* 5th ed. Philadelphia, PA: Lippincott Williams & Wilkins; 2007, with permission.)

- **Aortic transection**
  - **Signs** – widened mediastinum, 1st or 2nd rib fractures, apical capping, loss of aortopulmonary window, loss of aortic contour, left hemothorax, trachea deviation to right
  - Tear is usually at the **ligamentum arteriosum** (just distal to subclavian takeoff). Other areas include near the aortic valve and where the aorta traverses the diaphragm
  - CXR normal in 5% of patients with aortic tears – need aortic evaluation in patients with significant mechanism (head on car crash > 45 mph, fall > 15 ft)
  - Dx: CT angiogram of chest
  - Operative approach – **left thoracotomy and repair** with partial left heart bypass or place a **covered stent endograft** (distal transections only)
  - Important to treat other life-threatening injuries 1st → patient with positive DPL or other life-threatening injury needs to have that addressed before the aortic transection
- **Approach for specific injuries**
  - **Median sternotomy** – for injuries to ascending aorta, innominate artery, proximal right subclavian artery, innominate vein, proximal left common carotid
  - **Left thoracotomy** – for injuries to left subclavian artery, descending aorta
  - **Distal right subclavian artery** – midclavicular incision, resection of medial clavicle
- **Myocardial contusion** – V-tach and V-fib most common causes of death
  - Risk highest in 1st 24 hours
  - **Supra-ventricular tachycardia** (SVT) – most common arrhythmia overall in these patients
  - Need monitoring for 24–48 hours
- **Flail chest** – ≥ 2 consecutive ribs broken at ≥ 2 sites → results in paradoxical motion
  - Underlying **pulmonary contusion** – biggest pulmonary impairment
- **Aspiration** – may not produce CXR findings immediately

- **Penetrating chest injury** – start with a **CXR** if the patient is stable (place chest tube for pneumothorax or hemothorax)
  - **Penetrating "box" injuries** – borders are clavicles, xiphoid process, nipples
    - Need pericardial window, bronchoscopy, esophagoscopy, barium swallow
  - **Penetrating chest wound outside "box"** without pneumothorax or hemothorax
    - Need chest tube if patient requires intubation
    - Otherwise follow patient's serial CXRs
  - **Pericardial window** – if you find blood, need **median sternotomy** to fix possible injury to heart or great vessels; place pericardial drain
  - **Penetrating injuries anterior-medial to midaxillary line and below nipples**
    - Need laparotomy or laparoscopy
    - May also need evaluation for **penetrating "box" injury** depending on the exact location
  - Some are using FAST scan of the pericardium instead of pericardial window for "box" injuries
- **Traumatic causes of cardiogenic shock** – cardiac tamponade, cardiac contusion, tension pneumothorax
- **Tension pneumothorax** (one way valve effect causes air entry and pressure build up)
  - Hypotension, ↑ airway pressures, ↓ breath sounds, bulging neck veins, tracheal shift
  - Can see bulging diaphragm during laparotomy
  - Cardiac compromise secondary to ↓ venous return (IVC, SVC compression)
  - Tx: chest tube
- **Sternal fractures** – these patients are at high risk for cardiac contusion
- **1st** and **2nd rib fractures** – high risk for aortic transaction

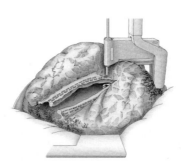

Pulmonary tractotomy. Dividing the pulmonary parenchyma between adjacent staple lines permits rapid direct access to injured vessels or bronchi along the tract of a penetrating injury. (From Johnson JL, Moore EE. Thoracic trauma. In: Fischer JE, Bland KI, et al, eds. *Mastery of Surgery.* 5th ed. Philadelphia, PA: Lippincott Williams & Wilkins; 2007, with permission.)

PELVIC TRAUMA
- Pelvic fractures can be a major source of **blood loss**.
- If hemodynamically unstable with pelvic fracture and negative DPL, negative CXR, and no other signs of blood loss or reasons for shock → stabilize pelvis (C-clamp, external fixator, or sheet) and go to angio for **embolization**
- These patients are at high risk for **genitourinary** and **abdominal injuries**

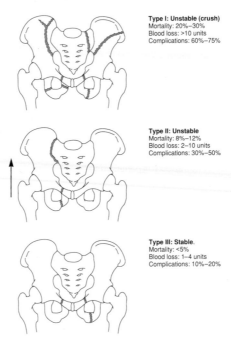

Type I: Unstable (crush)
Mortality: 20%–30%
Blood loss: >10 units
Complications: 60%–75%

Type II: Unstable
Mortality: 8%–12%
Blood loss: 2–10 units
Complications: 30%–50%

Type III: Stable.
Mortality: <5%
Blood loss: 1–4 units
Complications: 10%–20%

Classification of pelvic fractures with relative stability, mortality rates, and blood loss indicated.

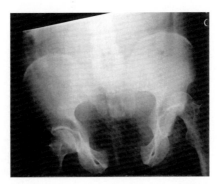

Wide pubic diastasis, characteristic of "open book" horizontally unstable pelvis (type B), with associated femoral head fracture and hip dislocation.

- **Anterior pelvic fractures** – more likely to have venous bleeding
- **Posterior pelvic fractures** – more likely to have arterial bleeding
- May need colostomy for open pelvic fractures with rectal tears and perineal lacerations
- Pelvic fracture repair itself may need to be delayed until other associated injuries are repaired
- Intra-op **penetrating injury pelvic hematomas** – open (some suggest going to angiography for these)
- Intra-op **blunt injury pelvic hematomas** – leave; if expanding or patient unstable → stabilize pelvic fracture, pack pelvis if in OR, and go to angiography for **embolization**; if packs are placed intra-op, remove after 24–48 hours when patient is stable

DUODENAL TRAUMA

- Usually from blunt trauma (crush or deceleration injury)
- **2nd portion of the duodenum** (descending portion, near ampulla of Vater) – most common area of injury
- Can also get tears near ligament of Treitz
- 80% of injuries requiring surgery can be treated with **debridement** and **primary closure**
- **Segmental resection** with primary end-to-end closure possible with **all segments** *except* **second portion of the duodenum**
- 25% mortality in these patients because of associated **shock**
- **Fistulas** are the major source of morbidity
- **Intra-op paraduodenal hematomas** (≥ **2 cm** considered significant; usually in third portion of duodenum overlying spine in blunt injury) – need to open for both blunt and penetrating injuries
- **Paraduodenal hematomas on CT scan** (or missed on initial CT scan)
  • Can present with high **small bowel obstruction** (SBO) 12–72 hours after injury
  • UGI study will show **"stacked coins"** or **"coiled spring"** appearance (make sure there is no extravasation of contrast)
  • Tx: **conservative** (NGT and TPN) - cures 90% over 2–3 weeks (hematoma is reabsorbed)
- If at laparotomy and duodenal injury suspected, perform **Kocher maneuver** and **open lesser sac** through the omentum; check for hematoma, bile, succus, and fat necrosis → if found, need formal inspection of the entire duodenum (also need to check for pancreatic injury)
- **Diagnosing suspected duodenal injury** – abdominal CT with contrast initially. UGI contrast study best. CT scan may show bowel wall thickening, hematoma, free air, contrast leak, or retroperitoneal fluid/air
  • If CT scan is worrisome for injury but nondiagnostic, can repeat the CT in 8–12 hours to see if the finding is getting worse
- Tx: Try to get **primary repair** or **anastomosis**; may need to divert with pyloric exclusion and gastrojejunostomy to allow healing. Place a distal feeding jejunostomy and possibly a proximal draining jejunostomy tube that threads back to duodenal injury site. **Place drains**
  • If in **2nd portion of duodenum** and can't get primary repair
    ◦ Place **jejunal serosal patch** over hole; may need Whipple in future
    ◦ Need pyloric exclusion and gastrojejunostomy
    ◦ Consider feeding and draining jejunostomies; leave drains
    ◦ Trauma Whipple is rarely if ever indicated (very high mortality)
  • **Drains** - remove when patient tolerating diet without an increase in drainage
  • **Fistulas** - often close with time; Tx: bowel rest, TPN, octreotide, conservative management for 4–6 weeks

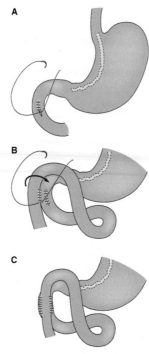

Jejunal serosal patch.

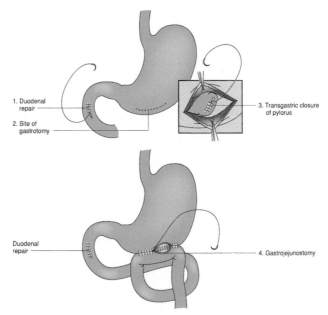

Gastro-jejunostomy and pyloric exclusion for complex duodenal injury.

SMALL BOWEL TRAUMA
- Most common organ injured with penetrating injury (some texts say liver)
- These injuries can be hard to diagnose early if associated with blunt trauma
- **Occult small bowel injuries**
  - Abdominal CT scan showing **intra-abdominal fluid not associated with a solid organ injury**, **bowel wall thickening**, or a **mesenteric hematoma** is suggestive of injury
  - **Need close observation and possibly repeat abdominal CT** after 8–12 hours or so to make sure finding is not getting worse
  - Need to make sure patients with these nonconclusive findings can **tolerate a diet before discharge**
- Repair lacerations **transversely → avoids stricture**
- **Large lacerations** that are **> 50% of the bowel circumference** or results in **lumen diameter < ⅓ normal →** perform resection and reanastomosis
- **Multiple close lacerations** – just resect that segment
- **Mesenteric hematomas** – open if expanding or large (> 2 cm)

COLON TRAUMA
- Most associated with penetrating injury
- **Right** and **transverse colon** injuries – perform primary repair/anastomosis
- **Left** colon – perform primary repair/anastomosis; place **diverting ileostomy** if patient is in **shock** or there is **gross contamination**
- Paracolonic hematomas – both blunt and penetrating need to be opened

RECTAL TRAUMA
- Most associated with penetrating injury
- **High rectal**
  - **Extraperitoneal** – generally not repaired because of inaccessibility
    - Tx: serial debridement; consider diverting ileostomy
  - **Intraperitoneal** – Tx: repair defect, presacral drainage, consider diverting ileostomy
  - Place **diverting ileostomy** with **shock**, **gross contamination**, or **extensive injury**
- **Low rectal** (< 5 cm) – can probably be repaired transanally

LIVER TRAUMA
- Most common organ injury with blunt abdominal trauma (some texts say spleen)
- Lobectomy rarely necessary
- **Common hepatic artery** – can be ligated with collaterals through gastroduodenal artery
- **Pringle maneuver** (clamping **portal triad**) does not stop bleeding from **hepatic veins**
- **Damage control peri-hepatic packing** – can pack severe penetrating liver injuries if patient becomes unstable in the OR and the injury is not easily fixed (eg retro-hepatic IVC injury). Go to the ICU and get the patient resuscitated and stabilized. Live to fight another day.
- **Atriocaval shunt** – for retrohepatic IVC injury, allows for control while performing repair
- **Portal triad hematomas** – need to be explored

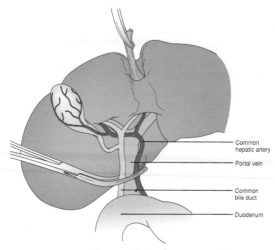

Common hepatic artery

Portal vein

Common bile duct

Duodenum

Pringle maneuver compression of the portal triad structures with a noncrushing vascular clamp for hepatic inflow control. If possible, clamp times should be limited to 15- to 20-minute intervals.

- **Common bile duct injury**
  - < 50% of circumference – **repair over stent**
  - > 50% circumference or complex injury – go with **choledochojejunostomy**
  - May need intraoperative cholangiogram to define injury
  - 10% of duct anastomoses leak – place drains intra-op
- **Portal vein injury** – need to repair
  - May need to transect through the pancreas to get to the injury in the portal vein
  - Will need to perform **distal pancreatectomy** with that maneuver
  - Ligation of portal vein associated with 50% mortality
- **Omental graft** – can be placed in liver laceration to help with bleeding and prevent bile leaks
- **Leave drains** with **liver injuries**
- **Conservative management of blunt liver injuries**
  - **Has failed if** patient becomes **unstable** despite aggressive resuscitation, including 4 units of PRBCs (HR > 120 or SBP < 90) or requires **> 4 units** of PRBCs to keep Hct > 25. **Go to OR**
  - **Active blush** on abdominal CT or **pseudoaneurysm** also indication for **OR**
    - If <u>posterior</u>, may be better off going to **angiogram** (when in doubt → OR)
    - If <u>anterior</u>, go to **OR**
  - With **conservative management**, need bed rest for **5 days**

SPLEEN TRAUMA
- Fully healed after 6 weeks
- Postsplenectomy sepsis greatest risk **within 2 years** of splenectomy
- Splenic salvage is associated with increased transfusions
- **Conservative management of blunt splenic injuries**
  - **Has failed if** patient becomes **unstable** despite aggressive resuscitation, including 2 units of PRBCs (HR > 120 or SBP ≤ 90) or requires **> 2 units** of PRBCs to keep Hct > 25. **Go to OR.**

- **Active blush** on abdominal CT or **pseudoaneurysm** also indication for **OR**
- With **conservative management**, need bed rest for **5 days**
- Threshold for splenectomy in **children** is much higher; hardly any children undergo splenectomy
- Need immunizations after trauma splenectomy

PANCREATIC TRAUMA

- **Penetrating injury** – accounts for 80% of all pancreatic injuries
- **Blunt injury** – can result in pancreatic duct fractures, usually perpendicular to the duct
- Edema or necrosis of peripancreatic fat usually indicative of injury
- **Pancreatic contusion** – leave if stable, place drains if in OR
- **Distal pancreatic duct injury** – distal pancreatectomy, can take up to 80% of the gland
- **Pancreatic head duct injury that is not reparable** – place drains initially; delayed Whipple or possible ERCP w/ stent may eventually be necessary
- Whipple vs. distal pancreatectomy based on duct injury in relation to the **SMV** (superior mesenteric vein)
- Kocher maneuver helps evaluate the pancreas operatively
- **Leave drains** with pancreatic injury
- **Pancreatic hematoma** – both penetrating and blunt need to be opened
- Persistent or rising **amylase** may indicate missed pancreatic injury
- CT scans poor at diagnosing pancreatic injuries initially
  - Delayed signs – fluid, edema, necrosis
- **ERCP** good at finding duct injuries and may be able to treat with temporary stent

VASCULAR TRAUMA

- **Vascular repair** (or vascular shunt) performed *before* **orthopaedic repair**
- **Major signs of vascular injury** – active hemorrhage, pulse deficit, expanding or pulsatile hematoma, distal ischemia, bruit, thrill → **go to OR for exploration** (may need angio in the OR to define injury)
- **Moderate/soft signs of vascular injury** – history of hemorrhage, deficit of anatomically related nerve, large stable/nonpulsatile hematoma, ABI < 0.9 → **go to angio**
- **Saphenous vein graft** – will be needed if segment > 2 cm missing
  - Use vein from the contralateral leg when fixing lower extremity arterial injuries
- Vein injuries that need repair – vena cava, femoral, popliteal, brachiocephalic, subclavian, and axillary
- Transection of single artery in the calf in an otherwise healthy patient → ligate
- Cover site of anastomosis with viable tissue and muscle
- Consider **fasciotomy** if ischemia > 4-6 hours (prevents compartment syndrome)
- **Compartment syndrome** – consider if compartment pressures are > 20 mm Hg or if clinical exam suggests elevated pressures (see Vascular Chapter)
  - Pain → paresthesia → anesthesia → paralysis → poikilothermia → pulselessness (late finding)
  - Most commonly occurs after supracondylar humeral fractures, tibial fractures, crush injuries, or other injuries that result in a disruption and then restoration of blood flow after 4-6 hours
  - Tx: **fasciotomy**

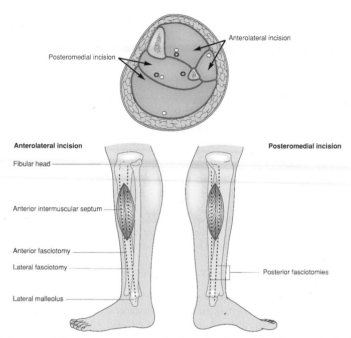

Surgical approach for four compartment fasciotomies through incisions on the medial and lateral aspects of the calf.

- ■ **IVC** – primary repair if residual stenosis is $<$ 50% the diameter of the IVC; otherwise place saphenous vein or synthetic patch
  - • Bleeding of IVC best controlled with proximal and distal pressure, <u>not</u> clamps → can tear it
  - • Repair posterior wall injury through the anterior wall (may need to cut through the anterior IVC to get to posterior IVC injuries)

ORTHOPAEDIC TRAUMA
- ■ Can have $>$ **2 L blood** loss from a **femur fracture**
- ■ Orthopaedic emergencies – pelvic fractures in unstable patients, spine injury with deficit, open fractures, dislocations or fractures with vascular compromise, compartment syndrome
- ■ Femoral neck fractures – high risk for **avascular necrosis**
- ■ Long bone fracture or dislocations with loss of pulse (or weak pulse) → immediate reduction of fracture or dislocation and reassessment of pulse:
  - • If pulse does not return → go to OR for vascular bypass or repair (may need angiography in OR to define injury)
  - • If pulse is weak → angiography
  - • All knee dislocations need to go to angiogram, unless pulse is absent, in which case you would just go to OR (may need angio in OR to define injury)
  - • **Upright falls** are associated with **calcaneus, lumbar,** and **distal forearm** (radius/ulnar) fractures

Orthopaedic Trauma	Concomitant Nerve/Artery Injury
UPPER EXTREMITY	
Anterior shoulder dislocation	Axillary nerve
Posterior shoulder dislocation	Axillary artery
Proximal humerus Fx	Axillary nerve
Midshaft humerus Fx (or spiral humerus Fx)	Radial nerve
Distal (supracondylar) humerus Fx	Brachial artery
Elbow dislocation	Brachial artery
Distal radius Fx	Median nerve
LOWER EXTREMITY	
Anterior hip dislocation	Femoral artery
Posterior hip dislocation	Sciatic nerve
Distal (supracondylar) femur Fx	Popliteal artery
Posterior knee dislocation	Popliteal artery
Fibula neck Fx	Common peroneal nerve
OTHER FRACTURES	
Temporal or parietal bone Fx	Epidural hematoma
Maxillofacial Fx	Cervical spine Fx
Sternal Fx	Cardiac contusion
First or second rib Fx	Aortic transection
Scapula Fx	Pulmonary contusion, aortic transection
Rib Fx's (left, 8-12)	Spleen laceration
Rib Fx's (right, 8-12)	Liver laceration
Pelvic Fx	Bladder rupture, urethral transaction

Modified from Engelhardt SL, Winchell RJ. Definitive care phase: orthopedic and spinal injuries. In: Greenfield LJ, et al, eds. *Surgery: Scientific Principles and Practice.* 3rd ed. Philadelphia, PA: Lippincott Williams & Wilkins; 2001:372.

RENAL TRAUMA

- **Hematuria** is the best indicator of renal trauma
- All patients with hematuria need an abdominal CT scan
- IVP can be useful if going immediately to OR without abdominal CT scan → will identify presence of functional contralateral kidney, which could affect intraoperative decision making
- **Left renal vein** - can be ligated near IVC; has **adrenal** and **gonadal vein collaterals** Right renal vein does <u>not</u> have these collaterals
- **Anterior** → **posterior** renal hilum structures - **vein**, **artery**, **pelvis** (VAP)
- 95% of injuries are treated nonoperatively
- Not all urine extravasation injuries require operation
- **Indications for operation**
  - **Acutely** - ongoing hemorrhage with instability
  - **After acute phase** - major collecting system disruption, non-resolving urine extravasation, severe hematuria
- With exploration, try to get control of the **vascular hilum 1st**
- Place **drains** intra-op, especially if collecting system is injured
- **Methylene blue dye** can be used at the end of the case to check for leak
- **When at exploration for another blunt injury or penetrating trauma:**
  - **Blunt renal injury with hematoma** - leave unless pre-op CT/IVP shows no function or significant urine extravasation
  - **Penetrating renal injury with hematoma** - open unless pre-op CT/IVP shows good function without significant urine extravasation
- **Trauma to flank and IVP shows no uptake in stable patient** - Tx: angiogram; can stent if flap present

BLADDER TRAUMA
- **Hematuria** best indicator of bladder trauma
- > 95% associated with pelvic fractures
- Signs and symptoms – meatal blood, sacral or scrotal hematoma
- Dx: **cystogram**
- **Extraperitoneal bladder rupture** – cystogram shows starbursts
  - Tx: Foley 7–14 days
- **Intraperitoneal bladder rupture** – more likely in kids, cystogram shows leak
  - Tx: operation and repair of defect, followed by Foley drainage

URETERAL TRAUMA
- Hematuria unreliable → **IVP** and **retrograde urethrogram** (RUG) best tests
- If **large ureteral segment** is missing (> 2 cm) and cannot perform reanastomosis:
  - **Upper ⅓ injuries** and **middle ⅓ injuries that won't reach bladder** (above pelvic brim)
    - Temporize with **percutaneous nephrostomy** (tie off both ends of the ureter); can go with <u>ileal interposition</u> or <u>trans-ureteroureterostomy</u> later
  - **Lower ⅓ injuries** – reimplant in the bladder; may need bladder hitch procedure
- If **small ureteral segment** is missing (< 2 cm):
  - **Upper ⅓ injuries** and **middle ⅓ injuries** – mobilize ends of ureter and perform **primary repair** over stent
  - **Lower ⅓ injuries** – re-implant in the bladder (easier anastomosis than primary repair)
- One-shot IVP does not evaluate the ureters sufficiently
- IV indigo carmine or IV methylene blue can be used to check for leaks
- Blood supply is medial in the upper ⅔ of the ureter and lateral in the lower ⅓ of the ureter
- **Leave drains** for all ureteral injuries

URETHRAL TRAUMA
- **Hematuria** or **blood at meatus best signs**; free-floating prostate gland; usually associated with pelvic fractures
- <u>No Foley</u> if this injury is suspected
- **Retrograde urethrogram** (RUG) best test
- Membranous portion at risk for transection
- **Significant tears** – Tx: **suprapubic cystostomy** and repair in 2–3 months *(safest method* – high stricture and impotence rate if repaired early)
- **Small, partial tears** – Tx: may get away with bridging urethral catheter across tear area and repair in 2–3 months
- **Genital trauma** – can get fracture in erectile bodies from vigorous sex
  - Need to repair the tunica and Buck's fascia
- **Testicular trauma** – get ultrasound to see if tunica albuginea is violated, then repair if necessary

PEDIATRIC TRAUMA
- Blood pressure is not a good indicator of blood loss in children – last thing to go
- Heart rate, respiratory rate, mental status, and clinical exam are best indicators of shock
- ↑ risk of **hypothermia** (↑ BSA compared with weight)
- ↑ risk of **head injury**

Normal Vital Signs by Age

Age Group	Pulse (beats/min)	SBP (mm Hg)	Respiratory Rate (breaths/min)
Infant (< 1 yr)	160	80	40
Preschool (< 5 yr)	140	90	30
Adolescent (> 10 yr)	120	100	20

TRAUMA DURING PREGNANCY

- At all costs, **save the mother**
- Pregnant patients can have up to a ⅓ total blood volume loss without signs
- Estimate pregnancy based on **fundal height** (20 cm = 20 wk = umbilicus). Place fetal monitor
- Try to avoid CT scan with early pregnancy. If life-threatening and needed, get CT scan.
- Ultrasound (FAST scan) may have a role in pregnant patients
- Check for vaginal discharge – blood, amnion; check for effacement, dilation, fetal station
- **Fetal maturity** – lecithin:sphingomyelin (LS) ratio > 2:1; positive **phosphatidylcholine** in amniotic fluid
- **Placental abruption** – > 50% results in almost 100% fetal death rate
  - > 50% of all traumatic placental abruptions result in fetal demise
  - Signs of abruption – uterine tenderness, contractions, fetal HR < 120
  - Can be caused by **shock** (most common mechanism) or **mechanical forces**
  - **Kleihauer–Betke test** – test for fetal blood in the maternal circulation → sign of placental abruption
- **Uterine rupture** – more likely to occur in the <u>posterior fundus</u>
  - If occurs after delivery of child, aggressive resuscitation even in the face of shock leads to the best outcome. The uterus will eventually clamp down after delivery; just have to aggressively resuscitate until then (fluids, blood)
- **Indications for C-section during exploratory laparotomy for trauma**
  - Persistent maternal shock or severe injuries and pregnancy near term (> 34 weeks)
  - Pregnancy a threat to the mother's life (hemorrhage, DIC)
  - Mechanical limitation to life-threatening vessel injury
  - Risk of fetal distress exceeds risk of immaturity
  - Direct intra-uterine trauma

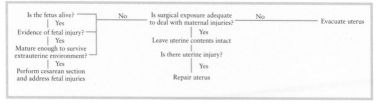

Assessment of the pregnant uterus during celiotomy.

Management of Hematomas

Hematoma (≥ 2 cm considered significant)	Penetrating Trauma	Blunt Trauma
Pelvic	Open	Leave
Paraduodenal	Open	Open
Portal triad	Open	Open
Retrohepatic	Leave if stable	Leave
Midline supramesocolic	Open	Open
Midline inframesocolic	Open	Open
Pericolonic	Open	Open
Perirenal	Open[a]	Leave[b]

[a]Unless preoperative CT scan or IVP shows no injury.
[b]Unless preoperative CT scan or IVP shows injury.

Zones of the Peritoneum

Zone	Location	Associated Injuries
1	Central retroperitoneum	Pancreaticoduodenal injuries or major abdominal vascular injury (usually <u>open</u> hematomas in these areas)
2	Flank or perinephric area	Injuries to the genitourinary tract or to the colon (ie with penetrating trauma; usually <u>open</u> hematomas in these areas)
3	Pelvis	Pelvic fractures (usually <u>leave</u> these hematomas alone)

- **Drains** – leave drains with pancreatic, liver, biliary system, urinary, and duodenal injuries
- **Snakebites** (symptoms depend on species) – shock, bradycardia, and arrhythmias can result; Tx: stabilize patient, anti-venin, tetanus shot

CARDIOVASCULAR SYSTEM

Normal Values

Parameter	Value
Cardiac output (CO) (L/min)	4–8
Cardiac index (CI) (L/min)	2.5–4
Systemic vascular resistance (SVR)	800–1,400
Pulmonary capillary wedge pressure (PCWP)	11 ± 4
Central venous pressure (CVP)	7 ± 2
Pulmonary artery pressure (PAP)	$25/10 \pm 5$
Mixed venous oxygen saturation (SvO2)	75 ± 5

- $\underline{MAP} = CO \times SVR$, $\underline{CI} = CO/BSA$
- <u>Kidney</u> gets 25% of CO, <u>brain</u> gets 15%, <u>heart</u> gets 5%
- **Preload** – left ventricular end-diastolic length, linearly related to left ventricular end-diastolic volume (LVEDV) and filling pressure

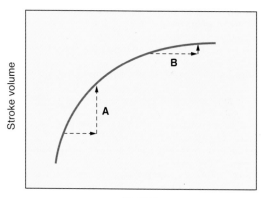

Preload

The concept of preload recruitable stroke volume is demonstrated. If the ventricle is on the steep part of the Starling curve (A), then a given increase in preload will lead to a significant increase in stroke volume. By contrast, on the flatter part of the curve (B), the stroke volume increases marginally if at all with the same increase in preload. Dynamic indices of preload-recruitable stroke volume are more accurate than static indices in identifying where on this curve the patient is at any point in time.

- **Afterload** – resistance against the ventricle contracting (**SVR**)
- **Stroke volume** determined by <u>LVEDV</u>, <u>contractility</u>, and <u>afterload</u>
  - Stroke volume = LVEDV – LVESV
- **Ejection fraction** = stroke volume/LVEDV
- **EDV** (end-diastolic volume) – determined by preload and distensibility of the ventricle
- **ESV** (end-systolic volume) – determined by contractility and afterload
- Cardiac output increases with HR up to 120–150 beats/min, then starts to go down because of **decreased diastolic filling time**

- **Atrial kick** – accounts for 20% of LVEDV
- **Anrep effect** – automatic increase in **contractility** secondary to ↑ **afterload**
- **Bowditch effect** – automatic increase in **contractility** secondary to ↑ **HR**
- **Arterial O_2 content** (CaO_2) = Hgb × 1.34 × O_2 saturation + (Po_2 × 0.003)
- **O_2 delivery** = CO × arterial O_2 content (CaO_2) × 10
- **O_2 consumption** (VO_2) = CO × (CaO_2 – CvO_2); CvO_2 = venous O_2 content
  - **Normal O_2 delivery-to-consumption ratio is 5:1.** CO increases to keep this ratio constant.
  - O_2 consumption is usually <u>supply independent</u> (consumption does not change until low levels of delivery are reached)
- Causes of **right shift** on **oxygen–Hgb dissociation curve** (O_2 unloading) – ↑ CO_2, ↑ temperature, ↑ ATP production, ↑ 2,3-DPG production, or ↓ pH
  - Opposite above causes left shift (increased O_2 binding)
  - Normal p50 (O_2 at which 50% of O_2 receptors are saturated) = 27 mm Hg
- ↑ **SvO_2** (saturation of venous blood, normally 75% ± 5%; used on some Swan–Ganz catheters) – occurs with ↑ shunting of blood or ↓ O_2 extraction (eg sepsis, cirrhosis, cyanide toxicity, hyperbaric O_2, hypothermia, paralysis, coma, sedation)
- ↓ **SvO_2** – occurs with ↑ O_2 extraction or ↓ O_2 delivery (eg ↓ O_2 saturation, ↓ CO, malignant hyperthermia)
- **Wedge** – may be thrown off by pulmonary hypertension, aortic regurgitation, mitral stenosis, mitral regurgitation, high PEEP, poor LV compliance
- **Swan–Ganz catheter** – should be placed in **zone III** (lower lung)
  - **Hemoptysis after flushing Swan–Ganz catheter** – increase PEEP, which will tamponade the pulmonary artery bleed, mainstem intubate non-affected side; can try to place Fogarty balloon down mainstem on affected side; may need thoracotomy and lobectomy
  - **Relative contraindications** – previous pneumonectomy, left bundle branch block
  - Approximate **Swan–Ganz catheter distances to wedge** – R SCV 45 cm, **R IJ** 50 cm, **L SCV** 55 cm, **L IJ** 60 cm
  - **Pulmonary vascular resistance** (PVR) can be measured only by using a **Swan–Ganz catheter** (ECHO does not measure PVR)
  - **Wedge pressure** measurements should be taken at **end-expiration** (for both ventilated and nonventilated patients)
- ↑ **Ventricular wall tension** (#1) and **HR** are the primary determinants of <u>myocardial O_2 consumption</u> → can lead to myocardial ischemia
- **Unsaturated bronchial blood** – empties into pulmonary veins; thus, LV blood is 5 mm Hg (Po_2) lower than pulmonary capillaries
- **Alveolar–arterial gradient** – is 10–15 mm Hg in a normal nonventilated patient
- Blood with the lowest venous saturation → coronary sinus blood (30%)

SHOCK
- **Shock** = inadequate tissue oxygenation (most basic definition)
  - **Tachypnea** and **mental status** changes occur with progressive shock
- **Adrenal insufficiency**
  - MCC – withdrawal of exogenous steroids
  - **Acute** – cardiovascular collapse; characteristically **unresponsive to fluids** and **pressors**; nausea and vomiting, abdominal pain, fever, lethargy, ↓ glucose, ↑ K
  - Tx: Dexamethasone
  - **Steroid potency**
    - 1× – cortisone, hydrocortisone
    - 5× – prednisone, prednisolone, methylprednisolone
    - 30× – dexamethasone

■ **Neurogenic shock** – loss of sympathetic tone; usually associated with spine or head injury
  • Usually have ↓ HR, ↓ BP, warm skin
  • Tx: give **volume 1st**, then **phenylephrine** after resuscitation
■ **Hemorrhagic shock** – initial alteration is ↑ <u>diastolic pressure</u>
■ **Cardiac tamponade** (causes cardiogenic shock)
  • Mechanism of hypotension is **decreased ventricular filling** due to fluid in the pericardial sac around the heart
  • Beck's triad – hypotension, jugular venous distention, and muffled heart sounds
  • Echocardiogram shows **impaired diastolic filling of right atrium initially** (1st sign of cardiac tamponade)
  • Pericardiocentesis blood does not form clot
  • Tx: fluid resuscitation to temporize situation; need **pericardial window** or **pericardiocentesis**

Types of Shock

Shock	CVP and PCWP	CO	SVR
Hemorrhagic	↓	↓	↑
Septic (hyperdynamic)[a]	↓ (usually)	↑	↓
Cardiogenic (eg MI, cardiac tamponade)	↑	↓	↑
Neurogenic (eg head or spinal cord injury)	↓	↓	↓
Adrenal insufficiency	↓ (usually)	↓	↓

[a]Severe septic shock that leads to cardiac dysfunction can cause a hypodynamic state, leading to ↓ CO and ↑ SVRI.

■ **Early sepsis triad** – hyperventilation, confusion, hypotension
  • **Early gram-negative sepsis** – ↓ insulin, ↑ **glucose** (impaired utilization)
  • **Late gram-negative sepsis** – ↑ insulin, ↑ **glucose** (secondary to insulin resistance)
  • **Hyperglycemia** – often occurs just before patient becomes clinically septic
■ **Neurohormonal response** to hypovolemia
  • **Rapid** – **epinephrine** and **norepinephrine** release (<u>adrenergic</u> release; results in vasoconstriction and increased cardiac activity)
  • **Sustained** – **renin** (from <u>kidney</u>; renin-angiotensin pathway activated resulting in vasoconstriction and water resorption), **ADH** (from <u>pituitary</u>; reabsorption of water), and **ACTH** release (from <u>pituitary</u>; increases cortisol)

EMBOLI
■ **Fat emboli** - petechia, hypoxia, and confusion (can also be similar to pulmonary embolism [PE])
  • **Sudan red stain** may show fat in sputum and urine
  • Most common with lower extremity (hip, femur) fractures/orthopaedic procedures
■ **Pulmonary emboli** (PE) – chest pain and dyspnea; ↓ Po_2 and Pco_2; respiratory alkalosis; ↑ HR and ↑ RR; hypotension and shock if massive
  • Most PEs arise from **iliofemoral region**
  • Tx: heparin, Coumadin; consider open or percutaneous (suction catheter) embolectomy if patient is in shock despite massive pressors and inotropes
■ **Air emboli** – place patient head down and roll to left (keeps air in RV and RA), then aspirate air out with central line or PA catheter to RA/RV

INTRA-AORTIC BALLOON PUMP (IABP)
■ <u>Inflates</u> on **T wave** (diastole); <u>deflates</u> on **P wave** (systole)
■ Aortic regurgitation is a contraindication to IABP

■ Place tip of the catheter just distal to left subclavian (1–2 cm below the top of the arch)
■ Used for **cardiogenic shock** (after CABG or MI) or in patients with **refractory angina** awaiting revascularization
■ **Decreases afterload** (deflation during ventricular systole)
■ **Improves diastolic BP** (inflation during ventricular diastole), which **improves diastolic coronary perfusion**

RECEPTORS
■ **Alpha-1** – vascular smooth muscle constriction; gluconeogenesis and glycogenolysis
■ **Alpha-2** – venous smooth muscle constriction
■ **Beta-1** – myocardial contraction and rate
■ **Beta-2** – relaxes bronchial smooth muscle, relaxes vascular smooth muscle; increases insulin, glucagon, and renin
■ **Dopamine receptors** – relax renal and splanchnic smooth muscle

CARDIOVASCULAR DRUGS
■ **Dopamine** (2–5 µg/kg/min initially)
  • 2–5 µg/kg/min – <u>dopamine receptors</u> (renal)
  • 6–10 µg/kg/min – <u>beta-adrenergic</u> (heart contractility)
  • >10 µg/kg/min – <u>alpha-adrenergic</u> (vasoconstriction and ↑ BP)
■ **Dobutamine** (3 µg/kg/min initially)
  • <u>Beta-1</u> (↑ contractility mostly, tachycardia with higher doses)
■ **Milrinone**
  • **Phosphodiesterase inhibitor** (↑ cAMP)
  • Results in ↑ Ca flux and ↑ myocardial contractility
  • Also causes vascular smooth muscle relaxation and **pulmonary vasodilation**
■ **Phenylephrine** (10 µg/min initially)
  • Alpha-1, vasoconstriction
■ **Norepinephrine** (5 µg/min initially)
  • <u>Low dose</u> – beta-1 (↑ contractility)
  • <u>High dose</u> – alpha-1 and alpha-2
  • Potent splanchnic vasoconstrictor
■ **Epinephrine** (1–2 µg/min initially)
  • <u>Low dose</u> – beta-1 and beta-2 (↑ contractility and vasodilation)
    • Can ↓ BP at low doses
  • <u>High dose</u> – alpha-1 and alpha-2 (vasoconstriction)
    • ↑ Cardiac ectopic pacer activity and myocardial O_2 demand
■ **Isoproterenol** (1–2 µg/min initially)
  • Beta-1 and beta-2, ↑ HR and contractility, vasodilates
  • Side effects: extremely arrhythmogenic; ↑ heart metabolic demand (rarely used); may actually ↓ BP
■ **Vasopressin**
  • V-1 receptors – vasoconstriction of vascular smooth muscle
  • V-2 receptors (intrarenal) – water reabsorption at collecting ducts
  • V-2 receptors (extrarenal) – mediate release of factor VIII and von Willebrand factor (vWF)
■ **Nipride** – arterial vasodilator
  • **Cyanide toxicity** at doses > 3 µg/kg/min for 72 hours; can check **thiocyanate levels** and signs of metabolic acidosis
  • **Tx for cyanide toxicity** – amyl nitrite, then sodium nitrite
■ **Nitroglycerin** – predominately venodilation with ↓ myocardial wall tension from ↓ preload; moderate coronary vasodilator
■ **Hydralazine** – α-blocker; lowers BP

PULMONARY SYSTEM

- **Compliance** – (change in volume)/(change in pressure)
  - High compliance means lungs easy to ventilate
  - Pulmonary compliance is *decreased* in patients with ARDS, fibrotic lung diseases, reperfusion injury, pulmonary edema, atelectasis
- **Aging** – ↓ FEV_1 and vital capacity, ↑ functional residual capacity (FRC)
- **V/Q ratio** (ventilation/perfusion ratio) – highest in upper lobes, lowest in lower lobes
- **Ventilator**
  - ↑ PEEP to improve oxygenation (alveoli recruitment) → **improves FRC**
  - ↑ Rate or volume to ↓ CO_2
  - **Normal weaning parameters** – negative inspiratory force (NIF) > 20, FiO_2 ≤ 40%, PEEP 5 (physiologic), pressure support 5, RR < 24/min, HR < 120 beats/min, Po_2 > 60 mm Hg, Pco_2 < 50 mm Hg, pH 7.35-7.45, saturations > 93%, off pressors, follows commands, can protect airway
  - **Pressure support** – decreases the work of breathing (inspiratory pressure is held constant until minimum volume is achieved)
  - **Keep FiO_2 ≤ 60%** – prevents O_2 radical toxicity
  - **Barotrauma** – high risk if plateaus > 30 and peaks > 50 → need to decrease TV; consider pressure control ventilation
  - **PEEP** – *improves FRC* and compliance by keeping alveoli open → best way to improve oxygenation
  - **Excessive PEEP complications** – ↓ RA filling, ↓ CO, ↓ renal blood flow, ↓ urine output, and ↑ pulmonary vascular resistance
  - **High-frequency ventilation** – used a lot in kids; tracheoesophageal fistula, bronchopleural fistula
- **Pulmonary function measurements**
  - **Total lung capacity** (TLC) – lung volume after maximal inspiration
    - TLC = FVC + RV
  - **Forced vital capacity** (FVC) – maximal exhalation after maximal inhalation
  - **Residual volume** (RV) – lung volume after maximal expiration (20% TLC)
  - **Tidal volume** (TV) – volume of air with normal inspiration and expiration
  - **Functional residual capacity** (FRC) – lung volume after normal exhalation
    - FRC = ERV + RV
    - Surgery (atelectasis), sepsis (ARDS), and trauma (contusion, atelectasis, ARDS) – all ↓ FRC
  - **Expiratory reserve volume** (ERV) – volume of air that can be forcefully expired after normal expiration
  - **Inspiratory capacity** – maximum air breathed in from FRC
  - **FEV_1** – forced expiratory volume in 1 second (after maximal inhalation)
  - **Minute ventilation** = TV × RR
  - **Restrictive lung disease** – ↓ TLC, ↓ RV, and ↓ FVC
    - FEV_1 can be normal or ↑
  - **Obstructive lung disease** – ↑ TLC, ↑ RV, and ↓ FEV_1
    - FVC can be normal or ↓
- **Dead space** – normally to the level of the bronchiole (150 mL)
  - Area of lung that is ventilated but not perfused
  - Dead space *increases* with drop in cardiac output, PE, pulmonary HTN, ARDS, and excessive PEEP; can lead to **high CO_2** buildup (hypercapnia)
- **COPD** – ↑ work of breathing due to **prolonged expiratory phase**
- **ARDS** – mediated primarily by PMNs; get ↑ proteinaceous material, ↑ A-a gradient, ↑ pulmonary shunt
  - Most common cause is **pneumonia**; other causes – sepsis, multi-trauma, severe burns, pancreatitis, aspiration, DIC

> ### Acute Respiratory Distress Syndrome (ARDS) Criteria
> Acute onset
> Bilateral pulmonary infiltrates
> $PaO_2/FiO_2 \leq 300$
> Absence of heart failure (wedge < 18 mm Hg)

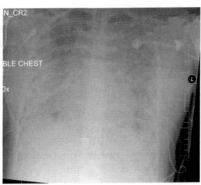
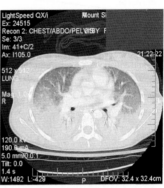

Characteristic chest radiograph (*A*) and CT scan (*B*) in a patient with severe ARDS following multiple trauma. (From Cheadle WG, Branson R, Franklin GA. Pulmonary risk and ventilatory support. In: Fischer JE, Bland KI, et al, eds. *Mastery of Surgery*. 5th ed. Philadelphia, PA: Lippincott Williams & Wilkins; 2007, with permission.)

- ■ **Aspiration** – pH < 2.5 and volume > 0.4 cc/kg is associated with ↑ degree of damage
  - • **Mendelson's syndrome** – chemical pneumonitis from **aspiration of gastric secretions**
  - • Most frequent site is **superior segment of the right lower lobe** (RLL)
- ■ **Atelectasis** – collapse of alveoli resulting in reduced oxygenation; usually caused by poor inspiration postop
  - • Most common cause of **fever** in first 48 hours after operation
  - • Sx's – fever, tachycardia, hypoxia
  - • Increased in patients with COPD, upper abdominal surgery, obesity
  - • Tx: incentive spirometer, pain control, ambulation
- ■ Lots of things can throw off a pulse oximeter → nail polish, dark skin, low-flow states, ambient light, anemia, vital dyes
- ■ **Pulmonary vasodilation** – PGE_1, prostacyclin (PGI_2), nitric oxide, bradykinin
- ■ **Pulmonary vasoconstriction** – **hypoxia** (#1), acidosis, histamine, serotonin, TXA_2
- ■ **Alkalosis** – pulmonary vasodilator
- ■ **Acidosis** – pulmonary vasoconstrictor
- ■ **Pulmonary shunting** – occurs with nitroprusside (Nipride), nitroglycerin, and nifedipine

RENAL SYSTEM
- ■ **Hypotension intra-op** – the most common cause of postoperative renal failure
- ■ 70% of nephrons need to be damaged before renal dysfunction occurs
- ■ Check serum and urine electrolytes; check urinary catheter for obstruction
- ■ **FeNa** (fractional excretion of sodium) = (urine Na/Cr)/(plasma Na/Cr) → **best test for azotemia**

Standard Measurements in the Diagnosis of Renal Failure

Test	Prerenal	Parenchymal
Urine osmolarity (mOsm)	> 500	250–350
U/P osmolality	> 1.5	< 1.1
U/P creatinine	> 20	< 10
Urine sodium	< 20	> 40
FE_{Na}	< 1%	> 3%

FE_{Na}, fraction of excreted sodium; U/P, urine-to-plasma ratio.

- **Oliguria**
  - 1st – make sure patient is volume loaded (CVP 11–15 mm Hg)
  - 2nd – try diuretic trial → furosemide (Lasix)
  - 3rd – dialysis if needed
- **Indications for dialysis** – fluid overload, ↑ K, metabolic acidosis, uremic encephalopathy, uremic coagulopathy, poisoning
- **Hemodialysis** – rapid, can cause large volume shifts
- **CVVH** – slower, good for ill patients who cannot tolerate the volume shifts (septic shock, etc.); Hct increases by 5–8 for each liter taken off with dialysis
- **Renin**
  - Released in response to ↓ pressure sensed by **juxtaglomerular apparatus** in kidney
  - Also released in response to ↑ Na concentrations sensed by the **macula densa**
  - Beta-adrenergic stimulation and hyperkalemia also cause release
  - Converts angiotensinogen (synthesized in the liver) to angiotensin I
  - **Angiotensin-converting enzyme** (lung) – converts angiotensin I to angiotensin II
  - **Adrenal cortex** – releases aldosterone in response to angiotensin II
  - **Aldosterone** acts at the **distal convoluted tubule** to **reabsorb water** by up-regulating the **Na/K ATPase** on the membrane (Na re-absorbed, K secreted)
  - **Angiotensin II** – also vasoconstricts as well as increases HR, contractility, glycogenolysis, and gluconeogenesis; inhibits renin release
- **Atrial natriuretic peptide** (or factor)
  - Released from **atrial wall** with atrial distention
  - **Inhibits Na and water resorption** in the collecting ducts
  - Also a **vasodilator**
- **Antidiuretic hormone** (ADH; vasopressin)
  - Released by **posterior pituitary gland** when osmolality is high
  - Acts on collecting ducts for **water resorption**
  - Also a **vasoconstrictor**
- **Efferent limb** of the kidney controls **GFR**
- **Renal toxic drugs**
  - **NSAIDs** – cause renal damage by **inhibiting prostaglandin synthesis**, resulting in renal arteriole vasoconstriction
  - **Aminoglycosides** – direct tubular injury
  - **Myoglobin** – direct tubular injury; Tx: **alkalinize urine**
  - **Contrast dyes** – direct tubular injury; Tx: **pre-hydration** before contrast exposure best; HCO3-, N-acetylcysteine

SYSTEMIC INFLAMMATORY RESPONSE SYNDROME (SIRS)
- **Causes** – shock, infection, burns, multi-trauma, pancreatitis, severe inflammatory responses
  - **Endotoxin** (lipopolysaccharide – **lipid A**) is the most potent stimulus for **SIRS**
  - Lipid A is a very potent stimulator of **TNF release**

- **Mechanism** – inflammatory response is activated systemically (**TNF-alpha** and IL-1 major components) and can lead to shock and eventually multi-organ dysfunction
  - Results in capillary leakage, microvascular thrombi, hypotension, and eventually end-organ dysfunction
- **Sepsis = SIRS + infection**

Definitions of Systemic Inflammatory Response Syndrome (SIRS), Shock, and Multisystem Organ Dysfunction (MOD)

SIRS →	Shock →	MOD

SIRS
- Temperature $> 38°C$ or $< 36°C$
- Heart rate > 90 beats/min
- Respiratory rate > 20/min or $Paco_2 < 32$
- White blood count $> 12,000/\mu L$ or $< 4,000/\mu L$

Shock
- Arterial hypotension despite adequate volume resuscitation (inadequate tissue oxygenation)

MOD
- Progressive but reversible dysfunction of 2 or more organs arising from an acute disruption of normal homeostasis

Modified from Awad SS, Gale SC. Multiple organ dysfunction syndrome: pathogenesis, management, and prevention. In: Fischer JE, Bland KI, et al, eds. *Mastery of Surgery*. 5th ed. Philadelphia, PA: Lippincott Williams & Wilkins; 2007, with permission.

Diagnostic Criteria for Significant Organ Dysfunction[a]

Organ System	Criteria
Pulmonary	Need for mechanical ventilation; $Pao_2:Fio_2$ ratio < 300 mm Hg for 24 hours
Cardiovascular	Need for inotropic drugs or CI < 2.5 L/min/m^2
Kidney	Creatinine > 2 times baseline on 2 consecutive days or need for dialysis
Liver	Bilirubin > 3 mg/dL on 2 consecutive days or PT > 1.5 control
Nutrition	10% reduction in lean body mass; albumin < 2.0, total lymphocyte count < 1
CNS	Glasgow Coma Scale score < 10 without sedation
Coagulation	Platelet count < 50, fibrinogen < 100, or need for factor replacement
Host defenses	WBC $< 1,000/\mu L$ or invasive infection including bacteremia

[a]Pao_2, partial pressure of oxygen in arterial blood; Fio_2, fraction of inspired oxygen; CI, cardiac index; PT, prothrombin time; WBC, white blood cell count. (From Awad SS, Gale SC. Multiple organ dysfunction syndrome: pathogenesis, management, and prevention. Modified from Fischer JE, Bland KI, et al, eds. *Mastery of Surgery*. 5th ed. Philadelphia, PA: Lippincott Williams & Wilkins; 2007, with permission.)

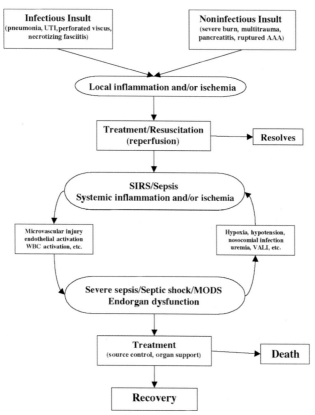

Pathophysiology of multisystem organ dysfunctions (MODS). UTI, urinary tract infection; AAA, abnormal aortic aneurysm; SIRS, systemic inflammatory response syndrome; WBC, white blood count; VALI, ventilator-associated lung injury. (From Cheadle WG, Branson R, Franklin GA. Pulmonary risk and ventilatory support. In: Fischer JE, Bland KI, et al, eds. *Mastery of Surgery*. 5th ed. Philadelphia, PA: Lippincott Williams & Wilkins; 2007, with permission.)

BRAIN DEATH

- **Precludes diagnosis** – temperature $< 32°C$, BP < 90 mm Hg, drugs (eg phenobarbital, pentobarbital, ETOH), metabolic derangements (hyperglycemia, uremia), desaturation with apnea test
- **Following must exist for 6–12 hours** → unresponsive to pain, absent cold caloric oculovestibular reflexes, absent oculocephalic reflex (patient doesn't track), no spontaneous respirations, no corneal reflex, no gag reflex, fixed and dilated pupils, positive apnea test
- **EEG** – shows electrical silence; **MRA** – will show no blood flow to brain
- **Apnea test** – the patient is pre-oxygenated, a catheter delivering O_2 at 8 L/min is placed at the carina through the ET-tube and CO_2 should be normal before the start of the test;
  - The patient is disconnected from ventilator for 10 minutes
  - A $CO_2 > 60$ mm Hg or **increase in CO_2 by 20 mm Hg** at the end of the test is a positive test for apnea (meets brain death criteria)

- If BP drops ($<$ 90 mm Hg), the patient desaturates ($<$ 85% on pulse oximeter), or spontaneous breathing occurs, the test is terminated (<u>negative test for apnea</u>) → place back on the ventilator (cannot declare brain death)
■ *Can still have deep tendon reflexes with brain death*

OTHER CONDITIONS
■ **Carbon monoxide**
  - Can **falsely** ↑ **oxygen saturation** reading on pulse oximeter
  - Binds hemoglobin directly (creates **carboxyhemoglobin** – HA, nausea, confusion, coma, death)
  - Can usually correct with **100% oxygen on ventilator** (displaces carbon monoxide); rarely need hyperbaric O_2
  - Abnormal carboxyhemoglobin $>$ 10%; in smokers $>$ 20%
■ **Methemoglobinemia** (from nitrites such as Hurricaine spray; nitrites bind Hgb) – O_2 **saturation reads 85%**
  - Tx: methylene blue
■ **Critical illness polyneuropathy** – motor $>$ sensory neuropathy; occurs with sepsis; can lead to failure to wean from ventilation
■ **Xanthine oxidase** – in endothelial cells, forms toxic **oxygen radicals** with reperfusion, involved in **reperfusion injury**
  - Also involved in the metabolism of purines and breakdown to **uric acid**
■ Most important mediator of **reperfusion injury** – **PMNs**
■ **DKA** – nausea and vomiting, thirst, polyuria, ↑ glucose, ↑ ketones, ↓ Na, ↑ K
  - Tx: **normal saline** and **insulin** initially
■ **ETOH withdrawal** – HTN, tachycardia, delirium, seizures after 48 hours
  - Tx: thiamine, folate, B_{12}, Mg, K, PRN lorazepam (Ativan)
■ **ICU** (or hospital) **psychosis** – generally occurs after third postoperative day and is frequently preceded by lucid interval
  - Need to rule out metabolic (hypoglycemia, DKA, hypoxia, hypercarbia, electrolyte imbalances) and organic (MI, CVA) causes

CHAPTER 17. BURNS

Burn Classification

Degree	Description
1st	Sunburn (epidermis)
2nd	
Superficial dermis (papillary)	Painful to touch; blebs and blisters; hair follicles intact; blanches (do <u>not</u> need skin grafts)
Deep dermis (reticular)	Decreased sensation; *loss of hair follicles* (need **skin grafts**)
3rd	Leathery (charred parchment); down to subcutaneous fat
4th	Down to bone; into adjacent adipose or muscle tissue

- 1st- and superficial 2nd-degree burns heal by **epithelialization** (primarily from **hair follicles**)
- **Extremely deep burns**, **electrical burns**, or **compartment syndrome** can cause **rhabdomyolysis** with **myoglobinuria** (Tx: hydration, alkalinize urine)

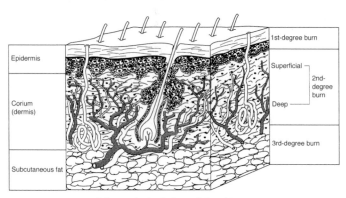

Schematic depiction of the skin.

ADMISSION CRITERIA[1]

- 2nd- and 3rd-degree burns > 10% BSA in patients aged < 10 or > 50 years
- 2nd- and 3rd-degree burns > 20% BSA in all other patients
- 2nd- and 3rd-degree burns to significant portions of hands, face, feet, genitalia, perineum, or skin overlying major joints
- 3rd-degree burns > 5% in any age group
- Electrical and chemical burns
- Concomitant inhalational injury, mechanical traumas, preexisting medical conditions
- Injuries in patients with special social, emotional, or long-term rehabilitation needs
- Suspected child abuse or neglect

BURN ASSESSMENT

- Deaths highest in children and elderly (trouble getting away)
- Scald burns – most common

[1]Modified from Feliciano DV, et al. *Trauma*. 3rd ed. Stamford, CT: Appleton & Lange; 1996:937.

- Flame burns – more likely to come to hospital and be admitted
- **Assessing percentage of body surface burned** (rule of 9s)
  - Head = 9, arms = 18, chest = 18, back = 18, legs = 36, perineum = 1
  - Can also use patient's palm to estimate injury (palm = 1%)
- **Parkland formula**
  - Use for **burns ≥ 20%** only – give 4 cc/kg × % burn in first 24 hours; give ½ the volume in the first 8 hours
  - Use **lactated Ringer's** solution (LR) in first 24 hours
    - Urine output best measure of resuscitation (0.5–1.0 cc/kg/h in adults, 2–4 cc/kg/h in children < 6 months)
  - Parkland formula can grossly underestimate volume requirements with inhalational injury, ETOH, electrical injury, post-escharotomy
  - **Important to use LR in first 24 hours**
  - Colloid (albumin) in 1st 24 hours causes ↑ pulmonary/respiratory complications → can use colloid after 24 hours

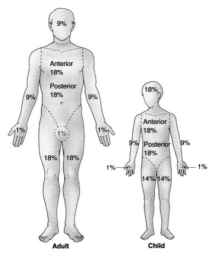

Estimating burn size accurately is essential for care of the burn patient. The rule of nines provides a simple algorithm for calculating the burned surface area.

- **Escharotomy indications** (perform within 4–6 hours):
  - Circumferential deep burns
  - Low temperature, weak pulse, ↓ capillary refill, ↓ pain sensation, or ↓ neurologic function in extremity
  - Problems ventilating patient with significant chest torso burns
  - May need fasciotomy if compartment syndrome suspected after escharotomy
- **Risk factors for burn injuries** - alcohol or drug use, age (very young/very old), smoking, low socioeconomic status, violence, epilepsy

CHILD ABUSE
- Accounts for 15% of burn injuries in children
- History and exam findings that suggest abuse:
  - **History** - delayed presentation for care, conflicting histories, previous injuries
  - **Exam** - sharply demarcated margins, uniform depth, absence of splash marks, stocking or glove patterns, flexor sparing, dorsal location on hands, very deep localized contact injury

LUNG INJURY
- Caused primarily by **carbonaceous materials** and **smoke**, <u>not</u> heat
- **Risk factors for airway injury** – ETOH, trauma, closed space, rapid combustion, extremes of age, delayed extrication
- **Signs and symptoms of possible airway injury** – facial burns, wheezing, carbonaceous sputum
- **Indications for intubation** – upper airway stridor or obstruction, worsening hypoxemia, massive volume resuscitation can worsen symptoms
- **Pneumonia** – most common infection in patients with > 30% BSA burns
  - Also most common cause of **death** after > 30% BSA burns

UNUSUAL BURNS
- **Acid and alkali burns** – copious water irrigation
  - Alkalis produce deeper burns than acid due to <u>liquefaction necrosis</u>
  - Acid burns produce <u>coagulation necrosis</u>
- **Hydrofluoric acid burns** – spread **calcium** on wound
- **Powder burns** – wipe away before irrigation
- **Tar burns** – cool, then wipe away with a **lipophilic solvent** (adhesive remover)
- **Electrical burns** – need cardiac monitoring
  - Can cause rhabdomyolysis and compartment syndrome
  - Other complications – polyneuritis, quadriplegia, transverse myelitis, cataracts, liver necrosis, intestinal perforation, gallbladder perforation, pancreatic necrosis
- **Lightning** – cardiopulmonary arrest secondary to electrical paralysis of brainstem

1ST WEEK – EARLY EXCISION OF BURNED AREAS
- **Caloric need**: 25 kcal/kg/day + (30 kcal × % burn)
- **Protein need**: 1 g/kg/day + (3 g × % burn)
- **Glucose** – best source of nonprotein calories in patients with burns
  - Burn wounds use glucose in an obligatory fashion
- **Excise burn wounds** in **< 72 hours** (but <u>not</u> until after appropriate fluid resuscitation)
  - Used for **deep 2nd-, 3rd-,** and some **4th-degree** burns
  - Viability is based on color, texture, punctate bleeding after removal
- Wounds to **face**, **palms**, **soles**, and **genitals** are **deferred** for the 1st week
- **For each burn wound excision** – want < 1 L blood loss, < 20% of skin excised, and < 2 hours in OR
  - Patients can get extremely sick if too much time is spent in OR
- **Skin grafts are contraindicated** if culture is positive for **beta-hemolytic strep** or **bacteria > 10^5**
- **Autografts** (split-thickness [STSG] or full-thickness [FTSG]) – <u>best</u>
  - ↓ Infection, desiccation, protein loss, pain, water loss, heat loss, and RBC loss compared to dermal substitutes
  - Donor skin site is regenerated from **hair follicles** and **skin edges** on STSGs
  - **Imbibition** (osmotic) – blood supply to skin graft for days 0–3
  - **Neovascularization** – starts around day 3
  - Poorly vascularized beds are unlikely to support skin grafting → includes tendon, bone without periosteum, XRT areas
  - **Split-thickness grafts** are 12–15 mm (includes epidermis and part of dermis)
- **Homografts** (allografts; cadaveric skin) – not as good as autografts
  - Can be a good temporizing material; last 2–4 weeks
  - Allografts vascularize and are eventually rejected at which time they must be replaced
- **Xenografts** (porcine) – not as good as homografts; last 2 weeks; these do not vascularize
- **Dermal substitutes** – not as good as homografts or xenografts

- **Meshed grafts** – use for back, flank, trunk, arms, and legs
  - **Reasons to delay autografting** – infection, not enough skin donor sites, patient septic or unstable, do not want to create any more donor sites with concomitant blood loss
  - **Most common reason for skin graft loss** – seroma or hematoma formation under graft
    - Need to apply pressure dressing (cotton balls) to the skin graft to prevent seroma and hematoma buildup underneath the graft
  - **STSGs** are more likely to survive – graft not as thick so easier for **imbibition** and subsequent revascularization to occur
  - **FTSGs** have less wound contraction – good for areas such as the palms and back of hands
- **Burn scar hypopigmentation** and **irregularities** can be improved with dermabrasion thin split-thickness grafts

2ND TO 5TH WEEKS – SPECIALIZED AREAS ADDRESSED, ALLOGRAFT REPLACED WITH AUTOGRAFT
- **Face** – topical antibiotics for 1st week, **FTSG** for unhealed areas (nonmeshed)
- **Hands**
  - **Superficial** – ROM exercises; splint in extension if too much edema
  - **Deep** – immobilize in extension for 7 days after skin graft (need **FTSG**), then physical therapy. May need wire fixation of joints if unstable or open.
- **Palms** – try to preserve specialized palmar attachments. Splint hand in extension for 7 days after **FTSG**
- **Genitals** – can use **STSG** (meshed)

BURN WOUND INFECTIONS
- Usually apply **bacitracin** or **Neosporin** immediately after burns
- No role for prophylactic IV antibiotics
- **Pseudomonas** is most common organism in burn wound infection (some texts say staph but *Pseudomonas* is the classic answer), followed by *Staphylococcus*, *E. coli*, and *Enterobacter*
- More common in burns > **30% BSA**
- Topical agents have decreased incidence of burn wound bacterial infections
- *Candida* infections have increased incidence secondary to topical antimicrobials
- Granulocyte chemotaxis and cell-mediated immunity are impaired in burn patients
- **Silvadene** (silver sulfadiazine) – can cause **neutropenia** and **thrombocytopenia**
  - Do not use in patients with sulfa allergy
  - Limited eschar penetration; can inhibit epithelialization
  - Ineffective against some *Pseudomonas*; effective for *Candida*
- **Silver nitrate** – can cause **electrolyte imbalances** (hyponatremia, hypochloremia, hypocalcemia, and hypokalemia)
  - Discoloration
  - Limited eschar penetration
  - Ineffective against some *Pseudomonas* species and GPCs
  - Can cause **methemoglobinemia** – contraindicated in patients with G6PD deficiency
- **Sulfamylon** (mafenide sodium) – painful application
  - Can cause **metabolic acidosis** due to carbonic anhydrase inhibition ($\downarrow$ renal conversion of $H_2CO_3 \rightarrow H_2O + CO_2$)
  - Good **eschar penetration**; good for burns overlying **cartilage**
  - Broadest spectrum against *Pseudomonas* and GNRs
- **Mupirocin** – good for MRSA; very expensive
- **Signs of burn wound infection** – peripheral edema, 2nd- to 3rd-degree burn conversion, hemorrhage into scar, erythema gangrenosum, green fat, black skin around wound, rapid eschar separation, focal discoloration

- **Burn wound sepsis** – usually due to *Pseudomonas*
- **HSV** – most common viral infection in burn wounds
- **< 10^5 organisms** – <u>not</u> a burn wound infection
- Best way to detect burn wound infection (and differentiate from colonization) – **biopsy of burn wound**

COMPLICATIONS AFTER BURNS

- **Seizures** – usually iatrogenic and related to **Na concentration**
- **Peripheral neuropathy** – secondary to small vessel injury and demyelination
- **Ectopia** – from contraction of burned adnexa. Tx: eyelid release
- **Eyes** – fluorescein staining to find injury. Tx: topical fluoroquinolone or gentamicin
- **Corneal abrasion** – Tx: topical antibiotics
- **Symblepharon** – eyelid stuck to conjunctiva. Tx: release with glass rod
- **Heterotopic ossification of tendons** – Tx: physical therapy; may need surgery
- **Fractures** – Tx: often need external fixation to allow for treatment of burns
- **Curling's ulcer** – gastric ulcer that occurs with burns
- **Marjolin's ulcer** – highly malignant **squamous cell CA** that arises in chronic non-healing burn wounds or unstable scars
- **Hypertrophic scar**
  - Usually occurs 3–4 months after injury secondary to ↑ **neovascularity**
  - More likely to be deep thermal injuries that take > 3 weeks to heal, heal by contraction and epithelial spread, or heal across flexor surfaces
  - Tx: **steroid injection into lesion** (best), silicone, compression; wait 1–2 years before scar modification surgery

ERYTHEMA MULTIFORME AND VARIANTS

- **Erythema multiforme** – least severe form (self-limited, target lesions)
- **Stevens–Johnson syndrome** (more serious) – < 10% BSA
- **Toxic epidermal necrolysis** (TEN) – most severe form
- **Staph scalded skin syndrome** (caused by *Staphylococcus aureus*)
- Skin <u>epidermal–dermal separation</u> seen in all
- Caused by a variety of drugs (Dilantin, Bactrim, penicillin) and viruses
- Tx: fluid resuscitation and supportive; need to prevent wound desiccation with homografts/xenografts wraps; topical antibiotics; IV antibiotics if due to *Staphylococcus*
- **No steroids**

SKIN
- **Epidermis** – primarily cellular
  - **Keratinocytes** – main cell type in epidermis; originate from basal layer; provide mechanical barrier
  - **Melanocytes** – neuroectodermal origin (neural crest cells); in basal layer of epidermis
    - Have dendritic processes that transfer melanin to neighboring keratinocytes via melanosomes
    - Density of melanocytes is the same among races; difference is in melanin production
- **Dermis** – primarily structural proteins (collagen) for the epidermis
- **Langerhans cells**
  - Act as antigen-presenting cells (MHC class II)
  - Originate from bone marrow
  - Have a role in contact hypersensitivity reactions (type IV)
- **Sensory nerves**
  - **Pacinian corpuscles** – pressure
  - **Ruffini's endings** – warmth
  - **Krause's end-bulbs** – cold
  - **Meissner's corpuscles** – tactile sense
- **Eccrine sweat glands** – aqueous sweat (thermal regulation, usually hypotonic)
- **Apocrine sweat glands** – milky sweat
  - Highest concentration of glands in palms and soles; most sweat is the result of sympathetic nervous system via acetylcholine
- **Lipid-soluble drugs** – ↑ skin absorption
- **Type I collagen** – predominant type in skin; 70% of dermis; gives tensile strength
- **Tension** – resistance to stretching (collagen)
- **Elasticity** – ability to regain shape (branching proteins that can stretch to 2× normal length)
- **Cushing's striae** – caused by loss of tensile strength and elasticity

FLAPS
- MCC of **pedicled** or **anastomosed free flap necrosis** – **venous thrombosis**
- **Tissue expansion** occurs by local recruitment, thinning of the dermis and epidermis, mitosis
- **TRAM flaps**
  - Complications – flap necrosis, ventral hernia, bleeding, infection, abdominal wall weakness
  - Rely on **superior epigastric vessels**
  - **Periumbilical perforators** most important determinant of **TRAM flap viability**

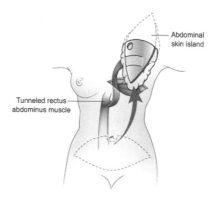

Abdominal skin island

Tunneled rectus abdominus muscle

Transverse rectus abdominis myocutaneous (TRAM) flap reconstruction.

Pressure Sores		
Stage	Description	Treatment
I	**Erythema** and pain, no skin loss	
II	**Partial skin loss** with yellow debris	Local treatment, keep pressure off
III	Full-thickness skin loss, **subcutaneous fat exposure**	Sharp debridement; likely need myocutaneous flap
IV	Involves **bony cortex, muscle**	Myocutaneous flaps

After Deziel DJ, et al. *Rush University Review of Surgery.* 3rd ed. Philadelphia, PA: WB Saunders; 2000:598.

UV RADIATION
- Damages DNA and repair mechanisms
- Both a promoter and initiator
- **Melanin** single best factor for protecting skin from UV radiation
- **UV-B** – responsible for chronic sun damage

MELANOMA
- Represents only 5% of skin CA but accounts for 65% of the deaths
- **Risk factors** for melanoma:
  - Dysplastic, atypical, or large **congenital nevi** – 10% lifetime risk for melanoma
  - Familial **BK mole syndrome** – almost 100% risk of melanoma
  - **Xeroderma pigmentosum**
  - Fair complexion, easy sunburn, intermittent sunburns, previous skin CA, previous XRT
  - 10% of melanomas familial
- **Most common melanoma site on skin** – back in men, legs in women
- **Prognosis worse** for men, ulcerated lesions, ocular and mucosal lesions
- **Signs of melanoma** (ABCDE) – <u>asymmetry</u> (angulations, indentation, notching, ulceration, bleeding), <u>borders</u> that are irregular, <u>color</u> change (darkening), <u>diameter</u> increase, <u>evolving</u> over time
- Originates from **neural crest cells** (melanocytes) in **basal layer** epidermis
- **Blue color** → most ominous
- **Lung** – most common location for distant melanoma metastases
- Most common metastasis to <u>small bowel</u> – **melanoma**
- **Dx:**
  - < **2 cm lesion** – <u>excisional</u> biopsy (tru-cut core needle biopsy) unless cosmetically sensitive area – need resection with margins if pathology comes back as melanoma

- > **2 cm lesions** or **cosmetically sensitive area** – <u>incisional</u> biopsy (or punch biopsy), will need to resect with margins if pathology shows melanoma
- **Types**:
  - **Melanoma in situ** or **thin lentigo maligna** (Hutchinson's freckle) – just in the superficial papillary dermis; 0.5-cm margins OK
  - **Lentigo maligna melanoma** – least aggressive, minimal invasion, radial growth 1st usual; elevated nodules
  - **Superficial spreading melanoma** – most common, intermediate malignancy; originates from nevus/sun-exposed areas
  - **Nodular** – *most aggressive*; most likely to have metastasized at time of diagnosis; deepest growth at time of diagnosis; vertical growth 1st; bluish-black with smooth borders; occurs anywhere on the body
  - **Acral lentiginous** – very aggressive; palms/soles of African Americans
- **Staging** – chest/abd/pelvic CT, LFTs, and LDH for all melanoma ≥ 1 mm; examine all possible draining lymph nodes
- **Tx for all stages** → 1) resection of primary tumor with appropriate margins and; 2) management of lymph nodes

Recommended Surgical Margins for Melanoma Excision	
Melanoma Thickness (mm)	Clinical Excision Margin (cm)
In situ	0.5–1.0
≤ 1.0	1.0
1.1–2.0	1.0–2.0
> 2.0	2.0

Margins may need to be modified based on anatomic considerations but still require histologic confirmation of tumor-free margins. For clinically ill-defined lentigo maligna melanoma, wider margins may be required for histologic confirmation of tumor-free margins.

- **Nodes**
  - Always need to **resect clinically positive nodes**
  - Perform **sentinel lymph node biopsy** if nodes clinically negative and tumor ≥ 1 mm deep
  - **Involved nodes** usually nontender, round, hard, 1–2 cm
  - Need to include **superficial parotidectomy** for all **anterior head/neck** melanomas ≥ 1 mm deep (20% metastasis rate to parotid)
- **Axillary node melanoma with no other primary** – Tx: complete axillary node dissection (remove Level I, II, and III nodes – unlike breast CA)
- **Resection of metastases** has provided some patients with long disease-free interval and is the best chance for cure
- **Isolated metastases** (ie lung or liver) that can be resected with a low-risk procedure should probably undergo resection
- **IL-2** and **tumor vaccines** can be used for systemic disease

BASAL CELL CARCINOMA
- **Most common malignancy in United States**; 4× more common than squamous cell skin CA
- 80% on head and neck
- Originates from **epidermis** – basal epithelial cells and hair follicles

- **Pearly** appearance, **rolled borders**, slow and indolent growth
- Pathology – **peripheral palisading of nuclei** and **stromal retraction**
- **Regional adenectomy** for **clinically positive nodes**
- **Morpheaform type** – most aggressive; has **collagenase** production
- Tx: **0.3–0.5-cm** margins
  - XRT and chemotherapy – may be of limited benefit for inoperable disease, metastases or neuro/lymphatic/vessel invasion

SQUAMOUS CELL CARCINOMA

- Overlying erythema, papulonodular with crust and ulceration; usually red-brown
- May have surrounding induration and satellite nodules
- Metastasizes more frequently than basal cell CA but less common than melanoma
- Can develop in post-XRT areas or in old burn scars
- **Risk factors** – actinic keratoses, xeroderma pigmentosum, Bowen's disease, atrophic epidermis, arsenics, hydrocarbons (coal tar), chlorophenols, HPV, immunosuppression, sun exposure, fair skin, previous XRT, previous skin CA
- Risk factors for metastasis – poorly differentiated, greater depth, recurrent lesions, immunosuppression
- Tx: **0.5–1.0-cm** margins for low risk
  - Can treat high risk with **Mohs surgery** (margin mapping using conservative slices; not used for melanoma) when trying to minimize area of resection (ie lesions on face)
  - **Regional adenectomy** for **clinically positive nodes**
  - XRT and chemotherapy – may be of limited benefit for inoperable disease, metastases or neuro/lymphatic/vessel invasion

SOFT TISSUE SARCOMA

- **Most common soft tissue sarcomas** – **#1 malignant fibrous histiosarcoma**, #2 liposarcoma
- 50% arise from extremities; 50% in children (arise from embryonic mesoderm)
- Most sarcomas are large, grow rapidly, and are painless
- Symptoms: asymptomatic mass (most common presentation), GI bleeding, bowel obstruction, neurologic deficit
- CXR – to R/O lung mets
- **MRI *before* biopsy** to R/O vascular, neuro, or bone invasion
- **Biopsy**
  - **Excisional biopsy** if mass < 4 cm
  - **Longitudinal incisional biopsy** for masses > 4 cm
  - Need to eventually resect biopsy skin site if biopsy shows sarcoma
- **Hematogenous spread**, not to lymphatics → metastasis to nodes is rare
  - **Lung** – most common site for metastasis
- **Staging** based on **grade**, not size
- Tx: Want at least **3-cm margins** and at least **1 uninvolved fascial plane** → try to perform limb-sparing operation
  - **Place clips** to mark site of likely recurrence → will XRT these later
  - **Postop XRT** – for high-grade tumors, close margins, or tumors > 5 cm
  - Chemotherapy is **doxorubicin** based
  - Tumors > 10 cm may benefit from preop chemo-XRT → may allow limb-sparing resection
  - **Isolated sarcoma metastases** without other evidence of systemic disease can be resected and are the best chance for survival; otherwise can palliate with XRT
  - Midline incision favored for pelvic and retroperitoneal sarcomas
  - With resection, try to preserve motor nerves and retain or reconstruct vessels

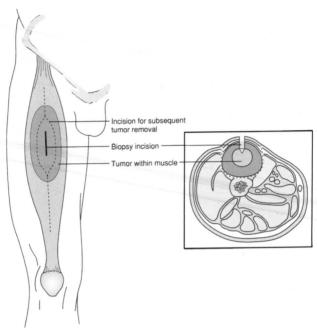

Incision for subsequent
tumor removal

Biopsy incision

Tumor within muscle

Technique for biopsy of an extremity soft-tissue mass suspected of being a sarcoma. The incision should be oriented along the long axis of the extremity, at the point where the lesion is closest to the surface, and situated so that it can be readily excised along with the tumor if a diagnosis of sarcoma is made. There should be no raising of flaps or disturbance of tissue planes superficial to the tumor. The mass should not be enucleated within the pseudocapsule; rather, incisional biopsy leaving the bulk of the lesion undisturbed should be carried out. Before wound closure, hemostasis should be achieved to avoid a hematoma, which could disseminate tumor cells through normal tissue planes. Drains are not used routinely.

- ■ **Poor prognosis overall**
  - Delay in diagnosis
  - Difficulty with total resection
  - Difficulty getting XRT to pelvic tumors
  - 40% 5-year survival rate with complete resection
- ■ **Head** and **neck sarcomas** – can occur in the pediatric population (usually rhabdomyosarcoma)
  - Hard to get margins because of proximity to vital structures
  - Postop XRT for positive or close margins as negative margins may be impossible to obtain
- ■ **Visceral** and **retroperitoneal sarcomas** – most commonly are leiomyosarcomas and liposarcomas
  - Ability to completely remove the tumor the most important prognostic factor in visceral and retroperitoneal sarcomas
- ■ **Risk factors**
  - **Asbestos** – mesothelioma
  - **PVC** and **arsenic** – angiosarcoma
  - **Chronic lymphedema** – lymphangiosarcoma
- ■ **Kaposi's sarcoma** (KS) – vascular sarcoma
  - Oral and pharyngeal mucosa are the most common sites; bleeding, dysphagia
  - Associated with immunocompromised state; most common malignancy in AIDS

- Rarely a cause of death in AIDS
- Tx: primary goal is **palliation**
  - **AIDS Tx** (HAART) shrinks AIDS-related KS – *best Tx*
  - Consider XRT or intra-lesional vinblastine for local disease
  - Interferon-alpha for disseminated disease
  - Surgery for severe intestinal hemorrhage
- **Childhood rhabdomyosarcoma**
  - #1 soft tissue sarcoma in kids
  - Head/neck, genitourinary, extremities, and trunk (poorest prognosis)
  - **Embryonal** subtype – most common
  - **Alveolar** subtype – worst prognosis
  - Tx: surgery; doxorubicin-based chemotherapy
- **Bone sarcomas**
  - Most are metastatic at the time of diagnosis
  - **Osteosarcoma**
    - Increased incidence around the knee
    - Originates from **metaphyseal cells**
    - Usually in children
- **Genetic syndromes for soft tissue tumors**
  - Neurofibromatosis – CNS tumors, peripheral sheath tumors, pheochromocytoma
  - Li–Fraumeni syndrome – childhood rhabdomyosarcoma, many others
  - Hereditary retinoblastoma – also includes other sarcomas
  - Tuberous sclerosis – angiomyolipoma
  - Gardner's syndrome – familial adenomatous polyposis and intra-abdominal desmoids tumors

OTHER CONDITIONS

- **Lip lacerations** – important to line up vermillion border
- **Xanthoma** – yellow, contains histiocytes. Tx: excision
- **Warts** (verruca vulgaris) – viral origin, contagious, autoinoculable, can be painful
  - Tx: liquid nitrogen initially
- **Lipomas** – common but rarely malignant; back, neck, between shoulders
- **Neuromas** – can be associated with neurofibromatosis and von Recklinghausen's disease (café-au-lait spots, axillary freckling; peripheral nerve and CNS tumors)
- **Keratoses**
  - **Actinic keratosis** – premalignant in sun-damaged areas; need excisional biopsy if suspicious
  - **Seborrheic keratosis** – <u>not</u> premalignant; trunk on elderly; can be dark
  - **Arsenical keratosis** – associated with squamous cell carcinoma
- **Merkel cell carcinoma** – are **neuroendocrine**
  - Very aggressive malignant tumor with early regional and systemic spread
  - Red to purple papulonodule or indurated plaque
  - Have **neuron-specific enolase** (NSE), **cytokeratin**, and **neurofilament protein**
- **Glomus cell tumor**
  - Painful tumor composed of **blood vessels** and **nerves**
  - **Benign**; most common in the **terminal aspect of the digit**
  - Tx: tumor excision
- **Desmoid tumors** – benign but locally very invasive; occur in fascial planes
  - **Anterior abdominal wall** (most common location) desmoids can occur during or following pregnancy; can also occur after trauma or surgery
  - **Intra-abdominal desmoids** associated with Gardner's syndrome and retroperitoneal fibrosis; often **encases bowel**, making it hard to get en bloc resection
  - High risk of local recurrences; no distant spread
  - Tx: surgery if possible; chemotherapy (**sulindac, tamoxifen**) if vital structure involved or too much bowel would be taken (high risk of short bowel syndrome with surgery)

- **Bowen's disease** – SCCA in situ; 10% turn into invasive SCCA; associated with **HPV**
  - Tx: **imiquimod,** cautery ablation, topical 5-FU, _**avoid wide local excision**_ if possible (high recurrence rate w/ HPV); regular biopsies to R/O CA
- **Keratoacanthoma**
  - Rapid growth, rolled edges, crater filled with **keratin**
  - Is <u>not</u> malignant but can be confused with SCCA
  - Involutes spontaneously over months
  - Always biopsy these to be sure
  - If small, excise; if large, biopsy and observe
- **Hyperhidrosis** – ↑ sweating, especially noticeable in the palms. Tx: **thoracic sympathectomy** if refractory to variety of antiperspirants
- **Hidradenitis** – infection of the apocrine sweat glands, usually in axilla and groin regions
  - Staph/strep most common organisms
  - Tx: antibiotics, improved hygiene 1st; may need surgery to remove skin and associated sweat glands
- **Benign cysts**
  - **Epidermal inclusion cyst** – most common; have completely mature epidermis with creamy **keratin** material
  - **Trichilemmal cyst** – in scalp, no epidermis
  - **Ganglion cyst** – over tendons, usually over wrist; filled with **collagen** material
  - **Dermoid cyst** – midline intra-abdominal and sacral lesions usual; need resection due to malignancy risk
  - **Pilonidal cyst** – congenital coccygeal sinus with ingrown hair; gets infected and needs to be excised

ANATOMY AND PHYSIOLOGY

- **Anterior neck triangle** – sternocleidomastoid muscle (SCM), sternal notch, inferior border of the digastric muscle; contains the **carotid sheath**
- **Posterior neck triangle** – posterior border of the SCM, trapezius muscle, and the clavicle; contains the **accessory nerve** (innervates SCM, trapezius, and platysma) and the **brachial plexus**
- **Parotid glands** – secrete mostly serous fluid
- **Sublingual glands** – secrete mostly mucin
- **Submandibular glands** – 50/50 serous/mucin
- In larynx, the false vocal cords are superior to the true vocal cords
- Trachea has U-shaped cartilage and a posterior portion that is membranous

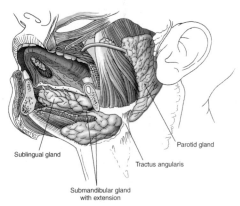

Sublingual gland

Parotid gland

Tractus angularis

Submandibular gland with extension

Major salivary glands. The lateral view, illustrating the tractus angularis and submandibular gland with extension under the mylohyoid muscle and the sublingual gland. (From Byers RM. Operations involving the submandibular and sublingual salivary glands. In: Fischer JE, Bland KI, et al, eds. *Mastery of Surgery.* 5th ed. Philadelphia, PA: Lippincott Williams & Wilkins; 2007, with permission.)

- **Vagus nerve** – runs between internal jugular (IJ) vein and carotid artery
- **Phrenic nerve** – runs on top of the anterior scalene muscle
- **Long thoracic nerve** – runs posterior to the middle scalene muscle
- **Trigeminal nerve** – ophthalmic, maxillary, and mandibular branches
  - Gives **sensation** to most of face
  - Mandibular branch – taste to anterior ⅔ of tongue, floor of mouth, and gingiva
- **Facial nerve** – temporal, zygomatic, buccal, marginal mandibular, and cervical branches
  - **Motor** function to face
- **Glossopharyngeal nerve** – taste to posterior ⅓ tongue
  - Motor to stylopharyngeus
  - Injury affects **swallowing**
- **Hypoglossal nerve** – motor to all of tongue except palatoglossus
  - Tongue deviates to the **same side** of a hypoglossal nerve injury
- **Recurrent laryngeal nerve** – innervates all of larynx except cricothyroid muscle
- **Superior laryngeal nerve** – innervates the cricothyroid muscle

- **Frey's syndrome** – occurs after parotidectomy; injury of **auriculotemporal nerve** that then cross-innervates with **sympathetic fibers** to sweat glands of skin
  - Symptom: **gustatory sweating**
- **Thyrocervical trunk** – "STAT": suprascapular artery, transverse cervical artery, ascending cervical artery, inferior thyroid artery
- **External carotid artery** – 1st branch is superior thyroid artery
- **Trapezius flap** – based on transverse cervical artery
- **Pectoralis major flap** – based on either the thoracoacromial artery or the internal mammary artery
- **Torus palatini** – congenital bony mass on upper palate of mouth. Tx: nothing
- **Torus mandibular** – similar to above but on lingual surface of mandible. Tx: nothing
- **Modified radical neck dissection** (MRND) – takes omohyoid, submandibular gland, sensory nerves C2–C5, cervical branch of facial nerve, and ipsilateral thyroid
  - No mortality difference compared with RND
- **Radical neck dissection** (RND) – same as MRND *plus* accessory nerve (CN XII), sternocleidomastoid, and internal jugular resection (rarely done anymore)
  - Most morbidity occurs from accessory nerve resection

ORAL CAVITY CANCER
- **Most common cancer of the oral cavity, pharynx, and larynx** – squamous cell CA
  - **Biggest risk factors** – tobacco and ETOH
  - **Erythroplakia** – considered more premalignant than leukoplakia
- **Oral cavity includes** mouth floor, anterior ⅓ tongue, gingiva, hard palate, anterior tonsillar pillars, and lips
- **Lower lip** – most common site for oral cavity CA (more common than upper lip due to sun exposure)
- **Survival rate lowest** for **hard palate tumors** – hard to resect
- **Oral cavity CA** increased in patients with **Plummer–Vinson syndrome** (glossitis, cervical dysphagia from esophageal web, spoon fingers, iron-deficiency anemia)
- **Treatment**
  - **Wide resection** (1 cm margins)
  - **MRND** for tumors > 4 cm, clinically positive nodes, or bone invasion
  - **Postop XRT** for advanced lesions (> 4 cm, positive margins, or nodal/bone involvement)
- **Lip CA** – may need **flaps** if more than ½ of the lip is removed
  - Lesions along the **commissure** are **most aggressive**
- **Tongue CA** – can still operate with jaw invasion (commando procedure)
- **Verrucous ulcer** – a well-differentiated SCCA; often found on the cheek; oral tobacco
  - Not aggressive, rare metastasis
  - Tx: full cheek resection ± flap; *__no MRND__*
- **Cancer of maxillary sinus** – Tx: maxillectomy
- **Tonsillar CA** – ETOH, tobacco, males; SCCA most common; asymptomatic until large; 80% have lymph node metastases at time of diagnosis
  - Tx: **tonsillectomy** best way to biopsy; wide resection with margins after that

PHARYNGEAL CANCER
- **Nasopharyngeal SCCA** – EBV; Chinese; presents with nose bleeding or obstruction
  - Goes to **posterior cervical neck nodes**
  - Tx: ***XRT primary therapy*** (*very sensitive*; give chemo-XRT for advanced disease – *no surgery*)
  - **Children** – <u>lymphoma</u> #1 tumor of nasopharynx. Tx: chemotherapy
  - **Papilloma** – most common benign neoplasm of nose/paranasal sinuses

- **Oropharyngeal SCCA** – neck mass, sore throat
  - Goes to **posterior cervical neck nodes**
  - Tx: **XRT** for tumors < **4 cm** and no nodal or bone invasion
  - Combined **surgery, MRND,** and **XRT** for **advanced tumors** (> 4 cm, bone invasion or nodal invasion)
- **Hypopharyngeal SCCA** – hoarseness; <u>early metastases</u>
  - Goes to **anterior cervical nodes**
  - Tx: **XRT** for tumors < **4 cm** and no nodal or bone invasion
  - Combined **surgery, MRND,** and **XRT** for **advanced tumors** (> 4 cm, bone invasion or nodal invasion)
- **Nasopharyngeal angiofibroma** – benign tumor
  - Presents in males < 20 years (obstruction or epistaxis)
  - Extremely **vascular**
  - Tx: angiography and **embolization** (usually internal maxillary artery), followed by **resection**

LARYNGEAL CANCER
- Hoarseness, aspiration, dyspnea, dysphagia
- Try to **preserve larynx**
- Tx: **XRT** (if vocal cord only) or **chemo-XRT** (if beyond vocal cord)
  - Surgery is <u>not</u> the primary Tx; try to **preserve larynx**
  - MRND needed if nodes clinically positive
  - Take **ipsilateral thyroid lobe** with MRND
- Papilloma – most common benign lesion of larynx

SALIVARY GLAND CANCERS
- Parotid, submandibular, sublingual, and minor salivary glands
- Submandibular or sublingual tumors – can present as a neck mass or swelling in the floor of the mouth
- **Mass in <u>large</u> salivary gland** → more likely mass is <u>benign</u>
- **Mass in <u>small</u> salivary gland** → more likely mass is <u>malignant</u>, although the parotid gland is the most frequent site for malignant tumor
- **Malignant tumors**
  - Often present as a painful mass but can also present with facial nerve paralysis or lymphadenopathy
  - Lymphatic drainage is to the intra-parotid and anterior cervical chain nodes
  - **Mucoepidermoid CA** – #1 malignant tumor of the salivary glands
    - Wide range of aggressiveness
  - **Adenoid cystic CA** – #2 malignant tumor of the salivary glands
    - Long, indolent course; propensity to invade nerve roots
    - Very sensitive to **XRT**
  - Tx for both: **resection of salivary gland** (eg total parotidectomy), **prophylactic MRND,** and **postop XRT** if <u>high grade</u> or <u>advanced disease</u>
    - If in parotid, need to take whole lobe; try to preserve facial nerve
- **Benign tumors**
  - Often present as a painless mass
  - **Pleomorphic adenoma** (mixed tumor) – #1 benign tumor of the salivary glands
    - **Malignant degeneration** in **5%**
    - Tx: superficial parotidectomy
    - If malignant degeneration, need total parotidectomy
  - **Warthin's tumor** – #2 benign tumor of the salivary glands
    - Males, bilateral in 10%
    - Tx: superficial parotidectomy

- Most common injured nerve with parotid surgery – **greater auricular nerve** (numbness over lower portion of ear)
- For submandibular gland resection – need to find <u>mandibular branch of facial nerve</u>, <u>lingual nerve</u>, and <u>hypoglossal nerve</u>
- Most common salivary gland tumor in children – **hemangiomas**

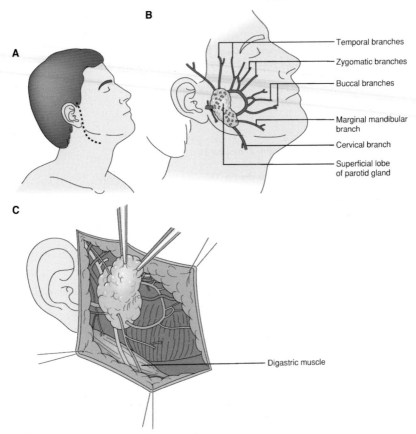

Superficial parotidectomy. *(A)* The standard Blair incision or the cosmetically superior facelift incision can be used. *(B)* Branches of the facial nerve course between the superficial and deep lobes of the parotid. *(C)* The main trunk of the facial nerve is identified 8 mm deep to the tympanomastoid suture line and at the same level as the digastric muscle.

EAR

- **Pinna lacerations** – need suture through involved cartilage
- **Cauliflower ear** – undrained hematomas that organize and calcify; need to be drained to avoid this
- **Cholesteatoma** – epidermal inclusion cyst of ear; slow growing but erode as they grow; present with conductive hearing loss and clear drainage from ear. Tx: surgical excision

■ **Chemodectomas** – vascular tumor of middle ear (paraganglionoma). Tx: surgery ± XRT

■ **Acoustic neuroma** – CN VIII, tinnitus, hearing loss, unsteadiness; can grow into cerebellar/pontine angle. Tx: craniotomy and resection; XRT is alternative to surgery

■ **Ear SCCA** – 20% metastasize to parotid gland. Tx: resection and parotidectomy, MRND for positive nodes or large tumors

■ **Rhabdomyosarcoma** – most common childhood aural malignancy (although rare) of the middle or external ear

NOSE

■ **Nasal fractures** – set after swelling decreases

■ **Septal hematoma** – need to drain to avoid infection and necrosis of septum

■ **CSF rhinorrhea** – usually a cribriform plate fracture (CSF has **tau protein**)
  • Repair of facial fractures may help leak; may need contrast study to help find leak
  • Tx: conservative 2–3 weeks; try epidural catheter drainage of CSF; may need transethmoidal repair

■ **Epistaxis** – 90% are <u>anterior</u> and can be controlled with packing; consider **internal maxillary artery** or **ethmoid artery embolization** for persistent <u>posterior</u> bleeding despite packing/balloon

NECK AND JAW

■ **Radicular cyst** – inflammatory cyst at the root of teeth; can cause bone erosion; lucent on X-ray; Tx local excision or curettage

■ **Ameloblastoma** – slow-growing malignancy of odontogenic epithelium (outside portion of teeth); soap bubble appearance on X-ray. Tx: wide local excision

■ **Osteogenic sarcoma** – poor prognosis. Tx: multimodality approach that includes surgery

■ **Maxillary jaw fractures** – most treated with wire fixation

■ **TMJ dislocations** – treated with closed reduction

■ **Lower lip numbness** – inferior alveolar nerve damage (branch of mandibular nerve)

■ **Stensen's duct laceration** – repair over catheter stent
  • Ligation can cause painful parotid atrophy and facial asymmetry

■ **Suppurative parotitis** – usually in elderly patients; occurs with **dehydration**; **staph** most common organism
  • Tx: fluids, salivation, antibiotics; drainage if abscess develops or patient not improving
  • Can be life-threatening

■ **Sialoadenitis** – acute inflammation of a salivary gland related to a stone in the duct; most calculi near orifice
  • 80% of the time affects the submandibular or sublingual glands
  • Recurrent sialoadenitis is due to ascending infection from the oral cavity
  • Tx: incise duct and remove stone
  • Gland excision may eventually be necessary for recurrent disease

ABSCESSES

■ **Peritonsillar abscess** – older kids (> 10 years)
  • Symptoms: trismus, odynophagia; usually does <u>not</u> obstruct airway
  • <u>Tx</u>: needle aspiration 1st, then drainage through <u>tonsillar bed</u> if no relief in 24 hours (may need to intubate to drain; will self-drain with swallowing once opened)

■ **Retropharyngeal abscess** – younger kids (< 10 years)
  • Symptoms: fever, odynophagia, drool; is an **airway emergency**
  • Can occur in elderly with Pott's disease

- Tx: intubate the patient in a calm setting; drainage through <u>posterior pharyngeal wall</u>; will self-drain with swallowing once opened
- **Parapharyngeal abscess** – all age groups; occurs with dental infections, tonsillitis, pharyngitis
  - Morbidity comes from vascular invasion and **mediastinal spread** via prevertebral and retropharyngeal spaces
  - Tx: <u>drain through lateral neck</u> to avoid damaging internal carotid and internal jugular veins; need to leave drain in
- **Ludwig's angina** – acute infection of the floor of the mouth, involves **mylohyoid muscle**
  - Most common cause is **dental infection** of the mandibular teeth
  - May rapidly spread to deeper structures and cause airway obstruction
  - Tx: airway control, surgical drainage, antibiotics

ASYMPTOMATIC HEAD AND NECK MASSES
- **Preauricular tumors**
  - All lumps near ear are parotid tumors until proved otherwise
  - Diagnosis is usually made after superficial lobectomy
  - 80% of all salivary tumors are in parotid
  - 80% of parotid tumors are benign
  - 80% of benign parotid tumors are pleomorphic adenomas
  - Most common distant metastases for head and neck tumors → **lung**
- **Posterior neck masses** – if no obvious malignant epithelial tumor, considered to have Hodgkin's lymphoma until proved otherwise. Need FNA or open biopsy
- **Neck mass workup**
  - 1st – H and P, laryngoscopy, and **_FNA (best test for Dx)_**; can consider antibiotics for 2 weeks with re-evaluation if thought to be inflammatory
  - 2nd – if above nondiagnostic → <u>panendoscopy</u> with multiple random biopsies, <u>neck and chest CT</u>
  - 3rd – still cannot figure it out → perform <u>excisional biopsy</u>; need to be prepared for MRND
  - Adenocarcinoma suggests breast, GI, or lung primary
- **Epidermoid CA** (SCCA variant) found in **cervical node _without_ known primary** →
  - 1st – <u>panendoscopy</u> to look for primary; get random biopsies
  - 2nd – <u>CT scan</u>
  - 3rd – still cannot find primary → <u>ipsilateral MRND</u>, <u>ipsilateral tonsillectomy</u> (most common location for occult head/neck tumor), <u>bilateral XRT</u>

OTHER CONDITIONS
- **Esophageal foreign body** – dysphagia; most just below the cricopharyngeus (95%)
  - Dx and Tx: **rigid EGD** under anesthesia
  - Perforation risk increases with <u>length of time in the esophagus</u>
- **Fever and pain** after EGD for foreign body → Gastrografin followed by barium swallow to rule out perforation
- **Laryngeal foreign body** – coughing; emergent cricothyroidotomy as a last resort may be needed to secure airway
- **Sleep apnea** – associated with MIs, arrhythmias, and death
  - More common in obese and those with micrognathia/retrognathia → have snoring and excessive daytime somnolence
  - Tx: CPAP, **uvulopalatopharyngoplasty** (best surgical solution), or permanent trach
- **Prolonged intubation** – can lead to subglottic stenosis, Tx: tracheal resection and reconstruction

- **Tracheostomy** – consider in patients who will require intubation for > 7–14 days
  - Decreases secretions, provides easier ventilation, decreases pneumonia risk
- **Median rhomboid glossitis** – failure of tongue fusion. Tx: none necessary
- **Cleft lip** (primary palate) – involves lip, alveolus, or both
  - Repair at 10 weeks, 10 lb, Hgb 10. Repair nasal deformities at same time
  - May be associated with poor feeding
- **Cleft palate** (secondary palate) – involves hard and soft palates; may affect speech and swallowing if not closed soon enough; may affect maxillofacial growth if closed too early → repair at 12 months
- **Hemangioma** – most common benign head and neck tumor in adults
- **Mastoiditis** – infection of the mastoid cells; can destroy bone
  - Rare; results as a complication of untreated **acute supportive otitis media**
  - Ear is pushed forward
  - Tx: antibiotics, may need emergency **mastoidectomy**
- **Epiglottitis**
  - Rare since immunization against *H. influenzae* type B
  - Mainly in children aged 3–5
  - Symptoms: stridor, drooling, leaning forward position, high fever, throat pain, thumbprint sign on lateral neck film
  - Can cause airway obstruction
  - Tx: early control of the airway; antibiotics

ANATOMY AND PHYSIOLOGY

- **Hypothalamus** – releases TRH, CRH, GnRH, GHRH, and dopamine into median eminence; passes through neurohypophysis on way to adenohypophysis
- **Dopamine** – inhibits prolactin secretion
- **Posterior pituitary** (neurohypophysis)
  - **ADH** – supraoptic nuclei, regulated by osmolar receptors in hypothalamus
  - **Oxytocin** – paraventricular nuclei in hypothalamus
  - Neurohypophysis does not contain cell bodies
- **Anterior pituitary** (80% of gland, adenohypophysis)
  - Releases ACTH, TSH, GH, LH, FSH, and prolactin
  - Does not have its own direct blood supply; passes through neurohypophysis 1st (portal venous system)
- **Bi-temporal hemianopia** – pituitary mass compressing optic nerve (CN II) at chiasm
- **Nonfunctional tumors** – almost always macroadenomas; present with mass effect and decreased ACTH, TSH, GH, LH, FSH. Tx: transsphenoidal resection
- **Contraindications to transsphenoidal approaches** – suprasellar extension, massive lateral extension, dumbbell-shaped tumor
- Most pituitary tumors respond to **bromocriptine** (dopamine agonist)

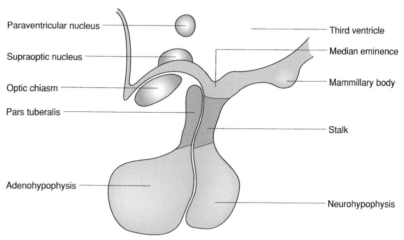

Schematic diagram of the pituitary and floor of the third ventricle as seen in a midline sagittal view. Anterior is to the left.

PROLACTINOMA

- **Most common pituitary adenoma**
- Mostly **microadenomas**
- Most patients do not need surgery. Prolactin is usually > 150 for symptoms to occur
- Symptoms: galactorrhea, irregular menses, ↓ libido, infertility
- Tx: **bromocriptine** (safe in pregnancy) or **cabergoline** (both are dopamine agonists) for most or transsphenoidal resection for failure of medical management
  - Macroadenomas – resection with hemorrhage, visual loss, wants pregnancy, CSF leak

ACROMEGALY (GROWTH HORMONE)

- Symptoms: HTN, DM, gigantism; can be life-threatening secondary to **cardiac symptoms** (valve dysfunction, cardiomyopathy)
- Usually macroadenomas
- Dx: **elevated IGF-1** *(best test)* growth hormone > 10 in 90%
- Tx: **octreotide** or **transsphenoidal resection**; XRT and bromocriptine can be used as secondary therapies

OTHER CONDITIONS

- **Sheehan's syndrome**
  - Post-partum **trouble lactating** – usually **1st sign**
  - Can also have amenorrhea, adrenal insufficiency, and hypothyroidism
  - Due to **pituitary ischemia** following hemorrhage and hypotensive episode during childbirth
  - Tx: **hormone replacement**
- **Craniopharyngioma** – benign calcified cyst, remnants of Rathke's pouch; grows along pituitary stalk to suprasellar location
  - Symptoms: most frequently presents with endocrine abnormalities, visual disturbances, headache, hydrocephalus
  - Tx: surgery to resect cyst
  - **Diabetes insipidus** – frequent complication postoperatively
- **Bilateral pituitary masses** – check pituitary axis hormones; if OK, probably metastases
- **Nelson's syndrome**
  - Occurs after **bilateral adrenalectomy**; ↑ CRH causes <u>pituitary enlargement</u>, resulting in **amenorrhea** and **visual problems** (bi-temporal hemianopia)
  - Also get **hyperpigmentation** from beta-MSH (melanocyte-stimulating hormone), a peptide byproduct of ACTH
  - Tx: **steroids**
- **Waterhouse–Friderichsen syndrome** – adrenal gland hemorrhage that occurs after meningococcal sepsis infection; can lead to adrenal insufficiency

- **Vascular supply**
  - **Superior adrenal** – inferior phrenic artery
  - **Middle adrenal** – aorta
  - **Inferior adrenal** – renal artery
  - **Left adrenal vein** goes to **left renal vein**
  - **Right adrenal vein** goes to **inferior vena cava**
- Made up of adrenal cortex and adrenal medulla
- No innervation to the cortex
- Medulla receives innervation from the sympathetic splanchnic nerves
- Lymphatics drain to subdiaphragmatic and renal lymph nodes

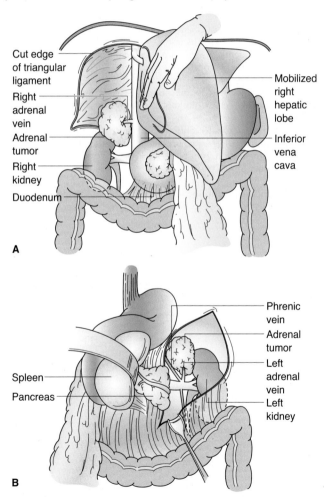

Anterior approach to right *(A)* and left *(B)* adrenalectomy. Note position of phrenic vein in relationship to the left adrenal vein and tumor.

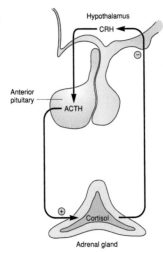

Schematic of hypothalamic–pituitary–adrenal axis for cortisol. Regulatory feedback relationships are designated with arrows.

ASYMPTOMATIC ADRENAL MASS
- 1%–2% of abdominal CT scans show incidentaloma (5% are metastases)
- Benign adenomas are common
- Adrenals are also common sites for metastases
- Dx: check for **functioning tumor** – urine metanephrines/VMA/catecholamines, urinary hydroxycorticosteroids, serum K with plasma renin and aldosterone levels
  - Consider CXR, colonoscopy, and mammogram to check for a primary tumor
- Surgery is indicated if mass has **ominous characteristics** (non-homogenous), is > **4–6 cm**, is **functioning**, or is **enlarging**
- If going to follow an incidentaloma, need repeat imaging every 3 months for 1 year, then yearly
- Anterior approach for adrenal CA resection
- **Common metastases to adrenal** – lung CA (#1), breast CA, melanoma, renal CA
- Cancer history with asymptomatic adrenal mass – **need biopsy**
- Some **isolated metastases** to the adrenal gland can be resected with adrenalectomy

ADRENAL CORTEX
- From mesoderm – remember GFR = salt, sugar, sex steroids
  - **Glomerulosa** – aldosterone; **fasciculata** – glucocorticoids; **reticularis** – androgens/estrogens
- Cholesterol → progesterone → androgens/cortisol/aldosterone
- All zones have **21-** and **11-beta hydroxylase**
- **Corticotropin-releasing hormone** (CRH) is released from the hypothalamus and goes to anterior pituitary gland
- **ACTH** is released from the anterior pituitary gland and causes the release of **cortisol**
- Cortisol has a diurnal peak at 4–6 a.m.
- **Cortisol** – inotropic, chronotropic, and increases vascular resistance; proteolysis and gluconeogenesis; decreases inflammation
- **Aldosterone** stimulates renal sodium resorption and secretion of potassium and hydrogen ion

- Aldosterone secretion is stimulated by **angiotensin II** and **hyperkalemia**, and to some extent ACTH
- **Excess estrogens** and **androgens** by adrenals – almost always cancer
- **Congenital adrenal hyperplasia** (enzyme defect in cortisol synthesis)
  - **21-Hydroxylase deficiency** (90%) – most common; precocious puberty in males, virilization in females
    - ↑ **17-OH progesterone** leads to ↑ production of testosterone
    - Is **salt wasting** (↓ sodium and ↑ potassium) and causes **hypotension**
    - Tx: cortisol, genitoplasty
  - **11-Hydroxylase deficiency** – precocious puberty in males, virilization in females
    - ↑ **11-Deoxycortisone**
    - Is **salt saving** (deoxycortisone acts as a mineralocorticoid) and causes **hypertension**
    - Tx: cortisol, genitoplasty
- **Hyperaldosteronism** (Conn's syndrome)
  - **Symptoms**: HTN secondary to sodium retention without edema; hypokalemia; also have weakness, polydipsia, and polyuria
  - **Primary disease** (renin is low) – adenoma (85%) → #1 cause of primary hyperaldosteronism, hyperplasia (15%), ovarian tumors (rare), cancer (rare)
  - **Secondary disease** (renin is high) – more common than primary disease; CHF, renal artery stenosis, liver failure, diuretics, Bartter's syndrome (renin-secreting tumor)
  - **Dx for primary hyperaldosteronism**
    - **Salt-load suppression test** (best, urine aldosterone will <u>stay high</u>)
    - **Aldosterone:renin ratio > 20**
    - Labs – ↓ serum K, ↑ serum Na, ↑ urine K, metabolic alkalosis
    - Plasma renin activity will be low
  - **Localizing studies** – MRI, NP-59 scintigraphy (shows hyperfunctioning adrenal tissue; differentiates adenoma from hyperplasia; 90% accurate); adrenal venous sampling if others nondiagnostic
  - Pre-op need **control of HTN** and **K replacement**
  - **Adenoma Tx** – adrenalectomy
  - **Hyperplasia Tx** – seldom cured (↑ morbidity with bilateral resection)
    - Try **medical therapy** first for hyperplasia using <u>spironolactone</u> (inhibits aldosterone), <u>calcium channel blockers</u>, and <u>potassium</u>
    - If **bilateral resection** is performed (usually done for **refractory hypokalemia**), patient will need **fludrocortisone** postoperatively
- **Hypocortisolism** (adrenal insufficiency, Addison's disease)
  - #1 cause – **withdrawal of exogenous steroids**
  - #1 primary disease – **autoimmune disease**
  - Also caused by pituitary disease, adrenal infection/hemorrhage/metastasis/resection
  - Causes ↓ **cortisol** (ACTH will be high) and ↓ **aldosterone**
  - Dx: **cosyntropin test** (ACTH given, urine cortisol measured) – cortisol will remain low
  - **Acute adrenal insufficiency** – hypotension, fever, lethargy, abdominal pain, nausea and vomiting, ↓ glucose, ↑ K
    - Tx: **dexamethasone**, fluids, and give **cosyntropin test** (dexamethasone does **not** interfere with test)
  - **Chronic adrenal insufficiency** – hyperpigmentation, weakness, weight loss, GI symptoms, ↑ K, ↓ Na; Tx: **corticosteroids**
- **Hypercortisolism** (Cushing's syndrome)
  - Most commonly **iatrogenic**
  - 1st – measure **24-hour urine cortisol** (most sensitive test) and **ACTH**
    - If **ACTH is low** (and cortisol is high), patient has a cortisol secreting lesion (eg **adrenal adenoma**, **adrenal hyperplasia**)
    - If **ACTH is high** (and cortisol is high), patient has a pituitary adenoma or an ectopic source of ACTH (eg small cell lung CA) → go to 2nd below

- 2nd – if **ACTH is high**, give **high-dose dexamethasone suppression test**
  - If urine cortisol is suppressed → **pituitary adenoma**
  - If urine cortisol is not suppressed → **ectopic producer of ACTH** (eg small cell lung CA)
- NP-59 scintography can help localize tumors and differentiate adrenal adenomas from hyperplasia
- **Pituitary adenoma** (Cushing's disease)
  - **#1 non-iatrogenic cause of Cushing's syndrome** → 80% of cases
  - Cortisol should be suppressed with either low- or high-dose dexamethasone suppression test
  - Mostly **microadenomas**
  - Need petrosal sampling to figure out which side; MRI can also help
  - Tx: most tumors removed with transsphenoidal approach; unresectable or residual tumors treated with XRT
- **Ectopic ACTH**
  - **#2 non-iatrogenic** cause of Cushing's syndrome
  - Most commonly from **small cell lung CA**
  - Cortisol is <u>not</u> suppressed with either low- or high-dose dexamethasone suppression test
  - Chest and abdominal CT can help localize
  - Tx: resection of primary if possible; medical suppression for inoperable lesions
- **Adrenal adenoma**
  - **#3 non-iatrogenic** cause of Cushing's syndrome
  - ↓ ACTH, unregulated steroid production
  - Tx: adrenalectomy
- **Adrenal hyperplasia** (macro or micro)
  - Tx: **metyrapone** (blocks cortisol synthesis) and **aminoglutethimide**; (inhibits steroid production); bilateral adrenalectomy if medical Tx fails
- **Adrenocortical carcinoma** – rare cause of Cushing's syndrome (see below)
- **Bilateral adrenalectomy** – consider in patients with ectopic ACTH from tumor that is unresectable (would need to be a slow growing tumor – rare) or ACTH from pituitary adenoma that cannot be found
- Give **steroids postop** when operating for Cushing's syndrome

■ **Adrenocortical carcinoma**
- Bimodal distribution (before age 5 and in the 5th decade); more common in females
- **50% are functioning tumors** – cortisol, aldosterone, sex steroids
- Children display virilization 90% of the time (precocious puberty in boys, virilization in females); feminization in men; masculinization in women can occur
- Symptoms: abdominal pain, weight loss, weakness
- 80% have advanced disease at the time of diagnosis
- Tx: radical adrenalectomy; debulking helps symptoms, prolongs survival
  - **Mitotane** (adrenal-lytic) for residual, recurrent, or metastatic disease
- 20% 5-year survival rate

ADRENAL MEDULLA
■ From **ectoderm** neural crest cells
■ Catecholamine production: **tyrosine** → **dopa** → **dopamine** → **norepinephrine** → **epinephrine**
■ **Tyrosine hydroxylase** – rate-limiting step (tyrosine to dopa)
■ **PNMT** (phenylethanolamine *N*-methyltransferase) – enzyme converts norepinephrine → epinephrine
- Enzyme is found only in the **adrenal medulla** (exclusive producers of epinephrine)
■ Only **adrenal pheochromocytomas** will produce **epinephrine**

- ■ **MAO** (monoamine oxidase) – breaks down catecholamines; converts norepinephrine to normetanephrine, epinephrine to metanephrine; **VMA** (vanillylmandelic acid) produced from these
- ■ **Extra-adrenal rests of neural crest tissue** can exist, usually in the retroperitoneum, most notably in the organ of Zuckerkandl at the aortic bifurcation
- ■ **Pheochromocytoma** (chromaffin cells)
  - Rare; usually slow growing; arise from sympathetic ganglia or ectopic neural crest cells
  - **10% rule** – malignant, bilateral, in children, familial, extra-adrenal
  - Can be associated with MEN IIa, MEN IIb, von Recklinghausen's disease, tuberous sclerosis, Sturge–Weber disease
  - **Right-sided** predominance
  - **Extra-adrenal tumors** are more likely **malignant**
  - Symptoms: HTN (frequently **episodic**), headache, diaphoresis, palpitations
  - Dx: **urine metanephrines** and **VMA**
    - **VMA** most sensitive test for Dx
    - **MIBG scan** (norepinephrine analogue) – can help identify location if having trouble finding tumor with CT scan/MRI
    - **Clonidine suppression test** – tumor doses not respond, keeps catecholamines ↑
    - **No** venography → can cause hypertensive crisis
  - Preoperatively: **volume replacement** and **α-blocker first** (phenoxybenzamine → avoids hypertensive crisis); then β-blocker if patient has tachycardia or arrhythmias
    - Need to be careful with β-blocker and give after α-blocker → can precipitate **hypertensive crisis** (unopposed alpha stimulation, can lead to **stroke**) and **heart failure**
  - Tx: **adrenalectomy** – ligate adrenal veins first to avoid spilling catecholamines during tumor manipulation
    - Debulking helps symptoms in patients with unresectable disease
    - **Metyrosine** – inhibits tyrosine hydroxylase causing ↓ synthesis of catecholamines
    - Should have Nipride, Neo-Synephrine, and antiarrhythmic agents (eg amiodarone) ready during the time of surgery
  - **Postop conditions** – persistent hypertension, hypotension, hypoglycemia, bronchospasm, arrhythmias, intracerebral hemorrhage, CHF, MI
  - **Other sites of pheochromocytomas** – vertebral bodies, opposite adrenal gland, bladder, aortic bifurcation
  - Most common site of extramedullary tissue – **organ of Zuckerkandl** (inferior aorta near bifurcation)
  - **Falsely elevated VMA** – coffee, tea, fruits, vanilla, iodine contrast, labetalol, α- and β-blockers
  - **Extra-medullary tissue** – responsible for **medullary CA of thyroid** and **extra-adrenal pheochromocytoma**
- ■ **Ganglioneuroma** – rare, benign, asymptomatic tumor of neural crest origin in the adrenal medulla or sympathetic chain; Tx: resection

ANATOMY AND PHYSIOLOGY

- From the 1st and 2nd pharyngeal <u>arches</u> (not from pouches)
- **Thyrotropin-releasing factor** (TRF) – released from the hypothalamus; acts on the anterior pituitary gland and causes release of TSH
- **Thyroid-stimulating hormone** (TSH) – released from the anterior pituitary gland; acts on the thyroid gland to release T3 and T4 (through a mechanism that involves ↑ cAMP)
- TRF and TSH release are controlled by T3 and T4 through a negative feedback loop
- **Superior thyroid artery** – 1st branch off external carotid artery
- **Inferior thyroid artery** – off thyrocervical trunk; supplies <u>both</u> the **inferior** and **superior parathyroids**
  - Ligate close to thyroid to avoid injury to parathyroid glands with thyroidectomy
- **Ima artery** – occurs in 1%, arises from the innominate or aorta and goes to the isthmus
- **Superior** and **middle thyroid veins** – drain into internal jugular vein
- **Inferior thyroid vein** – drains into innominate vein
- **Superior laryngeal nerve**
  - Motor to cricothyroid muscle
  - Runs lateral to thyroid lobes
  - Tracks close to superior thyroid artery but is variable
    Injury results in **loss of projection** and **easy voice fatigability** (opera singers)
- **Recurrent laryngeal nerves** (RLNs)
  - Motor to all of larynx except cricothyroid muscle
    Run posterior to thyroid lobes in the tracheoesophageal groove
  - Can track with inferior thyroid artery but are variable
  - Left RLN loops around aorta; right RLN loops around innominate artery
  - Injury results in **hoarseness**; bilateral injury can **obstruct airway** → need emergency tracheostomy
  - **Non-recurrent laryngeal nerve** – in 2%; more common on the right
  - **Risk of injury** is higher for a non-recurrent laryngeal nerve during thyroid surgery

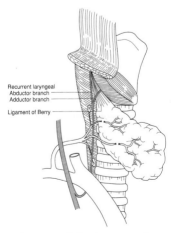

The ligament of Berry and distal recurrent laryngeal nerves.

- **Ligament of Berry** – posterior medial suspensory ligament close to RLNs; need careful dissection
- **Thyroglobulin** – stores T3 and T4 in colloid
  - Plasma T4:T3 ratio is 15:1; **T3** is the more active form (is tyrosine + iodine)
  - Most T3 is produced in periphery from T4 to T3 conversion by **deiodinases**
- **Peroxidases** link iodine and tyrosine together
- **Deiodinases** separate iodine from tyrosine
- **Thyroxine-binding globulin** – thyroid hormone transport; binds the majority of T3 and T4 in circulation
- **TSH** – most sensitive indicator of gland function
- **Tubercles of Zuckerkandl** – most lateral, posterior extension of thyroid tissue
  - Rotate medially to find RLNs
  - This portion is left behind with subtotal thyroidectomy because of proximity to RLNs
- **Parafollicular C cells** – produce **calcitonin**
- **Thyroxine treatment** – TSH levels should fall 50%; osteoporosis long-term side effect
- **Post-thyroidectomy stridor** – open neck and remove hematoma emergently → can result in airway compromise; can also be due to bilateral RLN injury → would need emergent tracheostomy

THYROID STORM
- Symptoms: ↑ HR, fever, numbness, irritability, vomiting, diarrhea, high-output cardiac failure (most common cause of death)
- Most common after surgery in patient with undiagnosed **Graves' disease**
- Can be precipitated by anxiety, excessive gland palpation, adrenergic stimulants
- Tx: **β-blockers** *(first line)*, PTU, Lugol's solution (KI), cooling blankets, oxygen, glucose
  - Emergent thyroidectomy rarely indicated
- **Wolff–Chaikoff effect** – very effective for thyroid storm; patient given high doses of iodine (Lugol's solution, potassium iodide), which inhibits TSH action on thyroid and inhibits organic coupling of iodide, resulting in less T3 and T4 release

ASYMPTOMATIC THYROID NODULE
- 90% of thyroid nodules are benign; female predominance
- Get **FNA** *(best initial test)* and **thyroid function tests**
  - **Determinant in 80%** → follow appropriate treatment
    - Shows **follicular cells** → lobectomy (10% CA risk; see Thyroid CA section)
    - Shows **thyroid CA** → thyroidectomy or lobectomy and appropriate treatment (see Thyroid CA section)
    - Shows **cyst fluid** → drain fluid
      - If it recurs or is bloody → lobectomy
    - Shows **colloid tissue** → most likely colloid goiter; low chance of malignancy (< 1%)
      - Tx: **thyroxine**; lobectomy if it enlarges
    - Shows **normal thyroid tissue** and **TFTs are elevated** → likely solitary toxic nodule
      - Tx: if asymptomatic can just monitor; **PTU** and ^{131}I if symptomatic
  - **Indeterminant in 20%** → get radionuclide study
    - **Hot nodule** → Tx: if asymptomatic can monitor; **PTU** and ^{131}I if symptomatic
    - **Cold nodule** → lobectomy (more likely malignant than hot nodule)
- **Goiter**
  - Any abnormal enlargement
  - Most identifiable cause is iodine deficiency; Tx: iodine replacement
  - Diffuse enlargement without evidence of functional abnormality = nontoxic colloid goiter
    - Unusual to have to operate unless goiter is causing **airway compression** or there is a **suspicious nodule**

- Tx: **subtotal** or **total thyroidectomy** for symptoms or if suspicious nodule; subtotal has decreased risk of RLN injury
- **Substernal goiter**
  - Usually secondary (vessels originate from superior and inferior thyroid arteries)
  - Primary substernal goiter – rare (vessels originate from innominate artery)
- **Mediastinal thyroid tissue** – most likely from acquired disease with inferior extensions of a normally placed gland (eg substernal goiter)

ABNORMALITIES OF THYROID DESCENT
- **Pyramidal lobe** – occurs in 10%, extends from the isthmus toward the thymus
- **Lingual thyroid**
  - Thyroid tissue that persists in foramen cecum at base of the tongue
  - Symptoms: dysphagia, dyspnea, dysphonia
  - 2% malignancy risk
  - Tx: thyroxine suppression; abolish with ^{131}I
    - Resection if worried about CA or if it does not shrink after medical therapy
  - Is the only thyroid tissue in 70% of patients who have it
- **Thyroglossal duct cyst**
  - Classically moves upward with swallowing
  - Susceptible to **infection** and may be **premalignant**
  - Tx: resection → need to take midportion or all of **hyoid bone** along with the **thyroglossal duct cyst** (Sistrunk procedure)

HYPERTHYROIDISM TREATMENT
- **Propylthiouracil** (PTU) and **methimazole** – good for young patients, small goiters, mild T3 and T4 elevation
- **PTU** (thioamides) – safe with pregnancy
  - **Inhibits peroxidases** and prevents iodine–tyrosine coupling
  - Side effects: **aplastic anemia, agranulocytosis** (rare)
- **Methimazole**
  - **Inhibits peroxidases** and prevents iodine–tyrosine coupling
  - Side effects: **cretinism** in newborns (crosses placenta), **aplastic anemia, agranulocytosis** (rare)
- **Radioactive iodine** (^{131}I)
  - Good for patients who are poor surgical risks or unresponsive to PTU
  - ^{131}I should <u>not</u> be used in <u>children</u> or during <u>pregnancy</u> → can traverse placenta
- **Thyroidectomy**
  - Good for cold nodules, toxic adenomas or multinodular goiters not responsive to medical therapy, pregnant patients not controlled with PTU, compressive symptoms
  - Best time to operate during pregnancy is **2nd trimester** (↓ risk of teratogenic events and premature labor)
  - Subtotal thyroidectomy can leave patient euthyroid

CAUSES OF HYPERTHYROIDISM
- **Graves' disease** (toxic diffuse goiter)
  - Women; exophthalmos, pretibial edema, atrial fibrillation, heat intolerance, thirst, ↑ appetite, weight loss, sweating, palpitations
  - Most common cause of hyperthyroidism (80%)
  - Caused by **IgG antibodies** to **TSH receptor** (long-acting thyroid stimulator [LATS], thyroid-stimulating immunoglobulin [TSI])
  - Dx: decreased TSH, increased T3 and T4; LATS level; ↑ ^{123}I uptake (thyroid scan) diffusely in thyrotoxic patient with goiter

- Medical therapy usually manages hyperthyroidism
- Tx: **thioamides** (50% recurrence), ^{131}I (5% recurrence), or **thyroidectomy** if medical therapy fails
- **Unusual to have to operate** on these patients (suspicious nodule most common reason)
  - **Preop preparation**: <u>PTU</u> until euthyroid, β-<u>blocker</u>, <u>Lugol's solution</u> for 14 days to decrease friability and vascularity (start only after euthyroid)
  - **Operation**: bilateral subtotal (5% recurrence) or total thyroidectomy (need lifetime thyroxine replacement)
  - **Indications for surgery**: noncompliant patient, recurrence after medical therapy, children, pregnant women not controlled with PTU, or concomitant suspicious thyroid nodule
- **Toxic multinodular goiter**
  - Women; age > 50 years, usually nontoxic 1st
  - Symptoms: tachycardia, weight loss, insomnia, airway compromise; symptoms can be precipitated by contrast dyes
  - Caused by hyperplasia secondary to chronic low-grade TSH stimulation
  - Tx: Most consider *surgery (subtotal or total thyroidectomy) the* **preferred initial Tx** for toxic multinodular goiter, but a **trial of** ^{131}I should be considered, especially in the elderly and frail
    - If compression or a suspicious nodule is present, need to go with surgery
- **Single toxic nodule**
  - Women; younger; usually > 3 cm to be symptomatic; function autonomously
  - Dx: **thyroid scan** (hot nodule) –20% of hot nodules eventually cause symptoms
  - Tx: **thioamides** and ^{131}I (95% effective); lobectomy if medical Tx ineffective
- **Rare causes of hyperthyroidism** – trophoblastic tumors, TSH-secreting pituitary tumors

CAUSES OF THYROIDITIS
- **Hashimoto's disease**
  - Most common cause of **hypothyroidism** in adults
  - Enlarged gland, painless, chronic thyroiditis
  - Women; history of childhood XRT
  - Can cause thyrotoxicosis in the acute early stage
  - Caused by both **humeral** and **cell-mediated autoimmune disease** (microsomal and thyroglobulin antibodies)
  - Goiter secondary to **lack of organification of trapped iodide inside gland**
  - Pathology shows a **lymphocytic infiltrate**
  - Tx: **thyroxine** *(first line)*; **partial thyroidectomy** if continues to grow despite thyroxine, if nodules appear, or if compression symptoms occur
  - Frequently, no surgery is necessary for Hashimoto's disease
- **Bacterial thyroiditis** (rare)
  - Usually secondary to **contiguous spread**
  - **Bacterial upper respiratory tract infection** (URI) usual precursor (staph/strep)
  - Normal thyroid function tests, fever, dysphagia, tenderness
  - Tx: **antibiotics**
    - May need **lobectomy** to rule out cancer in patients with unilateral swelling and tenderness
    - May need total thyroidectomy for persistent inflammation
- **De Quervain's thyroiditis**
  - Can be associated with hyperthyroidism initially
  - **Viral URI** precursor; tender thyroid, sore throat, mass, weakness, fatigue; women
  - Elevated **ESR**

- Tx: **steroids** and **ASA**
  - May need **lobectomy** to rule out cancer in patients with unilateral swelling and tenderness
  - May need total thyroidectomy for persistent inflammation
- **Riedel's fibrous struma** (rare)
  - <u>Woody, fibrous component</u> that can involve adjacent strap muscles and carotid sheath
  - Can resemble thyroid CA or lymphoma (need biopsy)
  - Disease frequently results in hypothyroidism and compression symptoms
  - Associated with sclerosing cholangitis, fibrotic diseases, methysergide Tx, and retroperitoneal fibrosis
  - Tx: **steroids** and **thyroxine**
    - May need **isthmectomy** or **tracheostomy** for airway symptoms
    - If resection needed, watch for RLNs

THYROID CANCER

- Most common endocrine malignancy in the United States
- **Follicular cells on FNA** – 5%–10% chance of malignancy (unable to differentiate between follicular cell adenoma, follicular cell hyperplasia, and follicular cell CA on FNA)
- **Worrisome for malignancy** – solid, solitary, cold, slow growing, hard; male, age > 50, previous neck XRT, MEN IIa or IIb
- **Sudden growth** – could be hemorrhage into previously undetected nodule or malignancy
- Patients can also present with **voice changes** or **dysphagia**
- **Follicular adenomas** – colloid, embryonal, fetal → no increase in cancer risk
  - Still need lobectomy to prove it is an adenoma
- **Papillary thyroid carcinoma**
  - Most common (85%) thyroid CA
  - Least aggressive, slow growing, has the best prognosis; women, children
  - Risk factors: childhood XRT (very ↑ risk) → most common tumor following neck XRT
  - Older age (> 40-50 years) predicts a worse prognosis
  - **Lymphatic spread 1st** but is not prognostic → prognosis based on **local invasion**
  - <u>Rare</u> metastases (**lung**)
  - **Children** are more likely to be **node positive** (80%) than are adults (20%)
  - Large, firm nodules in children are worrisome
  - Many are **multicentric**
  - Pathology – **psammoma bodies** (calcium) and **Orphan Annie nuclei**
  - Tx: minimal/incidental (< 1 cm) → **lobectomy**
    - **Total thyroidectomy** for bilateral lesions, multicentricity, history of XRT, positive margins, or tumors > 1 cm
    - **Clinically positive cervical nodes** – need ipsilateral MRND
    - **Extrathyroidal tissue involvement** – need ipsilateral MRND
    - **Metastatic disease, residual local disease, positive lymph nodes**, or **capsular invasion** → ^{131}I (4–6 weeks after surgery)
    - **XRT** only for unresectable disease not responsive to ^{131}I
  - 95% 5-year survival rate; death secondary to local disease
  - **Enlarged lateral neck lymph node** that shows normal-appearing thyroid tissue is **papillary thyroid CA with lymphatic spread** (lateral aberrant thyroid tissue)
    - Tx: total thyroidectomy and MRND; ^{131}I (4–6 weeks after surgery)
- **Follicular thyroid carcinoma**
  - **Hematogenous spread** (**bone** most common) → 50% have metastatic disease at the time of presentation

- More aggressive than thyroid papillary cell CA; older adults (50–60s), women
- If FNA shows just **follicular cells** – have 10% chance of malignancy, need lobectomy
- Tx: **lobectomy** → if pathology shows **adenoma** or **follicular cell hyperplasia**, nothing else needed
  - If **follicular CA** → total thyroidectomy for **lesions > 1 cm** or **extrathyroidal disease**
  - **Clinically positive cervical nodes** – need ipsilateral MRND
  - **Extrathyroidal tissue involvement** – need ipsilateral MRND
  - Patients with **lesions > 1 cm** or **extrathyroidal disease** – ^{131}I (4–6 weeks after surgery)
  - 70% 5-year survival rate; prognosis based on stage
- ■ **Medullary thyroid carcinoma**
  - Can be associated with MEN IIa or IIb
  - Usually the **1st manifestation** of MEN IIa and IIb (**diarrhea**)
  - Tumor arises from **parafollicular C cells** (which secrete calcitonin)
  - **C-cell hyperplasia** considered premalignant
  - **Pathology** – shows **amyloid** deposition
  - **Calcitonin** – can cause **flushing** and **diarrhea**
  - Need to screen for **hyperparathyroidism** and **pheochromocytoma**
  - **Lymphatic spread** – most have involved nodes at time of diagnosis
  - **Early metastases** to lung, liver, and bone
  - Tx: **total thyroidectomy** with **central neck node dissection**
    - **MRND** if patient has clinically positive nodes (bilateral MRND if both lobes have tumor) or if extrathyroidal disease present
    - Prophylactic thyroidectomy and central node dissection in MEN **IIa** (at age **6 years**) or **IIb** (at age **2 years**)
    - Liver and bone metastases prevent attempt at cure
    - XRT may be useful for unresectable local and distant metastatic disease
  - May be useful to **monitor calcitonin levels** for disease recurrence
  - More aggressive than follicular and papillary CA
  - 50% 5-year survival rate; prognosis based on presence of regional and distant metastases
- ■ **Hürthle cell carcinoma**
  - Most are **benign** (Hürthle cell adenoma); presents in older patients
  - Metastases go to bone and lung if malignant
  - Tx: total thyroidectomy; MRND for clinically positive nodes
- ■ **Anaplastic thyroid cancer**
  - Elderly patients with long-standing goiters
  - **Most aggressive thyroid CA**
  - Rapidly lethal (0% 5-year survival rate); usually beyond surgical management at diagnosis
  - Tx: total thyroidectomy for the rare lesion that can be resected
  - Can perform palliative thyroidectomy for compressive symptoms or give palliative chemo-XRT
- ■ **XRT effective** for papillary, follicular, medullary, and Hürthle cell thyroid CA
- ■ ^{131}**I effective** for papillary and follicular thyroid CA _only_
  - Can cure bone and lung metastases
  - Given 4–6 weeks after surgery when TSH levels are highest
  - Do not give thyroid replacement until _after_ treatment with ^{131}I → would suppress TSH and uptake of ^{131}I
  - **Indications** (used only for papillary and follicular thyroid CA)
    - **Recurrent CA**
    - **Primary inoperable tumors** due to **local invasion**
    - **Tumors that are** > 1 cm or have **extrathyroidal disease** (extra-capsular invasion, nodal spread, or metastases)

- Patients with papillary or follicular cell CA and metastases → need to perform total thyroidectomy to facilitate uptake of ^{131}I to the metastatic lesions (otherwise all gets absorbed by the thyroid gland)
- ^{131}**I Side effects** (rare): sialoadenitis, GI symptoms, infertility, bone marrow suppression, parathyroid dysfunction, leukemia

■ **Thyroxine** – can help suppress TSH and slow metastatic disease; administered only after ^{131}I therapy has finished

ANATOMY AND PHYSIOLOGY

- **Superior parathyroids – 4th** pharyngeal <u>pouch</u>; associated with thyroid complex
  - Found lateral to recurrent laryngeal nerves (RLNs), posterior surface of superior portion of gland, above inferior thyroid artery
- **Inferior parathyroids – 3rd** pharyngeal <u>pouch</u>; associated with thymus
  - Found medial to RLNs, more anterior, below inferior thyroid artery
  - Inferior parathyroids have more **variable location** and are more likely to be **ectopic**
  - Occasionally are found in the **tail of the thymus** (most common ectopic site) and can migrate to the anterior mediastinum
  - Other ectopic sites – intra-thyroid, mediastinal, near tracheoesophageal groove
- 90% have all 4 glands
- **Inferior thyroid artery** – blood supply to <u>both</u> **superior** and **inferior parathyroid glands**

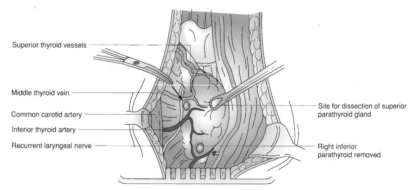

Superior thyroid vessels

Middle thyroid vein

Common carotid artery

Inferior thyroid artery

Recurrent laryngeal nerve

Site for dissection of superior parathyroid gland

Right inferior parathyroid removed

Lateral view of the right side of the neck after rotation of the thyroid lobe. The important anatomic landmarks are emphasized.

- **PTH** – *increases* <u>serum Ca</u>
  - $\uparrow$ kidney Ca reabsorption in the distal convoluted tubule, $\downarrow$ kidney PO_4 absorption
  - $\uparrow$ osteoclasts in bone to release Ca (and PO_4^-)
  - $\uparrow$ vitamin D production in kidney ($\uparrow$ 1-OH hydroxylation) $\rightarrow$ $\uparrow$ Ca-binding protein in intestine $\rightarrow$ $\uparrow$ intestinal Ca reabsorption
- **Vitamin D** – $\uparrow$ intestinal Ca and PO_4 absorption by increasing **calcium-binding protein**
- **Calcitonin** – *decreases* <u>serum Ca</u>
  - $\downarrow$ bone Ca resorption (osteoclast inhibition)
  - $\uparrow$ urinary Ca and PO_4 excretion
- **Normal Ca level**: 8.5–10.5 (ionized 4.4–5.5)
- **Normal PTH level**: 5–40 pg/mL
- **Normal PO_4 level**: 2.5–5.0
- **Normal Cl^- level**: 98–107
- Most common cause of hypoparathyroidism is **previous thyroid surgery**

PRIMARY HYPERPARATHYROIDISM

- Women, older age
- Due to autonomously high PTH
- Dx: ↑ Ca, ↓ PO_4^-; Cl^- to PO_4^- ratio > 33; ↑ renal cAMP; HCO_3^- secreted in urine
- Can get **hyperchloremic metabolic acidosis**
- **Osteitis fibrosa cystica** (brown tumors) – bone lesions from Ca resorption; characteristic of hyperparathyroidism
- Most patients **have no symptoms** – ↑ Ca found on routine lab work for some other problem or on checkup
- Symptoms: muscle weakness, myalgia, nephrolithiasis, pancreatitis, PUD, depression, bone pain, pathologic fractures, mental status changes, constipation, anorexia
- Hypertension can result from renal impairment

Diagnostic Workup for Primary Hyperparathyroidism

Take careful history, including records or medications, symptoms, prior head and neck radiotherapy, and other endocrinopathies in the patient and the patient's family.
Establish elevated calcium through 2 or 3 determinations.
Order a chest radiograph and search for bony metastases, sarcoidosis, and pulmonary tumors.
Order an excretory urogram and search for nephrolithiasis and, rarely, renal tumors.
Order a serum protein electrophoresis to rule out multiple myeloma.
Order a 24-hour urinary calcium determination (ie benign familial hypocalciuric hypercalcemia).
Rule out multiple endocrine neoplasia (usually multiple endocrine neoplasia type I).
Check the absolute or relative elevation of the parathyroid hormone level.

From Smith SL, Van Heerden JA. Conventional parathyroidectomy for primary hyperparathyroidism. In: Fischer JE, Bland KI, et al, eds. *Mastery of Surgery*. 5th ed. Philadelphia, PA: Lippincott Williams & Wilkins; 2007, with permission.

- **Indications for surgery**:
  - Symptomatic disease
  - Asymptomatic disease with Ca > 13, ↓ Cr clearance, kidney stones, substantially ↓ bone mass
- **Single adenoma** – occurs in 80% of patients
- **Multiple adenomas** – occur in 4% of patients
- **Diffuse hyperplasia** – occurs in 15%; patients with MEN I or IIa have 4-gland hyperplasia
- **Parathyroid adenocarcinoma** – very rare; can get very high Ca levels
- **Treatment**
  - **Adenoma** – resection; inspect other glands to rule out hyperplasia or multiple adenomas
  - **Parathyroid hyperplasia**
    - Do not biopsy all glands → risks hemorrhage and hypoparathyroidism
    - Tx: resect 3½ glands or total parathyroidectomy and autoimplantation
  - **Parathyroid CA** → need radical parathyroidectomy (need to take **ipsilateral thyroid lobe**)
  - **Pregnancy** – surgery in 2nd trimester; ↑ risk of stillbirth if not resected
- **Intraop frozen section** → can confirm that the tissue taken was indeed parathyroid
- **Intraop PTH levels** → can help determine if the causative gland is removed (PTH should go to $< ½$ of the preop value in 10 minutes)
- **Missing gland** – check inferiorly in thymus tissue (most common ectopic location, can remove tail of the thymus and see if PTH drops), near carotids, vertebral body, superior to pharynx, thyroid
- **Still cannot find gland** – close and follow PTH; if PTH still ↑, get **sestamibi scan** to localize

- **At reoperation for a missing gland**, the most common location for the gland is **normal anatomic position**
- **Hypocalcemia postop** – from bone hunger or failure of parathyroid remnant/graft
  - **Bone hunger** – normal PTH, decreased HCO_3^-
  - **Aparathyroidism** – decreased PTH, normal HCO_3^-
- **Persistent hyperparathyroidism** (1%) – most commonly due to missed adenoma remaining in the neck
- **Recurrent hyperparathyroidism** – occurs after a period of hypocalcemia or normocalcemia
  - Can be due to new adenoma formation
  - Can be due to tumor implants at the original operation that have now grown
  - Need to consider recurrent parathyroid CA
- **Reoperation** associated with ↑ risk of RLN injury, permanent hypoparathyroidism
- **Sestamibi scan**
  - Will have preferential uptake by the overactive parathyroid gland
  - Good for picking up adenomas but not 4-gland hyperplasia
  - Best for trying to pick up ectopic glands

SECONDARY HYPERPARATHYROIDISM
- Seen in patients with **renal failure**
- ↑ **PTH** in response to **low Ca**
- Most do <u>not</u> need surgery (95%)
- Ectopic calcification and osteoporosis can occur
- Tx: **Ca supplement**, vitamin D, control diet PO_4, PO_4-binding gel, ↓ aluminum
  - Surgery for **bone pain** (most common indication), fractures, or pruritus (80% get relief)
  - Surgery involves total parathyroidectomy with autotransplantation or subtotal parathyroidectomy

TERTIARY HYPERPARATHYROIDISM
- Renal disease now corrected with transplant but still overproduces PTH
- Has similar lab values as primary hyperparathyroidism (hyperplasia)
- Tx: subtotal (3½ glands) or total parathyroidectomy with autoimplantation

FAMILIAL HYPERCALCEMIC HYPOCALCIURIA
- Patients have ↑ serum Ca and ↓ urine Ca (should be ↑ if hyperparathyroidism)
- Caused by defect in PTH receptor in distal convoluted tubule of the kidney that causes ↑ resorption of Ca
- Dx: Ca 9–11, have normal PTH (30–60), ↓ urine Ca
- Tx: nothing (Ca generally not that high in these patients); **no parathyroidectomy**

PSEUDOHYPOPARATHYROIDISM
- Because of defect in PTH receptor in the kidney, does not respond to PTH

PARATHYROID CANCER
- Rare cause of hypercalcemia
- ↑ Ca, PTH, and alkaline phosphatase (can have extremely high Ca levels)
- **Lung** most common location for metastases
- Tx: wide en bloc excision (parathyroidectomy and ipsilateral thyroidectomy)
- 50% 5-year survival rate
- Mortality is due to **hypercalcemia**
- Recurrence in 50%

MULTIPLE ENDOCRINE NEOPLASIA SYNDROMES

- ■ Derived from APUD cells
- ■ Neoplasms can develop synchronously or metachronously
- ■ Autosomal dominant, 100% penetrance
- ■ **MEN I**
  - • **Parathyroid hyperplasia**
    - ◦ Usually the 1st part to become symptomatic; urinary symptoms
    - ◦ Tx: 4-gland resection with autotransplantation
  - • **Pancreatic islet cell tumors**
    - ◦ Gastrinoma #1 – 50% multiple, 50% malignant; major morbidity of syndrome
  - • **Pituitary adenoma**
    - ◦ Prolactinoma #1
  - • Need to correct hyperparathyroidism 1st if simultaneous tumors
- ■ **MEN IIa**
  - • **Parathyroid hyperplasia**
  - • **Medullary CA of thyroid**
    - ◦ Nearly all patients; diarrhea most common symptom; often bilateral
    - ◦ #1 cause of death in these patients
    - ◦ Usually 1st part to be symptomatic
  - • **Pheochromocytoma**
    - ◦ Often bilateral, nearly always benign
  - • Need to correct pheochromocytoma 1st if simultaneous tumors
- ■ **MEN IIb**
  - • **Medullary CA of thyroid**
    - ◦ Nearly all patients; diarrhea most common symptoms; often bilateral
    - ◦ #1 cause of death in these patients
    - ◦ Usually 1st part to be symptomatic
  - • **Pheochromocytoma**
    - ◦ Often bilateral, nearly always benign
  - • **Mucosal neuromas**
  - • **Marfan's habitus, musculoskeletal abnormalities**
  - • Need to correct pheochromocytoma 1st if simultaneous tumors
- ■ **MEN I** – MENIN gene
- ■ **MEN IIa and IIb** – RET proto-oncogene

Disease Phenotypes Related to Mutation of the RET Proto-Oncogene			
Phenotype	**Genetic Defect**	**Clinical Features**	**Prevalence (%)**
MEN 2A (60%)	Germline mutations in cysteine codons of extracellular and transmembrane domains of RET	Medullary thyroid carcinoma Pheochromocytoma Hyperparathyroidism	100 10–60 5–20
MEN 2B (5%)	Germline activating mutation in tyrosine kinase domain or RET	Medullary thyroid carcinoma Pheochromocytoma Marfanoid habitus Mucosal neuromas (gut) and ganglioneuromatosis	100 50 100 100
FMTC (35%)	Germline mutations in cysteine codons of extra-cellular or transmembrane domains of RET	Medullary thyroid carcinoma	100

FMTC, familial medullary thyroid carcinoma; MEN, multiple endocrine neoplasia.

HYPERCALCEMIA
- Causes:
  - Malignancy
    - Hematologic (25%) – lytic bone lesions
    - Nonhematologic (75%) – cancers that release PTHrP (small cell lung CA, breast CA)
  - Hyperparathyroidism
  - Hyperthyroidism
  - Familial hypercalcemic hypocalciuria
  - Immobilization
  - Granulomatous disease (sarcoidosis or tuberculosis)
  - Excess vitamin D
  - Milk–alkali syndrome (excessive intake of milk and calcium supplements)
  - Thiazide diuretics
- **Mithramycin** – inhibits osteoclasts (used with malignancies or failure of conventional treatment); has hematologic, liver, and renal side effects
- **Hypercalcemic crisis** – usually secondary to another surgery in patients with pre-existing hyperparathyroidism; Tx: **fluids** (normal saline) and **furosemide** (Lasix)
- **Breast CA metastases to bone** – release **PTHrP** (rP = related peptide); can cause **hypercalcemia**
  - Small cell lung CA and other nonhematologic cancers can do this as well → this is <u>not</u> due to bone destruction
  - Associated with ↑ urinary cAMP (from action of **PTHrP on kidney**)
- **Hematologic malignancies** – these can cause bone destruction with ↑ Ca (urinary cAMP will be low)

ANATOMY AND PHYSIOLOGY
- ■ **Breast development**
  - Breast formed from ectoderm milk streak
  - **Estrogen** – duct development (double layer of columnar cells)
  - **Progesterone** – lobular development
  - **Prolactin** – synergizes estrogen and progesterone
- ■ **Cyclic changes**
  - **Estrogen** – ↑ breast swelling, growth of glandular tissue
  - **Progesterone** – ↑ maturation of glandular tissue; withdrawal causes menses
  - **FSH, LH surge** – cause ovum release
  - After menopause, lack of estrogen and progesterone results in atrophy of breast tissue
- ■ **Nerves**
  - **Long thoracic nerve** – innervates **serratus anterior**; injury results in winged scapula
    - **Lateral thoracic artery** supplies serratus anterior
  - **Thoracodorsal nerve** – innervates **latissimus dorsi**; injury results in weak arm pull-ups and adduction
    - **Thoracodorsal artery** supplies latissimus dorsi
  - **Medial pectoral nerve** – innervates pectoralis major and pectoralis minor
  - **Lateral pectoral nerve** – pectoralis major only
  - **Intercostobrachial nerve** – lateral cutaneous branch of the 2nd intercostal nerve; provides sensation to medial arm and axilla; encountered just below axillary vein when performing axillary dissection
    - Can transect without serious consequences
- ■ Branches of **internal thoracic artery**, **intercostal arteries**, **thoracoacromial artery**, and **lateral thoracic artery** supply breast

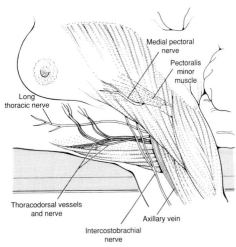

Major neurovascular structures to be preserved in an axillary dissection.

■ **Batson's plexus** – valveless vein plexus that allows direct hematogenous metastasis of breast CA to spine
■ **Lymphatic drainage**
  • 97% is to the axillary nodes
  • 2% is to the internal mammary nodes
  • Any quadrant can drain to the internal mammary nodes
  • Supraclavicular nodes – considered **N3 disease**
  • Primary axillary adenopathy – **#1 is lymphoma**
■ **Cooper's ligaments** – suspensory ligaments; divide breast into segments
  • Breast CA involving these strands can dimple the skin

BENIGN BREAST DISEASE
■ **Abscesses** – usually associated with breastfeeding. *Staphylococcus aureus* most common, strep
  • Tx: percutaneous or incision and drainage; discontinue breastfeeding; breast pump, antibiotics
■ **Infectious mastitis** – most commonly associated with breastfeeding
  • *S. aureus* most common in nonlactating women can be due to chronic inflammatory diseases (eg actinomyces) or autoimmune disease (eg SLE) → may need to rule out **necrotic cancer** (need incisional biopsy including the skin)
■ **Periductal mastitis** (mammary duct ectasia or **plasma cell mastitis**)
  • Symptoms: **noncyclical mastodynia**, **erythema**, nipple retraction, creamy discharge from nipple; can have sterile or infected <u>subareolar abscess</u>
  • Risk factors – smoking, nipple piercings
  • Biopsy – dilated mammary ducts, inspissated secretions, marked periductal inflammation
  • Tx: if typical creamy discharge is present that is not bloody and not associated with nipple retraction, give **antibiotics and reassure**; if not or if it recurs, need to rule out inflammatory CA (incisional biopsy including the skin)
■ **Galactocele** – breast cysts filled with milk; occurs with breastfeeding
  • Tx: ranges from aspiration to incision and drainage
■ **Galactorrhea** – can be caused by ↑ prolactin (pituitary prolactinoma), OCPs, TCAs, phenothiazines, metoclopramide, alpha-methyl dopa, reserpine
  • Is often associated with amenorrhea
■ **Gynecomastia** – 2-cm pinch; can be associated with cimetidine, spironolactone, marijuana; idiopathic in most
  • Tx: will likely regress; may need to resect if cosmetically deforming or causing social problems
■ **Neonatal breast enlargement** – due to circulating maternal estrogens; will regress
■ **Accessory breast tissue** (polythelia) – can present in axilla (most common location)
■ **Accessory nipples** – can be found from axilla to groin (most common breast anomaly)
■ **Breast asymmetry** – common
■ **Breast reduction** – ability to lactate frequently compromised
■ **Poland's syndrome** – hypoplasia of chest wall, amastia, hypoplastic shoulder, no pectoralis muscle
■ **Mastodynia** – pain in breast; rarely represents breast CA
  • Dx: history and breast exam; bilateral mammogram
  • Tx: danazol, OCPs, NSAIDs, evening primrose oil, bromocriptine
  • Discontinue caffeine, nicotine, methylxanthines
  • **Cyclic mastodynia** – pain before menstrual period; most commonly from fibrocystic disease
  • **Continuous mastodynia** – continuous pain, most commonly represents acute or subacute infection; continuous mastodynia is **more refractory** to treatment than cyclic mastodynia

- **Mondor's disease** – superficial vein thrombophlebitis of breast; feels cordlike, can be painful
  - Associated with trauma and strenuous exercise
  - Usually occurs in lower outer quadrant
  - Tx: NSAIDs
- **Fibrocystic disease**
  - Lots of types: papillomatosis, sclerosing adenosis, apocrine metaplasia, duct adenosis, epithelial hyperplasia, ductal hyperplasia, and lobular hyperplasia
  - **Symptoms:** breast pain, nipple discharge (usually yellow to brown), lumpy breast tissue that varies with hormonal cycle
  - Only **cancer risk** is <u>atypical</u> **ductal** or **lobular hyperplasia** – *need to resect these lesions*
    - Do not need to get negative margins with atypical hyperplasia; just remove all suspicious areas (ie calcifications) that appear on mammogram
- **Intraductal papilloma**
  - Most common cause of **bloody nipple discharge**
  - Are usually small, nonpalpable, and close to the nipple
  - These lesions are <u>not</u> premalignant → get **contrast ductogram** to find papilloma, then needle localization
  - Tx: subareolar resection of the involved duct and papilloma

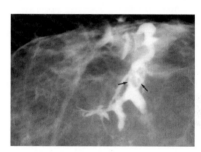

Ductogram. A large defect *(arrow)* represents an intraductal papilloma.

- **Fibroadenoma**
  - Most common breast lesion in adolescents and young women; 10% multiple
  - Usually painless, slow growing, well circumscribed, firm, and rubbery
  - Often grows to several cm in size and then stops
  - Can change in size with menstrual cycle and can enlarge in pregnancy
  - Giant fibromas can be > 5 cm (treatment is the same)
  - Prominent **fibrous tissue compressing epithelial cells** on pathology
  - Can have large, coarse calcifications (popcorn lesions) on mammography from degeneration
  - **In patients < 40 years old:**
    1) Mass needs to feel clinically benign (firm, rubbery, rolls, not fixed)
    2) Ultrasound or mammogram needs to be consistent with fibroadenoma
    3) Need FNA or core needle biopsy to show fibroadenoma
    - **Need all 3** of the above to be able to observe, otherwise need excisional biopsy
    - If the fibroadenoma continues to **enlarge**, need **excisional biopsy**
    - Avoid resection of breast tissue in teenagers and younger children → can affect breast development
  - **In patients > 40 years old** → excisional biopsy to ensure diagnosis

NIPPLE DISCHARGE
■ Most nipple discharge is **benign**
■ All need a history, breast exam, and bilateral mammogram
■ Try to find the trigger point or mass on exam
■ **Green discharge** – usually due to fibrocystic disease
   • Tx: if cyclical and nonspontaneous, **reassure patient**
■ **Bloody discharge** – most commonly intraductal papilloma; occasionally ductal CA
   • Tx: need **ductogram** and excision of that ductal area
■ **Serous discharge** – worrisome for cancer, especially if coming from only 1 duct or spontaneous
   • Tx: excisional biopsy of that ductal area
■ **Spontaneous discharge** – no matter what the color or consistency is, this is worrisome for CA → all these patients need excisional biopsy of duct area causing the discharge
■ **Nonspontaneous discharge** (occurs only with pressure, tight garments, exercise, etc.) – not as worrisome but may still need excisional biopsy (eg if bloody)
■ May have to do a complete subareolar resection if the area above cannot be properly identified (no trigger point or mass felt)

DUCTAL CARCINOMA IN SITU (DCIS)
■ **Malignant cells of the ductal epithelium *without* invasion of basement membrane**
■ 50% get cancer if not resected (ipsilateral breast)
■ 5% get cancer in contralateral breast
■ Considered a **premalignant lesion**
■ Usually not palpable and presents as a cluster of calcifications on mammography
■ Can have solid, cribriform, papillary, and comedo patterns
   • **Comedo pattern** – most aggressive subtype; has necrotic areas
      ◦ High risk for multicentricity, microinvasion, and recurrence
      ◦ Tx: simple mastectomy
■ ↑ recurrence risk with **comedo type** and **lesions > 2.5 cm**
■ Tx: **Lumpectomy** and **XRT**; need **1 cm margins**; *No ALND or SLNB*; possibly **tamoxifen**
   • **Simple mastectomy** if high grade (eg comedo type, multicentric, multifocal), if a large tumor not amenable to lumpectomy, or if not able to get good margins; *No ALND*

LOBULAR CARCINOMA IN SITU (LCIS)
■ 40% get cancer (either breast)
■ Considered a marker for the development of breast CA, **not premalignant itself**
■ Has no calcifications; is not palpable
■ Primarily found in premenopausal women
■ Patients who develop breast CA are more likely to develop a **ductal CA** (70%)
■ Usually an incidental finding; multifocal disease is common
■ 5% risk of having a synchronous breast CA at the time of diagnosis of LCIS (most likely ductal CA)
■ **Do not** need negative margins
■ Tx: nothing, tamoxifen, or bilateral subcutaneous mastectomy (no ALND)

Indications for Surgical Biopsy After Core Biopsy
Atypical ductal hyperplasia
Atypical lobular hyperplasia
Radial scar
Lobular carcinoma in situ
Columnar cell hyperplasia with atypia
Papillary lesions
Lack of concordance between appearance of mammographic lesion and histologic diagnosis
Nondiagnostic specimen (including absence of calcifications on specimen radiograph when biopsy is performed for calcifications)

BREAST CANCER
■ Breast CA decreased in economically poor areas
■ Japan has lowest rate of breast CA worldwide
■ U.S. breast CA risk – **1 in 8 women (12%)**; 5% in women with no risk factors
■ **Screening** decreases mortality by 25%
■ Untreated breast cancer – median survival 2–3 years
■ 10% of breast CAs have negative mammogram and negative ultrasound
■ **Clinical features of breast CA** – distortion of normal architecture; skin/nipple distortion or retraction; hard, tethered, indistinct borders
■ **Symptomatic breast mass workup**
  • **< 40 years old** – need **U/S** and **core needle Bx** (CNBx; consider FNA)
    • Need mammogram in patients < 40 if clinical exam or U/S is indeterminate or suspicious for CA although in general want to avoid excess radiation in this group
  • **> 40 years old** – need **bilateral mammograms, U/S,** and **CNBx**
  • If **CNBx or FNA** is <u>indeterminate</u>, <u>non-diagnostic</u>, or <u>non-concordant</u> with exam findings/imaging studies → will need **excisional biopsy**
  • Clinically **indeterminate** or **suspect solid masses** will eventually need **excisional biopsy** unless CA diagnosis is made prior to that
  • **Cyst fluid** – if **bloody**, need cyst <u>excisional biopsy</u>; if **clear and recurs**, need cyst <u>excisional biopsy</u>; if **complex cyst**, need cyst <u>excisional biopsy</u>
  • **CNBx** – gives architecture
  • **FNA** – gives cytology (just the cells)

Management of Breast Masses Based on FNA or CNBx

Diagnosis	Treatment
Malignant	Definitive therapy
Suspicious	Surgical biopsy
Atypia	Surgical biopsy
Nondiagnostic	Repeated FNA/CNBx or surgical biopsy
Benign	Possible observation – exam and imaging studies need to concordant with benign disease, otherwise need excisional biopsy

■ **Mammography**
  • Has 90% sensitivity/specificity
  • Sensitivity increases with age as the dense parenchymal tissue is replaced with fat
  • Mass needs to be ≥ 5 mm to be detected
  • **Suggestive of CA** – irregular borders; spiculated; multiple clustered, small, thin, linear, crushed-like and/or branching calcifications; ductal asymmetry, distortion of architecture

BI-RADS Classification of Mammographic Abnormalities

Category	Assessment	Recommendation
1	Negative	Routine screening
2	Benign finding	Routine screening
3	Probably benign finding	Short-interval follow-up mammogram
4	Suspicious abnormality (eg indeterminate calcifications or architecture)	Definite probability of CA; get **CNBx**
5	Highly suggestive of CA (suspicious calcifications or architecture)	High probability of CA; get **CNBx**

BI-RADS, breast imaging, reporting, and data system.

- **BI-RADS 4** lesion CNBx shows:
  - **Malignancy** → follow appropriate Tx
  - **Non-diagnostic, indeterminate,** or **benign and non-concordant** with mammogram → need needle localization excisional biopsy
  - **Benign and concordant** with mammogram → 6-month follow-up
- **BI-RADS 5** lesion CNBx shows:
  - **Malignancy** → follow appropriate Tx
  - ***Any other finding*** (nondiagnostic, indeterminate, or benign) → all need needle localization excisional biopsy
- CNBx *without* excisional biopsy allows **appropriate staging with SLNBx** (mass is still present) and **one-step surgery** (avoids 2 surgeries) for patients diagnosed with breast CA

■ **Screening**
  - **Mammogram every 2–3 years after age 40,** then **yearly after 50**
  - **High-risk screening** – mammogram 10 years before the youngest age of diagnosis of breast CA in first-degree relative
  - <u>No</u> **mammography in patients** < 40 unless high risk → hard to interpret because of dense parenchyma
  - Want to **decrease radiation dose** in young patients

■ **Node levels**
  - **I** – lateral to pectoralis minor muscle
  - **II** – beneath pectoralis minor muscle
  - **III** – medial to pectoralis minor muscle
  - Rotter's nodes – between the pectoralis major and pectoralis minor muscles
  - Need to take **level I** and **II nodes** (take level III nodes only if grossly involved)

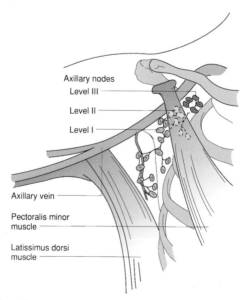

The axillary lymph nodes are divided into three levels by the pectoralis minor muscle. The level I nodes are inferior and lateral to the pectoralis minor, the level II nodes are below the axillary vein and behind the pectoralis minor, and the level III nodes are medial to the muscle against the chest wall.

- **Nodes** are the most important **prognostic staging factor**. Other factors include tumor size, tumor grade, progesterone, and estrogen receptor status
  - Survival is directly related to the number of positive nodes
    - 0 nodes positive   75% 5-year survival
    - 1–3 nodes positive   60% 5-year survival
    - 4–10 nodes positive   40% 5-year survival
- ■ **Bone** – most common site for distant metastasis (can also go to lung, liver, brain)
- ■ Takes approximately 5–7 years to go from single malignant cell to 1-cm tumor
- ■ **Central** and **subareolar tumors** have increased risk of multicentricity

TNM Definitions

Tx	Primary tumor cannot be assessed
T0	No evidence of primary tumor
Tis	Carcinoma in situ, ductal, or lobular or Paget's disease of the nipple with no tumor
T1	Tumor 2 cm or less in greatest dimension
T2	Tumor more than 2 cm but not more than 5 cm in greatest dimension
T3	Tumor more than 5 cm in greatest dimension
T4	Tumor of any size with direct extension to the chest wall (not including pectoralis muscle), skin edema, skin ulceration, satellite skin nodules, or inflammatory carcinoma

REGIONAL LYMPH NODES (PATHOLOGIC)

Nx	Nodes cannot be assessed
N0	No regional node metastases histologically, no additional examination for isolated tumor cells (ITCs)
N1	Metastasis to one to three axillary nodes or in internal mammary (IM) nodes with microscopic disease detected by sentinel node biopsy, which is not clinically apparent
N2	Metastases in four to nine axillary nodes or in clinically apparent IM nodes in the absence of axillary node metastasis
N3	Metastases in 10 or more axillary nodes, or in infraclavicular nodes, or in IM nodes in the presence of one or more positive axillary nodes; or in more than three axillary nodes with IM metastases, or in supraclavicular nodes

DISTANT METASTASES

Mx	Distant metastasis cannot be assessed
M0	No distant metastasis
M1	Distant metastasis

STAGE GROUPING

Stage 0	Tis	N0	M0
Stage 1	TI	N0	M0
Stage IIA	T0	N1	M0
	T1	N1	M0
	T2	N0	M0
Stage IIB	T2	N1	M0
	T3	N0	M0
Stage IIIA	T0	N2	M0
	T1	N2	M0
	T2	N2	M0
	T3	N1	M0
	T3	N2	M0
Stage IIIB	T4	N0	M0
	T4	N1	M0
	T4	N2	M0
Stage IIIC	Any T	N3	M0
Stage IV	Any T	Any N	M1

- **Breast cancer risk**
  - **Greatly increased risk** (relative risk > 4)
    - BRCA gene in patient with family history of breast CA
    - ≥ 2 primary relatives with bilateral or premenopausal breast CA
    - DCIS (ipsilateral breast at risk) and LCIS (both breasts have same high risk)
    - Fibrocystic disease with atypical hyperplasia
  - **Moderately increased risk** (relative risk 2–4) – prior breast cancer, radiation exposure, first-degree relative with breast cancer, age > 35 first birth
  - **Lower increased risk** (relative risk < 2) – early menarche, late menopause, nulliparity, proliferative benign disease, obesity, alcohol use, hormone replacement therapy
- **BRCA I and II** (+ family history of breast CA) and **CA risk**:
  - **BRCA I:**
    - Female breast CA   **60%** lifetime risk
    - Ovarian CA   **40%** lifetime risk
    - Male breast CA   **1%** lifetime risk
  - **BRCA II:**
    - Female breast CA   **60%** lifetime risk
    - Ovarian CA   **10%** lifetime risk
    - Male breast CA   **10%** lifetime risk
  - Consider **total abdominal hysterectomy** (TAH) and **bilateral salpingo-oophorectomy** (BSO) in BRCA families with history of breast CA
  - **First-degree relative with bilateral**, **premenopausal breast cancer** increases breast CA risk to 50%
  - **Considerations for prophylactic mastectomy**
    - Family history + BRCA gene
    - LCIS
    - **Also need one of the following**: high patient anxiety, poor patient access for follow-up exams and mammograms, difficult lesion to follow on exam or with mammograms, or patient preference for mastectomy
- **Receptors**
  - **Positive receptors** – better response to hormones, chemotherapy, surgery, and better overall prognosis
    - Receptor-positive tumors are more common in **postmenopausal women**
  - **Progesterone receptor–positive tumors** have better prognosis than estrogen receptor–positive tumors
  - Tumors that are both progesterone receptor and estrogen receptor positive have the best prognosis
  - 10% of breast CA is negative for both receptors
- **Male breast cancer**
  - < 1% of all breast CAs; usually **ductal**
  - Poorer prognosis because of late presentation
  - Have ↑ pectoral muscle involvement
  - Associated with steroid use, previous XRT, family history, Klinefelter's syndrome
  - Tx: modified radical mastectomy (MRM)
- **Ductal CA**
  - 85% of all breast CA
  - Various subtypes
    - **Medullary** – smooth borders, ↑ **lymphocytes**, bizarre cells, more favorable prognosis
    - **Tubular** – small **tubule** formations, more favorable prognosis
    - **Mucinous** (colloid) – produces an abundance of **mucin**, more favorable prognosis
    - **Scirrhotic** – worse prognosis
  - Tx: **MRM or BCT with postop XRT**

■ **Lobular cancer**
- 10% of all breast CAs
- Does not form calcifications; extensively infiltrative; ↑ bilateral, multifocal, and multicentric disease
- **Signet ring cells** confer worse prognosis
- Tx: **MRM** or **BCT with postop XRT**

■ **Inflammatory cancer**
- Considered T4 disease
- Very aggressive → median survival of 36 months
- Has **dermal lymphatic invasion,** which causes peau d'orange lymphedema appearance on breast; erythematous and warm
- Tx: **neoadjuvant chemo,** then **MRM,** then **adjuvant chemo-XRT** (most common method)

■ **Surgical options**
- **Subcutaneous mastectomy** (simple mastectomy)
  ◦ Leaves 1%–2% of breast tissue, preserves the nipple
  ◦ Not indicated for breast CA treatment
  ◦ Used for DCIS and LCIS
- **Breast-conserving therapy** (BCT = lumpectomy, quadrectomy, etc. plus ALND or SLNB); combined with **postop XRT**; need **1-cm margin**
- **Modified radical mastectomy**
  ◦ Removes all breast tissue, including the nipple areolar complex
  ◦ Includes axillary node dissection (level I nodes)

Contraindications to Breast-Conserving Therapy in Invasive Carcinoma

ABSOLUTE CONTRAINDICATIONS
■ Two or more primary tumors in separate quadrants of the breast
■ Persistent positive margins after reasonable surgical attempts
■ Pregnancy is an absolute contraindication to the use of breast irradiation. When cancer is diagnosed in the third trimester; it may be possible to perform breast-conserving surgery and treat the patient with irradiation after delivery
■ A history of prior therapeutic irradiation to the breast region that would result in retreatment to an excessively high radiation dose
■ Diffuse malignant-appearing microcalcifications

RELATIVE CONTRAINDICATIONS
■ A history of scleroderma or active systemic lupus erythematosus
■ Large tumor in a small breast that would result in cosmesis unacceptable to the patient
■ Very large or pendulous breasts if reproducibility of patient setup and adequate dose homogeneity cannot be ensured

---

- **SLNB**
  ◦ Fewer complications than ALND
  ◦ Indicated only for malignant tumors > 1 cm
  ◦ Not indicated in patients with clinically positive nodes; they need ALND
  ◦ Accuracy best when primary tumor is present (finds the right lymphatic channels)
  ◦ Well suited for small tumors with low risk of axillary metastases
  ◦ Lymphazurin blue dye or radiotracer is injected directly into tumor area
  ◦ **Type I hypersensitivity reactions** have been reported with Lymphazurin blue dye

- Usually find 1–3 nodes; 95% of the time, the sentinel node is found
- During **SLNB** – if no radiotracer or dye is found, need to do a formal ALND
- **Contraindications** – pregnancy, multicentric disease, neoadjuvant therapy, clinically positive nodes, prior axillary surgery, inflammatory or locally advanced disease
- **ALND** – take **level I and II nodes**
- **Complications of MRM** – infection, flap necrosis, seromas
- **Complications of ALND**
  - Infection, lymphedema, lymphangiosarcoma
  - **Axillary vein thrombosis** – sudden, early, postop swelling
  - **Lymphatic fibrosis** – slow swelling over 18 months
  - **Intercostal brachiocutaneous nerve injury** – hyperesthesia of inner arm and lateral chest wall; most commonly injured nerve after mastectomy; no significant sequelae
  - **Drains** – leave in until drainage < 40 cc/day
■ Radiotherapy
- Usually consists of **5,000 rad** for **BCT and XRT**
- **Complications of XRT** – edema, erythema, rib fractures, pneumonitis, ulceration, sarcoma, contralateral breast CA
- **Contraindications to XRT** – scleroderma (results in severe fibrosis and necrosis), previous XRT and would exceed recommended dose, SLE (relative), active rheumatoid arthritis (relative)
- **Indications for XRT after <u>mastectomy</u>:**
  - > 4 nodes
  - Skin or chest wall involvement
  - Positive margins
  - Tumor > 5 cm (T3)
  - Extracapsular nodal invasion
  - Inflammatory CA
  - Fixed axillary nodes (N2) or internal mammary nodes (N3)
- **BCT with XRT**
  - Need to have **negative margins** (1 cm) following BCT before starting XRT
  - 10% chance of local recurrence, usually within 2 years of 1st operation, need to re-stage with recurrence
  - Need **salvage MRM** for local recurrence
■ Chemotherapy
- **TAC** (taxanes, Adriamycin, and cyclophosphamide) for 6–12 weeks
- **Positive nodes** – everyone gets chemo *except* <u>postmenopausal women with positive estrogen receptors</u> → they can get hormonal therapy only with **aromatase inhibitor** (anastrozole)
- **> 1 cm** and **negative nodes** – everyone gets chemo *except* patients with <u>positive estrogen receptors</u> → they can get hormonal therapy only with **tamoxifen** if they are <u>premenopausal</u> or **aromatase inhibitor** (anastrozole) if they are <u>postmenopausal</u>
- **< 1 cm *and* negative nodes** – no chemo; hormonal therapy as above if positive estrogen receptors
- **After chemo**, patients positive for **estrogen receptors** should receive **appropriate hormonal therapy**
- Both chemotherapy and hormonal therapy have been shown to decrease recurrence and improve survival
- Taxanes – docetaxel, paclitaxel
- **Tamoxifen** – decreases risk of breast CA by 50%
  - 1% risk of blood clots; 0.1% risk of endometrial CA
■ **Almost all women with recurrence die of disease**
■ Increased recurrences and metastases occur with **positive nodes, large tumors, negative receptors, unfavorable subtype**

- **Metastatic flare** – pain, swelling, erythema in metastatic areas; XRT can help
  - XRT is good for bone metastases
- **Occult breast CA** – breast CA that presents as axillary metastases with unknown primary; Tx: **MRM** (70% are found to have breast CA)
- **Paget's disease**
  - Scaly skin lesion on nipple; biopsy shows Paget's cells
  - Patients have DCIS or ductal CA in breast
  - Tx: need MRM if cancer present; otherwise simple mastectomy (need to include the **nipple-areolar complex** with Paget's)
- **Cystosarcoma phyllodes**
  - 10% malignant, based on mitoses per high-power field (> 5–10)
  - **No nodal metastases**, hematogenous spread if any (rare)
  - Resembles giant fibroadenoma; has stromal and epithelial elements (mesenchymal tissue)
  - Can often be large tumors
  - Tx: WLE with negative margins; **no** ALND
- **Stewart–Treves syndrome**
  - **Lymphangiosarcoma** from **chronic lymphedema** following axillary dissection
  - Patients present with dark purple nodule or lesion on arm 5–10 years after surgery
- **Pregnancy with mass**
  - Tends to present late, leading to worse prognosis
  - Mammography and ultrasound do not work as well during pregnancy
  - Try to use ultrasound to avoid radiation
  - If **cyst,** drain it and send FNA for cytology
  - If **solid,** perform core needle biopsy or FNA
  - If core needle and FNA equivocal, need to go to excisional biopsy
  - If breast CA
    - 1st trimester – MRM
    - 2nd trimester – MRM
    - 3rd trimester – MRM or if late can perform lumpectomy with ALND and postpartum XRT
    - No XRT while pregnant; no breastfeeding after delivery

CHAPTER 25. **THORACIC**

ANATOMY AND PHYSIOLOGY
- **Azygous vein** runs along the right side and dumps into superior vena cava
- **Thoracic duct** runs along the right side, crosses midline at T4–5, and dumps into left subclavian vein at junction with internal jugular vein
- **Phrenic nerve** – runs anterior to hilum
- **Vagus nerve** – runs posterior to hilum
- Right lung volume 55% (3 lobes: RUL, RML, and RLL)
- Left lung volume 45% (2 lobes: LUL and LLL and lingula)
- Quiet inspiration – diaphragm 80%, intercostals 20%
- Greatest change in dimension superior/inferior
- Accessory muscles – sternocleidomastoid muscle (SCM), levators, serratus posterior, scalenes
- **Type I pneumocytes** – gas exchange
- **Type II pneumocytes** – surfactant production
- **Pores of Kahn** – direct air exchange between alveoli

PULMONARY FUNCTION TESTS
- Need predicted postop **FEV_1 > 0.8** (or > 40% of the predicted postop value)
  - If it is close → get qualitative V/Q scan to see contribution of that portion of lung to overall FEV_1 → if low, may still be able to resect
- Need predicted postop **DLCO > 10** mL/min/mm Hg CO (or > 40% of the predicted postop value)
  - Measures **carbon monoxide diffusion** and represents **oxygen exchange capacity**
  - This value depends on pulmonary capillary surface area, hemoglobin content, and alveolar architecture
- No resection if preop **pCO_2 > 50** or **pO_2 < 60** at rest
- No resection if preop VO_2 max **< 10–12 mL/min/kg** (maximum oxygen consumption)
- **Persistent air leak** – most common after segmentectomy/wedge
- **Atelectasis** – most common after lobectomy
- **Arrhythmias** – most common after pneumonectomy

LUNG CANCER
- Symptoms: can be asymptomatic with finding on routine CXR; cough, hemoptysis, atelectasis, PNA, pain, weight loss
- **Most common cause of cancer-related death in the United States**
- **Nodal involvement** has strongest influence on survival
- **Brain** – single most common site of metastasis
  - Can also go to supraclavicular nodes, other lung, bone, liver, and adrenals
- **Recurrence** usually appears as disseminated metastases
  - 80% of recurrences are within the 1st 3 years
- Lung CA overall 5-year survival rate 10%; 30% with resection for cure
- Stage I and II disease resectable; T3,N1,M0 (stage IIIa) possibly resectable
- Lobectomy or pneumonectomy most common procedure; sample suspicious nodes
- **Non–small cell carcinoma**
  - **80%** of lung CA
  - **Squamous cell carcinoma** usually more central
  - **Adenocarcinoma** usually more peripheral
  - **Adenocarcinoma** is the most common lung CA (<u>not</u> squamous)

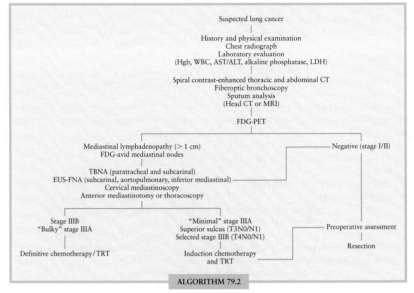

ALGORITHM 79.2

Evaluation of the patient who presents with a pulmonary mass.

TNM STAGING SYSTEM FOR LUNG CANCER

- **T1**: < 3 cm. **T2**: > 3 cm but > 2 cm away from carina. **T3**: invasion of chest wall, pericardium, diaphragm, or < 2 cm from carina. **T4**: mediastinum, esophagus, trachea, vertebra, heart, great vessels, malignant effusion (all indicate <u>unresectability</u>)
- **N1**: ipsilateral hilum nodes. **N2**: ipsilateral mediastinal or subcarinal (<u>unresectable</u>). **N3**: contralateral mediastinal or supraclavicular (<u>unresectable</u>)
- **M1**: distant metastasis

Stage	TNM Status
I	T1–2,N0,M0
IIa	T1,N1,M0
IIb	T2,N1,M0 or T3,N0,M0
IIIa	T1–3,N2,M0 or T3,N1,M0
IIIb	Any T4 or N3
IV	M1

Modified from AJCC. *Cancer Staging Handbook*. 6th ed.
New York, NY: Springer-Verlag; 2002:197–198.

■ **Small cell carcinoma**
- **20%** of lung CA; **neuroendocrine** in origin
- Usually unresectable at time of diagnosis (< 5% candidates for surgery)
- Overall 5-year survival rate < 5% (very poor prognosis)
- Stage T1,N0,M0 5-year survival rate – 50%
- Most get just chemo-XRT

- **Paraneoplastic syndromes**
  - **Squamous cell CA** – PTH-related peptide
  - **Small cell CA** – ACTH and ADH
  - Small cell **ACTH** – most common paraneoplastic syndrome
- **Mesothelioma**
  - Most malignant lung tumor
  - Aggressive local invasion, nodal invasion, and distant metastases common at the time of diagnosis
  - Asbestos exposure
- **Non–small cell** CA chemotherapy (stage II or higher) – carboplatin, Taxol
- **Small cell lung** CA chemotherapy – cisplatin, etoposide
- **XRT** can be used for lung CA as well
- **Chest and abdominal CT scan** – single best test for clinical assessment of **T and N status**
- **PET scan** – best test for **M status**
- **Mediastinoscopy**
  - Use for **centrally located tumors** and patients with **suspicious adenopathy** (> 0.8 cm or subcarinal > 1.0 cm) on chest CT
  - Does not assess aorto-pulmonary (AP) window nodes (left lung drainage)
  - Assesses **ipsilateral** (N2) and **contralateral** (N3) **mediastinal nodes**
  - If **mediastinal nodes** are **positive**, tumor is **unresectable**
  - Looking into **middle mediastinum** with mediastinoscopy
    - Left-side structures – RLN, esophagus, aorta, main pulmonary artery (PA)
    - Right-side structures – azygous and SVC
    - Anterior structures – innominate vein, innominate artery, right PA
- **Chamberlain procedure** (anterior thoracotomy or parasternal mediastinotomy) – assesses enlarged **AP window nodes**; go through left 2nd rib cartilage
- **Bronchoscopy** – needed for centrally located tumors to check for airway invasion
- **For lung CA**, patients need to 1) be **operable** (eg have appropriate FEV_1 and DLCO values) and 2) be **resectable** (ie can't have T4, N2, N3, or M disease)
- **Pancoast tumor** – tumor invades apex of chest wall and patients have **Horner's syndrome** (invasion of sympathetic chain → ptosis, miosis, anhidrosis) or **ulnar nerve** symptoms
- **Coin lesion**
  - Overall, 10% are malignant
  - Age < 50 → < 5% malignant; age > 50 → > 50% malignant
  - No growth in 2 years, and smooth contour suggests benign disease
  - If suspicious, will need either guided biopsy or wedge resection
- **Asbestos exposure** increases lung CA risk 90×
- **Bronchoalveolar CA** – can look like pneumonia; grows along alveolar walls; multifocal
- **Metastases to the lung** – if isolated and not associated with any other systemic disease, may be resected for colon, renal cell CA, sarcoma, melanoma, ovarian, and endometrial CA

CARCINOIDS

- **Neuroendocrine** tumor, usually central
  - 5% have metastases at time of diagnosis; 50% have symptoms (cough, hemoptysis)
- **Typical** carcinoid – 90% 5-year survival rate
- **Atypical** carcinoid – 60% 5-year survival
- Tx: resection; treat like cancer; outcome closely linked to histology
- Recurrence increased with positive nodes or tumors > 3 cm

BRONCHIAL ADENOMAS
- **Mucoepidermoid adenoma**, mucous gland adenoma, and **adenoid cystic adenoma** → all are *__malignant__ tumors*
- **Mucoepidermoid adenoma** and **mucous gland adenoma**
  - Slow growth, <u>no</u> metastases
  - Tx: resection
- **Adenoid cystic adenoma**
  - From submucosal glands; spreads along **perineural lymphatics**, well beyond endoluminal component; *very XRT sensitive*
  - Slow growing; can get 10-year survival with incomplete resection
  - Tx: resection; if unresectable, XRT can provide good palliation

HAMARTOMAS
- Most common **benign** adult lung tumor
- Have **calcifications** and can appear as a **popcorn lesion** on chest CT
- Diagnosis can be made with CT
- **Do not require resection**
- Repeat chest CT in 6 months to confirm diagnosis

MEDIASTINAL TUMORS IN ADULTS
- Most are asymptomatic; can present with chest pain, cough, dyspnea
- **Neurogenic tumors** – most common mediastinal tumor in adults and children, usually in posterior mediastinum
- 50% of symptomatic mediastinal masses are malignant
- 90% of asymptomatic mediastinal masses are benign
- **Location**
  - **Anterior** (thymus) – most common site for mediastinal tumor; **T's** →
    - **T**hymoma (#1 anterior mediastinal mass in adults)
    - **T**hyroid CA and goiters
    - **T**-cell lymphoma
    - **T**eratoma (and other germ cell tumors)
    - **P**arathyroid adenomas
  - **Middle** (heart, trachea, ascending aorta)
    - Bronchiogenic cysts
    - Pericardial cysts
    - Enteric cysts
    - Lymphoma
  - **Posterior** (esophagus, descending aorta)
    - Enteric cysts
    - Neurogenic tumors
    - Lymphoma
- **Thymoma**
  - All thymomas require resection
  - Thymus too big or associated with refractory myasthenia gravis → resection
  - 50% of thymomas are **malignant**
  - 50% of patients with thymomas have **symptoms**
  - 50% of patients with thymomas have **myasthenia gravis**
  - 10% of patients with myasthenia gravis have thymomas
- **Myasthenia gravis** – fatigue, weakness, diplopia, ptosis; antibodies to acetylcholine receptors
  - Tx: anticholinesterase inhibitors (neostigmine); steroids, plasmapheresis
  - 80% get improvement with thymectomy, including patients who do not have thymomas

- **Germ cell tumors**
  - Need to **biopsy** (often done with mediastinoscopy)
  - **Teratoma** – most common germ cell tumor in mediastinum
    - Can be benign or malignant
    - Tx: resection; possible chemotherapy
  - **Seminoma** – most common malignant germ cell tumor in mediastinum
    - 10% are beta-HCG positive; should <u>not</u> have AFP (alpha-fetoprotein)
    - Tx: **XRT** *(extremely sensitive);* chemotherapy reserved only for metastases or bulky nodal disease; surgery for residual disease after that
  - **Non-seminoma** – 90% have elevated beta-HCG and AFP
    - Tx: *chemo (cisplatin, bleomycin, VP-16)*; surgery for residual disease
- **Cysts**
  - **Bronchiogenic** – usually posterior to carina. Tx: **resection**
  - **Pericardial** – usually at right costophrenic angle. Tx: **can leave alone** (benign)
- **Neurogenic tumors** – have pain, neurologic deficit. Tx: resection
  - 10% have intra-spinal involvement that requires simultaneous spinal surgery
  - **Neurolemmoma** (schwannoma) – most common
  - **Paraganglioma** – can produce **catecholamines**, associated with von Recklinghausen's disease
  - Can also get **neuroblastomas** and **neurofibromas**

TRACHEA

- Benign tumors: adults – **papilloma**; children – **hemangioma**
- Malignant – **squamous cell carcinoma**
- Most common late complication after tracheal surgery – granulation tissue formation
- Most common early complication after tracheal surgery – laryngeal edema
  - Tx: reintubation, racemic epinephrine, steroids
- **Post-intubation stenosis** – at stoma site with tracheostomy, at cuff site with ET tube
  - Serial dilatation, bronchoscopic resection, or laser ablation if minor
  - Tracheal resection with end-to-end anastomosis if severe or if it keeps recurring
- **Tracheo-innominate artery fistula** – occurs after tracheostomy, can have rapid exsanguination
  - Tx: place finger in tracheostomy hole and hold pressure → **median sternotomy** with **ligation and resection of innominate artery**
  - This complication is avoided by keeping tracheostomy above the 3rd tracheal ring
- **Tracheo-esophageal fistula**
  - Usually occurs with prolonged intubation
  - Place large-volume cuff endotracheal tube below fistula
  - May need decompressing gastrostomy
  - Attempt repair after the patient is weaned from ventilator
  - Tx: tracheal resection, reanastomosis, close hole in esophagus, sternohyoid flap between esophagus and trachea

LUNG ABSCESS

- Necrotic area; most commonly associated with aspiration
- Most commonly in the **superior segment of RLL**
- Tx: *antibiotics alone (95% successful)*; CT-guided drainage if that fails
  - Surgery if above fails or cannot rule out cancer (> 6 cm, failure to resolve after 6 weeks)
- Chest CT can help differentiate empyema from lung abscess

EMPYEMA

- Usually secondary to **pneumonia** and **subsequent parapneumonic effusion** (staph, strep)
- Can also be due to esophageal, pulmonary, or mediastinal surgery

- Symptoms: pleuritic chest pain, fever, cough, SOB
- Pleural fluid often has WBCs > 500 cells/cc, bacteria, and a positive Gram stain
- **Exudative phase** (1st week) – Tx: chest tube, antibiotics
- **Fibro-proliferative phase** (2nd week) – Tx: chest tube, antibiotics; possible VATS (video-assisted thoracoscopic surgery) deloculation
- **Organized phase** (3rd week) – Tx: likely need **decortication**; fibrous peel occurs around lung
  - Some are using **intra-pleural tPA** (tissue plasminogen activator) to try and dissolve the peel
  - May need **Eloesser flap** (open thoracic window – direct opening to external environment) in frail/elderly

CHYLOTHORAX
- Milky white fluid; has ↑ lymphocytes and TAGs (> 110 mL/μL); Sudan red stains fat
- **Fluid is resistant to infection**
- 50% secondary to trauma or iatrogenic injury
- 50% secondary to tumor (lymphoma most common, due to tumor burden in the lymphatics)
- Injury **above T5–6** results in **left**-sided chylothorax
- Injury **below T5–6** results in **right**-sided chylothorax
- Tx: 2–3 weeks of conservative therapy (chest tube, octreotide, low-fat diet or TPN)
  - If above fails and chylothorax secondary to **trauma** or **iatrogenic injury**, need **ligation of thoracic duct** on **right side** low in mediastinum (80% successful)
  - For **malignant causes**, need **talc pleurodesis** and possible **chemo and/or XRT** (less successful than above)

MASSIVE HEMOPTYSIS
- **> 600 cc/24 h**; bleeding usually from high-pressure **bronchial arteries**
- Most commonly secondary to **infection**, death is due to asphyxiation
- Tx: place bleeding side down; mainstem intubation to side opposite of bleeding to prevent drowning in blood; rigid bronchoscopy to identify site and possibly control bleeding; may need lobectomy or pneumonectomy to control; bronchial artery embolization if not suitable for surgery

SPONTANEOUS PNEUMOTHORAX
- Tall, healthy, thin, young males; more common on the right
- Recurrence risk after 1st pneumothorax is 20%, after 2nd pneumothorax is 60%, after 3rd pneumothorax is 80%
- Results from rupture of a bleb usually in the apex of the upper lobe of the lung
- Tx: **chest tube**
- Surgery for recurrence, air leak > 7 days, non-reexpansion, high-risk profession (airline pilot, diver, mountain climber), or patients who live in remote areas
- Surgery consists of thoracoscopy, **apical blebectomy**, and **mechanical pleurodesis**

OTHER CONDITIONS
- **Tension pneumothorax** – most likely to cause arrest after blunt trauma; impaired venous return
- **Catamenial pneumothorax** – occurs in temporal relation to menstruation
  - Caused by **endometrial implants** in the visceral lung pleura
- **Residual hemothorax despite 2 good chest tubes** → OR for thoracoscopic drainage
- **Clotted hemothorax** – surgical drainage if > 25% of lung, air–fluid levels, or signs of infection (fever, ↑ WBCs); surgery in 1st week to avoid peel

■ **Broncholiths** – usually secondary to infection
■ **Mediastinitis** – usually occurs after cardiac surgery
■ **Whiteout on chest x-ray**
  • Midline shift toward whiteout – most likely collapse → need bronchoscopy to remove plug
  • No shift – CT scan to figure it out
  • Midline shift away from whiteout – most likely effusion → place chest tube
■ **Bronchiectasis** – acquired from infection, tumor, **cystic fibrosis**
  • Diffuse nature prevents surgery in most patients
■ **Tuberculosis** – lung apices; get calcifications, **caseating granulomas**
  • Ghon complex → parenchymal lesion + enlarged hilar nodes
  • Tx: INH, rifampin, pyrazinamide
■ **Sarcoidosis** – has **non-caseating granulomas**

Evaluation of Pleural Fluid			
Test	Transudate	Exudate	Empyema
WBC	< 1,000	> 1,000	> 1,000
			> 50,000 most specific
pH	7.45–7.55	≤ 7.45	< 7.30
Pleural fluid protein to serum ratio	< 0.5	> 0.5	> 0.5
Pleural fluid LDH to serum ratio	< 0.6	> 0.6	> 0.6

From Knight C, Paauw D. Respiratory tract infections. In: Shah SS, Hu KK, Crane HM, eds. *Blueprints Infectious Diseases*. Philadelphia, PA: Lippincott Williams & Wilkins; 2006, with permission.

■ **Recurrent pleural effusions** can be treated with mechanical pleurodesis
  • Talc pleurodesis for malignant pleural effusions
■ **Airway fires** – usually associated with the laser
  • Tx: stop gas flow, remove ET tube, re-intubate for 24 hours; bronchoscopy
■ **AVMs** – connections between the pulmonary arteries and pulmonary veins; usually in **lower lobes**; can occur with Osler–Weber–Rendu disease
  • Symptoms: hemoptysis, SOB, neurologic events
  • Tx: **embolization**
■ **Chest wall tumors**
  • **Benign** – **osteochondroma** most common
  • **Malignant** – **chondrosarcoma** most common

CONGENITAL HEART DISEASE

- **R → L shunts** cause **cyanosis**
  - Children squat to *increase* SVR and *decrease* R → L shunts
  - **Cyanosis** – can lead to polycythemia, strokes, brain abscess, endocarditis
  - **Eisenmenger's syndrome**: shift from **L → R shunt** to **R → L shunt**
    - Sign of increasing pulmonary vascular resistance (PVR) and **pulmonary HTN**; this condition is generally <u>irreversible</u>
- **L → R shunts** cause **CHF** – manifests as failure to thrive, ↑ HR, tachypnea, hepatomegaly; CHF in **children** – ***hepatomegaly*** 1st sign
- **L → R shunts** (CHF) – VSD, ASD, PDA
- **R → L shunts** (cyanosis) – tetralogy of Fallot
- **Ductus arteriosus** – connection between descending aorta and left pulmonary artery (PA); blood shunted away from lungs in utero
- **Ductus venosum** – connection between portal vein and IVC; blood shunted away from liver in utero
- **Fetal circulation to placenta** – 2 umbilical arteries
- **Fetal circulation from placenta** – 1 umbilical vein

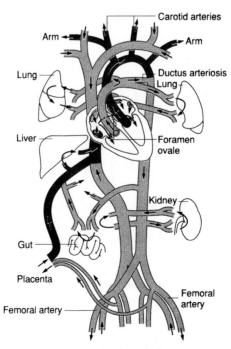

Persistent fetal circulation.

- **Ventricular septal defect** (VSD)
  - **Most common congenital heart defect**
  - **L → R shunt**
  - **80% close spontaneously** (usually by age 6 months)
  - Large VSDs – usually cause symptoms after 4–6 weeks of life, as PVR ↓ and shunt ↑
  - Can get **CHF** (tachypnea, tachycardia) and **failure to thrive**
  - Medical Tx: diuretics and digoxin
  - <u>Usual timing of repair</u>:
    - **Large** VSDs (shunt > 2.5) – **1 year** of age
    - **Medium** VSDs (shunt 2–2.5) – **5 years** of age
    - *Failure to thrive – most common reason for earlier repair*
- **Atrial septal defect** (ASD)
  - **L → R shunt**
  - **Ostium secundum** – most common (80%); centrally located
  - **Ostium primum** (or atrioventricular canal defects or endocardial cushion defects); can have mitral valve and tricuspid valve problems; frequent in **Down's syndrome**
  - Usually symptomatic when **shunt > 2** → CHF (SOB, recurrent infections)
  - Can get **paradoxical emboli** in adulthood
  - Medical Tx: diuretics and digoxin
  - <u>Usual timing of repair</u> – **1–2 years** of age (age 3–6 months with canal defects)
- **Tetralogy of Fallot** (4 parts)
  - VSD, pulmonic stenosis, overriding aorta, right ventricular (RV) hypertrophy
  - **R → L shunt**
  - **Most common congenital heart defect that results in cyanosis**
  - Medical Tx: **β-blocker**
  - <u>Usual timing of repair</u> – 3–6 months of age
  - Repair: RV outflow tract obstruction (RVOT) removal, RVOT enlargement, and VSD repair

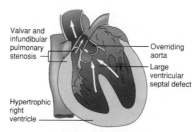

Valvar and infundibular pulmonary stenosis

Overriding aorta

Large ventricular septal defect

Hypertrophic right ventricle

The four anatomic features of the tetralogy of Fallot. The primary morphologic abnormality, anterior and superior displacement of the infundibular septum, results in a malalignment ventricular septal defect, overriding of the aortic valve, and obstruction of the right ventricular outflow. Right ventricular hypertrophy is a secondary occurrence.

- **Patent ductus arteriosus** (PDA)
  - **L → R shunt**
  - Indomethacin – causes the PDA to close; rarely successful beyond neonatal period
  - Requires surgical repair through left thoracotomy if it persists

ADULT CARDIAC DISEASE
- **Coronary artery disease**
  - Most common cause of death in the United States
  - Risk factors – smoking, HTN, male gender, family history, hyperlipidemia, diabetes
  - Medical Tx: nitrates, smoking cessation, weight loss, statin drugs, ASA

- Left main coronary artery branches into left anterior descending (LAD) and circumflex (Cx) arteries
- Most atherosclerotic lesions are **proximal**
- **Complications of myocardial infarction**:
  - **VSR** (ventricular septal rupture) – hypotension, pansystolic murmur, usually occurs **3–7 days** after MI; have a **step-up in oxygen content** between right atrium and pulmonary artery secondary to L → R shunt; Dx: **echo**; Tx: IABP to temporize, **patch over septum**
  - **Papillary muscle rupture** – get severe mitral regurgitation with hypotension and pulmonary edema; usually occurs **3–7 days** after MI; Dx: **echo**; Tx: IABP to temporize, **replace valve**
- **Drug-eluting stent** – restenosis in 20% at 1 year
- **Saphenous vein graft** – 80% 5-year patency
- **Internal mammary artery** – off subclavian artery
  - **Best conduit for CABG** (> 95% 20-year patency when placed to **LAD**)
  - Collateralizes with **superior epigastric artery**
- **CABG procedure**
  - **Potassium** and **cold solution cardioplegia** – causes arrest of the heart in diastole; keeps the heart protected and still while grafts are placed
- **Best indications for CABG** (> 70% stenosis significant for most areas except left main disease)
  - Left main disease (> 50% stenosis considered significant)
  - 3-vessel disease (LAD, Cx, and right coronary artery)
  - 2-vessel disease involving the LAD
  - Lesions not amenable to stenting
- **High mortality risk factors**: *pre-op cardiogenic shock* (#1 risk factor), emergency operations, age, low EF

VALVE DISEASE

- **Aortic stenosis** – most common valve lesion; **calcification** produces stenosis
- **Bioprosthetic tissue valves** (do not require anticoagulation)
  - For patients who want pregnancy, have contraindication to anticoagulation, are older (> 65) and unlikely to require another valve in their lifetime, or have frequent falls
  - Tissue valves **last 10–15 years** – not as durable as mechanical valves
  - Because of rapid calcification in children and young patients, use of tissue valves is contraindicated in those populations
- **Aortic stenosis** (AS) – most from degenerative calcification
  - **Cardinal symptoms**:
    - **Dyspnea** on exertion – mean survival 5 years
    - **Angina** – mean survival 4 years
    - **Syncope** (*worst of the cardinal symptoms*) – mean survival 3 years
  - Indications for operation – when **symptomatic** (usually have a peak gradient > 50 mm Hg and a valve area < 1.0 cm^2)
- **Mitral regurgitation** (MR)
  - Left ventricle becomes dilated
  - **Ventricular function** – key index of disease progression in patients with MR
  - **Atrial fibrillation** is common; in end-stage disease, **pulmonary congestion** occurs
  - Indications for operation – when **symptomatic** or if **severe mitral regurgitation**
- **Mitral stenosis** – rare now; most from rheumatic fever
  - Get **pulmonary edema** and **dyspnea**
  - Indications for operation – when **symptomatic** (usually have valve area < 1 cm^2)
  - **Balloon commissurotomy** to open valve often used as 1st procedure (not as invasive)

ENDOCARDITIS
- Fever, chills, sweats
- **Aortic valve** – most common site of prosthetic valve infections
- **Mitral valve** – most common site of native valve infections
- *Staphylococcus aureus* responsible for 50% of cases
- Most commonly left sided except in **drug abusers** (*Pseudomonas* most common organism for drug abusers)
- Medical therapy first – successful in 75%; sterilizes valve in 50%
- Indications for surgery – **failure of antimicrobial therapy, severe valve failure, perivalvular abscesses, pericarditis**

OTHER CARDIAC CONDITIONS
- **Most common tumors of heart**
  - Most common benign tumor – **myxoma**; 75% in LA
  - Most common malignant tumor – **angiosarcoma**
  - Most common metastatic tumor to the heart – **lung CA**
- Coming off cardiopulmonary bypass and aortic root vent, blood is dark and aortic perfusion cannula blood is red
  - Tx: **ventilate the lungs**
- **Coronary veins** have the **lowest oxygen tension** of any tissue in the body due to high oxygen extraction by myocardium
- **Superior vena cava** (SVC) **syndrome** – swelling of the upper extremities and face
  - Most cases secondary to lung CA invading the SVC
  - These tumors are unresectable since the tumor has invaded the mediastinum
  - Tx: **emergent XRT**
- **Mediastinal bleeding** – > 500 cc for 1st hour or > 250 cc/h for 4 hours → need to re-explore after cardiac procedure
- **Risk factors for mediastinitis** – obesity, use of bilateral internal mammary arteries, diabetes
  - Tx: debridement with pectoralis flaps; can also use omentum
- **Post-pericardiotomy syndrome** – pericardial friction rub, fever, chest pain, SOB
  - EKG – diffuse ST-segment elevation in multiple leads
  - Tx: **NSAIDs, steroids**

- **Most common congenital hypercoagulable disorder** – resistance to activated protein C (Leiden factor)
- **Most common acquired hypercoagulable disorder** – smoking

ATHEROSCLEROSIS STAGES
- **1st** – **foam cells** → macrophages that have absorbed fat and lipids in the vessel wall
- **2nd** – **smooth muscle cell proliferation** → caused by growth factors released from macrophages; results in wall injury
- **3rd** – **intimal disruption** (from smooth muscle cell proliferation) → leads to exposure of collagen in vessel wall and eventual **thrombus formation** → fibrous plaques then form in these areas with underlying atheromas
- Risk factors: smoking, HTN, hypercholesterolemia, DM, hereditary factors

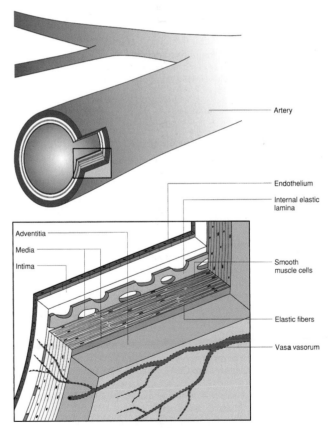

The artery wall is made of multiple layers (intima, media, and adventitia) that vary in composition depending on the artery.

CEREBROVASCULAR DISEASE

- Stroke 3rd most common cause of death in the United States
- **HTN** – most important risk factor for stroke
- Carotids supply 85% of blood flow to brain
  - **Carotid bifurcation** – most common site of stenosis
- Normal internal carotid artery (ICA) has **continuous forward flow**
  - 1st branch of internal carotid artery – **ophthalmic artery**
- Normal external carotid artery (ECA) has **triphasic flow**
  - 1st branch of external carotid artery – **superior thyroid artery**
- Communication between the ICA and ECA occurs through the **ophthalmic artery** (off ICA) and **internal maxillary artery** (off ECA)
- **Middle cerebral artery** – most commonly diseased <u>intracranial artery</u>
- **Cerebral ischemic events** – most commonly from **arterial embolization** from the ICA (not thrombosis)
  - Can also occur from a **low-flow state** through a severely stenotic lesion
  - **Heart** is the 2nd most common source of cerebral emboli
- **Anterior cerebral artery events** – mental status changes, release, slowing
- **Middle cerebral artery events** – contralateral motor and speech (if dominant side); contralateral facial droop
- **Posterior cerebral artery events** – vertigo, tinnitus, drop attacks, incoordination
- **Amaurosis fugax** – occlusion of the ophthalmic branch of the ICA (visual changes → shade coming down over eyes); visual changes are transient
  - See **Hollenhorst plaques** on ophthalmologic exam
- **Carotid traumatic injury with major fixed deficit**
  - If occluded, do <u>not</u> repair → can exacerbate injury with bleeding
  - If not occluded – repair with carotid stent or open procedure
- **Carotid endarterectomy** (CEA)
  - **Repair indications**: <u>symptomatic</u> > 70% stenosis, <u>asymptomatic</u> > 80% stenosis
  - **Recent completed stroke** → wait 4–6 weeks and then perform CEA if it meets criteria (bleeding risk if performed earlier)
  - **Emergent CEA** may be of benefit with <u>fluctuating neurologic symptoms</u> or <u>crescendo/evolving TIAs</u>
  - Use a **shunt** during CEA for **stump pressures < 50** or if **contralateral side is tight**
  - Repair the **tightest side first** if the patient has bilateral stenosis
  - Repair the **dominant side first** if the patient has equally tight carotid stenosis bilaterally
  - **Complications from repair**
    - **Vagus nerve injury – *most common cranial nerve injury with CEA*** → secondary to **vascular clamping** during endarterectomy; patients get ***hoarseness*** (recurrent laryngeal nerve comes off vagus)
    - **Hypoglossal nerve injury** – tongue deviates to the side of injury → ***speech and mastication difficulty***
    - **Glossopharyngeal nerve injury** – rare; occurs with really high carotid dissection → causes ***difficulty swallowing***
    - **Ansa cervicalis** – innervation to strap muscles; no serious deficits
    - **Mandibular branch of facial nerve** – affects corner of mouth (smile)
    - **Acute event immediately after CEA** → back to OR to check for flap or thrombosis
    - **Pseudoaneurysm** – pulsatile, bleeding mass after CEA; Tx: drape and prep before intubation, intubate, then repair
    - **20% have hypertension following CEA** – caused by injury to carotid body; Tx: **Nipride** to avoid bleeding

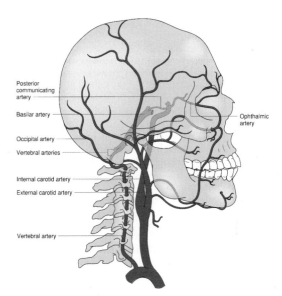

The paired carotid and vertebral arteries supply blood to the brain. Extensive extracranial collaterals between the external carotid and vertebral systems allow for antegrade perfusion when a proximal occlusion develops in either vessel. Likewise, periorbital collaterals allow for retrograde flow through the ophthalmic artery to the internal carotid artery in the presence of a cervical internal carotid artery occlusion. Extensive side-to-side collaterals are found between the right and left external carotid arteries and right and left vertebral arteries.

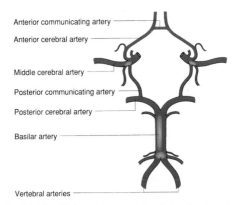

The circle of Willis is a highly efficient intracranial collateral network; however, multiple important variations occur, and an incomplete circle producing an isolated hemisphere is not uncommon.

- **Myocardial infarction** – most common cause of non-stroke morbidity and mortality following CEA
- **15% restenosis** rate after CEA
- **Carotid stenting** – for high-risk patients (eg patients with previous CEA and restenosis, multiple medical comorbidities, previous neck XRT)
■ **Vertebrobasilar artery disease**
  - Anatomy: the two **vertebral arteries** arise from the **subclavian arteries** and combine to form a single **basilar artery**; the basilar then splits into two **posterior cerebral arteries**.
  - Usually need basilar artery or bilateral vertebral artery disease to have symptoms
  - Caused by atherosclerosis, spurs, bands; get vertebrobasilar insufficiency
  - Symptoms: diplopia, vertigo, tinnitus, drop attacks, incoordination
  - Tx: PTA with stent
■ **Carotid body tumors** – present as a painless neck mass, usually near bifurcation, neural crest cells; are *extremely vascular*; Tx: resection

THORACIC AORTIC DISEASE

■ Anatomy – aortic arch vessels include the **innominate artery** (which branches into the right subclavian and right common carotid arteries), the **left common carotid artery**, and the **left subclavian artery**
■ **Ascending aortic aneurysms**
  - Often asymptomatic and picked up on routine CXR
  - Can get compression of vertebra (back pain), RLN (voice changes), bronchi (dyspnea or PNA), or esophagus (dysphagia)
  - Indications for repair: **acutely symptomatic**, ≥ **5.5 cm** (with Marfan's > 5.0 cm), or **rapid ↑ in size** (> 0.5 cm/yr)
■ **Descending aortic aneurysms** (also thoracoabdominal aneurysms)
  - Indications for repair
    - If **endovascular repair** possible – > **5.5 cm**
    - If **open repair** needed – > **6.5 cm**
  - Risk of mortality or paraplegia is less with endovascular repair (2%–3%) compared to open repair (20%)
  - Reimplant intercostal arteries below T8 to help prevent paraplegia with open repair
■ **Aortic dissections**
  - **Stanford classification** – based on presence or absence of involvement of ascending aorta
    - **Class A** – any ascending aortic involvement
    - **Class B** – descending aortic involvement only
  - **DeBakey classification** – based on the site of tear and extent of dissection
    - **Type I** – ascending and descending
    - **Type II** – ascending only
    - **Type III** – descending only
  - Most dissections start in the **ascending aorta**
  - Can mimic myocardial infarction
  - Symptoms: tearing-like chest pain; can have unequal pulses (or BP) in upper extremities
  - 95% of patients have **severe HTN** at presentation
  - Other risk factors: Marfan's syndrome, previous aneurysm, atherosclerosis
  - CXR – usually normal; may have wide mediastinum
  - Dx: chest CT with contrast
  - Dissection occurs in **medial layer** of blood vessel wall
  - **Aortic insufficiency** occurs in 70%, caused by annular dilatation or when aortic valve cusp is sheared off

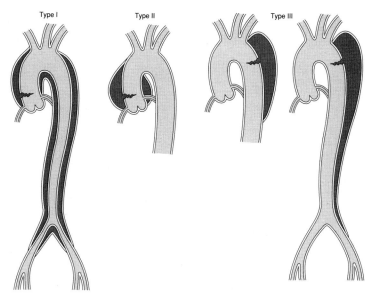

DeBakey classification of aortic dissection.

- Can also have occlusion of the coronary arteries and major aortic branches
- Death with ascending aortic dissections usually secondary to **cardiac failure** from aortic insufficiency, **cardiac tamponade**, or **rupture**
- Medical Tx initially → **control BP** with IV **β-blockers** (eg esmolol) and **Nipride**
- Tx:
    - Operate on *all ascending* aortic dissections – Tx: need **open repair**; graft is placed to eliminate flow to the false lumen
    - Only operate on **descending** aortic dissections with **visceral** or **extremity ischemia** or if **contained rupture** – Tx: **endograft** or **open repair**; can also just place **fenestrations** in the dissection flap to restore blood flow to viscera or extremity if ischemia is the problem
    - Follow these patients with lifetime serial scans (MRI to decrease radiation exposure); 30% eventually get aneurysm formation requiring surgery
- Postop complications for thoracic aortic surgery – **MI**, **renal failure**, **paraplegia** (descending thoracic aortic surgery)
- **Paraplegia** caused by spinal cord ischemia due to occlusion of intercostal arteries and artery of Adamkiewicz that occurs with descending thoracic aortic surgery

ABDOMINAL AORTIC DISEASE
- ■ **Abdominal aortic aneurysms** (AAAs)
    - Normal aorta 2-3 cm
    - Result from degeneration of the **medial layer**
    - Risk factors: males, age, smoking, family history
    - Usually found incidentally
    - Can present with rupture, distal embolization, or compression of adjacent organs

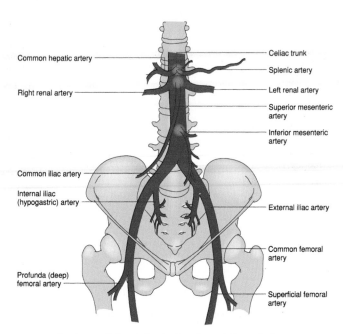

Common hepatic artery

Right renal artery

Common iliac artery

Internal iliac
(hypogastric) artery

Profunda (deep)
femoral artery

Celiac trunk

Splenic artery

Left renal artery

Superior mesenteric
artery

Inferior mesenteric
artery

External iliac artery

Common femoral
artery

Superficial femoral
artery

Anatomy of the abdominal aorta and iliac arteries.

- **Rupture**
  - Leading cause of death without an operation
  - Symptoms: back or abdominal pain; can have profound hypotension
  - Dx: ultrasound or abdominal CT
  - CT shows **fluid** in retroperitoneal space and **extraluminal contrast** with rupture
  - Most likely to rupture on **left posterolateral wall, 2–4 cm below renals**
  - More likely to rupture in presence of diastolic **HTN** or **COPD** (thought to be predictors of expansion)
  - **50% mortality with rupture** if patient reaches hospital alive
- Tx: repair if **symptomatic, > 5.5 cm**, or **growth > 0.5 cm/yr**
  - **Reimplant inferior mesenteric artery** (IMA) if backpressure < 40 mm Hg (ie poor backbleeding), previous colonic surgery, stenosis at the superior mesenteric artery, or flow to left colon appears inadequate
  - **Ligate bleeding lumbar arteries**
  - Usually use a straight tube Dacron graft for repair of AAAs
  - If performing an aorto-bifemoral repair instead of a straight tube graft, you should ensure flow to at least **one internal iliac artery** (hypogastric artery) to avoid **vasculogenic impotence**
- **Complications:**
  - **Major vein injury with proximal cross-clamp** – retro-aortic left renal vein
  - **Impotence** in ⅓ secondary to disruption of autonomic nerves and blood flow to the pelvis
  - 5% mortality with elective repair
  - **#1 cause of <u>acute</u> death after surgery** – MI
  - **#1 cause of <u>late</u> death after surgery** – renal failure
  - RFs for **mortality** – creatinine > 1.8 (#1), CHF, EKG ischemia, pulmonary dysfunction, older age, females

- **Graft infection rate** – 1%
- **Pseudoaneurysm** after graft placement – 1%
- **Atherosclerotic occlusion** – most common late complication after aortic graft placement
- **Diarrhea** (especially **bloody**) after AAA repair worrisome for **ischemic colitis**:
    - **Inferior mesenteric artery** (IMA) often sacrificed with AAA repair and can cause ischemia (most commonly the **left colon**)
    - Dx: endoscopy or abdominal CT; middle and distal rectum are spared from ischemia (middle and inferior rectal arteries are branches off internal iliac artery)
    - If patient has peritoneal signs, mucosa is black on endoscopy, or part of the colon looks dead on CT scan → take to OR for colectomy and colostomy placement

Ideal Criteria for Abdominal Aortic Aneurysm (AAA) Endovascular Repair

AAA Morphology	Criteria
Neck length	> 15 mm
Neck diameter	20–30 mm
Neck angulation	< 60 degrees
Common iliac artery length	> 10 mm
Common iliac artery diameter	8–18 mm
Other	Non-tortuous, noncalcified iliac arteries
	Lack of neck thrombus

Modified from Schermerhorn ML, Simosa HF. Type IV thoracoabdominal, infrarenal, and pararenal aortic aneurysms. In: Fischer JE, Bland KI, et al, eds. *Mastery of Surgery*. 5th ed. Philadelphia, PA: Lippincott Williams & Wilkins; 2007, with permission.

Endoleak Type	Failure Site	Tx
Type I	Proximal or distal graft **attachment sites**	**Extension cuffs**
Type II	**Collaterals** (eg patent lumbar, IMA, intercostals, accessory renal)	**Observe** most; percutaneous coil embolization if pressurizing aneurysm
Type III	**Overlap sites** when using multiple grafts or fabric tear	**Secondary endograft** to cover overlap site or tear
Type IV	**Graft wall porosity** or suture holes	**Observe**; can place nonporous stent if that fails
Type V (Endotension)	**Expansion of aneurysm without evidence of leak**	**Repeat EVAR** or **open repair**

- ■ **Inflammatory aneurysms**
    - Occurs in 10% of patients with AAA; males
    - <u>Not</u> secondary to infection – just an inflammatory process
    - Can get adhesions to the 3rd and 4th portions of the **duodenum**
    - **Ureteral entrapment** in 25%
    - Weight loss, ↑ ESR, thickened rim above calcifications on CT scan
    - May need to place preoperative **ureteral stents** to help avoid injury
    - Inflammatory process resolves after aortic graft placement
- ■ **Mycotic aneurysms**
    - ***Salmonella #1***, *Staphylococcus* #2
    - Bacteria infect atherosclerotic plaque, cause aneurysm
    - Pain, fevers, positive blood cultures in 50%

- Periaortic fluid, gas, retroperitoneal soft tissue edema, lymphadenopathy
- Usually need extra-anatomic bypass (axillary–femoral with femoral-to-femoral crossover) and resection of infrarenal abdominal aorta to clear infection

■ **Aortic graft infections**
  - ***Staphylococcus #1***, *E. coli #2*
  - See fluid, gas, thickening around graft
  - Blood cultures negative in many patients
  - Tx: bypass through non-contaminated field (eg axillary-femoral bypass with femoral-to-femoral crossover) and then resect the infected graft
  - More common with grafts going to the **groin** (eg aorto-bifemoral grafts)

■ **Aortoenteric fistula**
  - Usually occurs > 6 months after abdominal aortic surgery
  - **Herald bleed with hematemesis**, then blood per rectum
  - Graft erodes into 3rd or 4th portion of duodenum near proximal suture line
  - Tx: bypass through non-contaminated field (eg axillary-femoral bypass with femoral-to-femoral crossover), resect graft, and then close hole in the duodenum

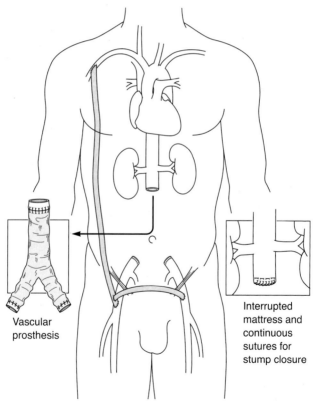

Vascular prosthesis

Interrupted mattress and continuous sutures for stump closure

Standard treatment for an infected aortic vascular prosthesis. An axillobifemoral bypass is performed first. This is followed a few days later by removal of the infected aortic prosthesis and careful oversewing of the aortic stump as illustrated.

PERIPHERAL ARTERIAL DISEASE (PAD)

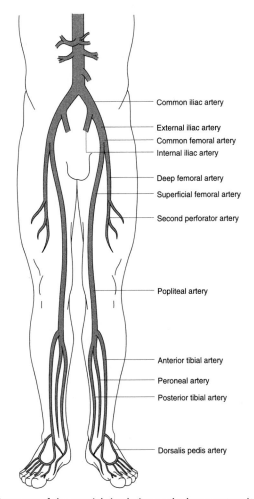

Common iliac artery

External iliac artery
Common femoral artery
Internal iliac artery

Deep femoral artery
Superficial femoral artery

Second perforator artery

Popliteal artery

Anterior tibial artery
Peroneal artery
Posterior tibial artery

Dorsalis pedis artery

Anatomy of the arterial circulation to the lower extremity.

- ■ **Leg compartments**
  - **Anterior** – deep peroneal nerve (dorsiflexion, sensation between 1st and 2nd toes), anterior tibial artery
  - **Lateral** – superficial peroneal nerve (eversion, lateral foot sensation)
  - **Deep posterior** – tibial nerve (plantar flexion), posterior tibial artery, peroneal artery
  - **Superficial posterior** – sural nerve
- ■ **Signs of PAD** – pallor, dependent rubor, hair loss, slow capillary refill
  - Most commonly due to **atherosclerosis**
- ■ **Statin drugs** (lovastatin) – #1 preventive agent for atherosclerosis
- ■ **Homocystinuria** can ↑ risk of atherosclerosis; Tx: **folate** and **B$_{12}$**

- **Claudication**: medical therapy first → ASA, smoking cessation, exercise until pain occurs to improve collaterals
- **Symptoms** occur **one level below** occlusion:
  - **Buttock** claudication – aortoiliac disease
  - **Mid-thigh** claudication – external iliac
  - **Calf** claudication – common femoral artery or proximal superficial femoral artery disease
  - **Foot** claudication – distal superficial femoral artery or popliteal disease
- **Lumbar stenosis** can mimic claudication
- **Diabetic neuropathy** can mimic rest pain
- **Leriche syndrome**
  - No femoral pulses
  - Buttock or thigh claudication
  - Impotence (from ↓ flow in the internal iliacs)
  - Lesion at aortic bifurcation or above
  - Tx: aorto-bifemoral bypass graft
- **Most common atherosclerotic occlusion in lower extremities** – Hunter's canal (**distal superficial femoral artery** exits here); the **sartorius muscle** covers Hunter's canal
- **Collateral circulation** – forms from abnormal pressure gradients
  - Circumflex iliacs to subcostals
  - Circumflex femoral arteries to gluteal arteries
  - Geniculate arteries around the knee
- **Postnatal angiogenesis** – budding from preexisting vessels; angiogenin involved
- **Ankle–brachial index** (ABI)
  - **< 0.9** - start to get claudication (typically occurs at same distance each time)
  - **< 0.5** - start to get rest pain (usually across the distal arch and foot)
  - **< 0.4** - ulcers (usually starts in toes)
  - **< 0.3** - gangrene
  - ABIs can be very **inaccurate in patients with diabetes** secondary to incompressibility of vessels; often have to go off Doppler waveforms in these patients
  - In patients with claudication, the ABI in the extremity drops with walking (ie resting ABI may be 0.9 but can drop to < 0.6 with exercise, resulting in pain)
- **Pulse volume recordings** (PVRs) – used to find significant occlusion and at what level
- **Arteriogram** is indicated if PVRs suggest significant disease – can also at times treat the patient with percutaneous intervention; gold standard for vascular imaging
- **Surgical indications for PAD** - rest pain, ulceration or gangrene, lifestyle limitation, atheromatous embolization
  - **PTFE** (Gortex) - _only_ for bypasses **above the knee**; need to use vein for below the knee bypasses
  - **Dacron** - good for aorta and large vessels
  - **Aortoiliac occlusive disease** - most get aorto-bifemoral repair
    - Need to ensure flow to at least **1 internal iliac artery** (hypogastric artery; want to see **good back-bleeding** from at least 1 of the arteries, otherwise need a bypass to an internal iliac artery) when performing aorto-bifemoral repair to prevent **vasculogenic impotence** and **pelvic ischemia**
  - **Isolated iliac lesions** - PTA with stent 1st choice; if that fails, consider femoral-to-femoral crossover
  - **Femoropopliteal grafts**
    - 75% 5-year patency
    - Improved patency rate with surgery for claudication as opposed to limb salvage
    - Popliteal artery exposure below knee - posterior muscle is **gastrocnemius** and anterior muscle is **popliteus**
  - **Femoral-distal grafts** (peroneal, anterior tibial, or posterior tibial artery)
    - 50% 5-year patency; patency not influenced by level of distal anastomosis
    - Distal lesions more limb threatening because of lack of collaterals

- Bypasses to **distal vessels** are usually used only for **limb salvage**
- Bypassed vessel needs to have **run-off below the ankle** for this to be successful
- **Synthetic grafts** have **decreased patency below the knee** → need to use saphenous vein
- **Extra-anatomic grafts** can be used to avoid hostile conditions in the abdomen (multiple previous operations in a frail patient)
- **Femoral-to-femoral crossover graft** – doubles blood flow to donor artery; can get vascular steal in donor leg
- ■ **Swelling** following lower extremity bypass:
  - <u>Early</u> – **reperfusion injury** and **compartment syndrome** (Tx: fasciotomies)
  - <u>Late</u> – DVT (Dx: U/S, Tx: **heparin, Coumadin**)
- ■ Complications of reperfusion of ischemic tissue – **compartment syndrome**, **lactic acidosis, hyperkalemia, myoglobinuria**
- ■ **Technical problem** – #1 cause of early failure of reversed saphenous vein grafts
- ■ **Atherosclerosis** – #1 cause of late failure of reversed saphenous vein grafts
- ■ **Patients with heel ulceration to bone** → Tx: amputation
- ■ **Dry gangrene** – noninfectious; can allow to autoamputate if small or just toes
  - Large lesions should be amputated
  - See if patient has correctable vascular lesion
- ■ **Wet gangrene** – infectious; need to remove infected necrotic material; antibiotics
  - Can be a surgical emergency if **extensive infection** (eg swollen red toe with pus coming out and red streaks up leg) or **systemic complications** occur (eg septic) – *may need **emergency amputation***
- ■ **Mal perforans ulcer**
  - At metatarsal heads – 2nd MTP joint most common
  - Diabetics; can have **osteomyelitis**
  - Tx: non-weightbearing, debridement of metatarsal head (need to remove cartilage), antibiotics; assess need for revascularization
- ■ **Percutaneous transluminal angioplasty** (PTA)
  - Excellent for common iliac artery stenosis
  - Best for short stenoses
  - Intima usually ruptured and media stretched, pushes the plaque out
  - Requires passage of wire first
- ■ **Compartment syndrome**
  - Is caused by **reperfusion injury** to the extremity (mediated by **PMNs**; occurs with cessation of blood flow to extremity and reperfusion > 4–6 hours later)
  - Reperfusion injury leads to **swelling of the muscle compartments** → raising compartment pressures, which can lead to ischemia
  - Symptoms: pain with passive motion; extremity feels tight and swollen
  - Most likely to occur in the **anterior compartment** of leg (get foot drop)
  - Dx: often based on clinical suspicion; compartment pressure > 20–30 mm Hg abnormal
  - Tx: **fasciotomies** (get all 4 compartments if in lower leg) → leave open 5–10 days
- ■ **Popliteal entrapment syndrome**
  - Most present with mild intermittent claudication
  - Men, 40s; *loss of pulses with plantar flexion*
  - Have medial deviation of artery around medial head of **gastrocnemius muscle**
  - Tx: **resection of medial head of gastrocnemius muscle**; may need arterial reconstruction
- ■ **Adventitial cystic disease**
  - Men, 40s; **popliteal fossa** most common area
  - *Often **bilateral*** – ganglia originate from adjacent joint capsule or tendon sheath
  - Symptoms: intermittent claudication; changes in symptoms with knee flexion/extension
  - Dx: angiogram
  - Tx: **resection of cyst**; vein graft if the vessel is occluded
- ■ **Arterial autografts** - radial artery grafts for CABG, IMA for CABG

AMPUTATIONS
- For gangrene, large non-healing ulcers, or unrelenting rest pain not amenable to surgery
- 50% mortality within 3 years for leg amputation
- **BKA** – 80% heal, 70% walk again, 5% mortality
- **AKA** – 90% heal, 30% walk again, 10% mortality
- Emergency amputation for **systemic complications** or **extensive infection**

ACUTE ARTERIAL EMBOLI

Clinical Distinctions Between Acute Arterial Embolism and Acute Arterial Thrombosis	
Embolism	Thrombosis
Arrhythmia	No arrhythmia
No prior claudication or rest pain	History of claudication or rest pain
Normal contralateral pulses	Contralateral pulses absent
No physical findings of chronic limb ischemia	Physical findings of chronic limb ischemia

- Usually do <u>not</u> have collaterals, signs of chronic limb ischemia, or history of claudication with emboli (do have collaterals with thrombosis)
- Contralateral leg usually has no chronic signs of ischemia and pulses are usually normal
- Symptoms: pain, paresthesia, poikilothermia, paralysis
- Extremity ischemia evolution: pallor (white) → cyanosis (blue) → marbling
- **Most common cause** – **atrial fibrillation**, recent MI with left ventricular thrombus, myxoma, aorto-iliac disease
- **Common femoral artery** most common site of peripheral obstruction from emboli
- Tx: **embolectomy** usual; need to get pulses back; postop angiogram
  - Consider fasciotomy if ischemia > 4-6 hours
  - Aortoiliac emboli (loss of both femoral pulses) can be treated with bilateral femoral artery cutdowns and bilateral embolectomies
- **Atheroma embolism** – cholesterol clefts that can lodge in small arteries
  - **Renals** most common site of atheroma embolization
  - **Blue toe syndrome** – flaking atherosclerotic emboli off abdominal aorta or branches
    - Patients typically have good distal pulses
    - **Aortoiliac disease** most common source
  - Dx: **chest/abdomen/pelvis CT scan** (look for aneurysmal source) and **ECHO** (clot or myxoma in heart)
  - Tx: may need aneurysm repair or arterial exclusion with bypass

ACUTE ARTERIAL THROMBOSIS
- These patients usually do <u>not</u> have arrhythmias
- Do have a history of claudication and have signs of chronic limb ischemia and poor pulses in the contralateral leg
- Tx: <u>**threatened limb**</u> (loss of sensation or motor function) → give heparin and go to OR for **thrombectomy**; if <u>**limb is not threatened**</u> → angiography for **thrombolytics**
- **Thrombosis of PTFE graft** → thrombolytics and anticoagulation; if limb threatened → OR for thrombectomy

RENAL VASCULAR DISEASE
- Right renal artery runs posterior to IVC
- Accessory renal arteries in 25%
- **Renovascular HTN** (renal artery stenosis) – bruits, diastolic blood pressure > 115, HTN, in children or premenopausal women, HTN resistant to drug therapy
  - **Renal atherosclerosis** – left side, proximal ⅓, men
  - **Fibromuscular dysplasia** – right side, distal ⅓, women

- Dx: angiogram
- Tx: **PTA** (percutaneous transluminal angioplasty); place **stent** if due to atherosclerotic disease
■ **Indications for nephrectomy with renal HTN** → atrophic kidney < 6 cm with persistently high renin levels

UPPER EXTREMITY
■ **Occlusive disease** – proximal lesions usually asymptomatic secondary to ↑ collaterals
  - **Subclavian artery** most common site of upper extremity stenosis
  - Tx: **PTA with stent**; common carotid to subclavian artery bypass if that fails
■ **Subclavian steal syndrome** – proximal subclavian artery stenosis resulting in reversal of flow through ipsilateral vertebral artery into the subclavian artery
  - Operate with limb or neurologic symptoms (usually vertebrobasilar symptoms)
  - Tx: **PTA with stent to subclavian artery**; common carotid to subclavian artery bypass if that fails
■ **Thoracic outlet syndrome** (TOS)
  - **Normal anatomy**
    - **Subclavian vein** – passes over the 1st rib <u>anterior</u> to the anterior scalene muscle, then behind clavicle
    - **Brachial plexus** and **subclavian artery** – pass over the 1st rib <u>posterior</u> to the anterior scalene muscle and anterior to the middle scalene muscle
  - General symptoms: back, neck, and/or arm pain/weakness/tingling (often worse with palpation/manipulation)
  - Dx: cervical spine and chest MRI, duplex U/S (vascular etiology), electromyelogram (EMG; neurologic etiology)

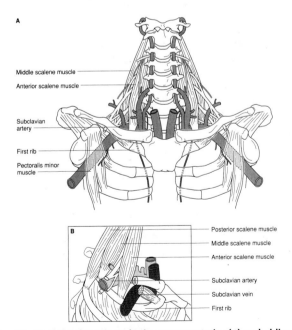

The normal anatomy of the thoracic outlet in anteroposterior (A) and oblique (B) views. The brachial plexus and subclavian artery traverse the narrow triangle formed by the anterior and middle scalene muscles and the first rib. The subclavian vein lies anteriorly.

- **Neurologic involvement** – much more common than vascular
- **#1 anatomic abnormality** – cervical rib
- **#1 cause of pain** – brachial plexus irritation
- **Brachial plexus irritation**
  - Usually have normal neurologic exam; tapping can reproduce symptoms (Tinsel's test)
  - **Ulnar nerve** distribution (C8–T1) most common (inferior portion of brachial plexus) → tricep muscle weakness and atrophy, weakness of intrinsic muscles of hand, weak wrist flexion
  - Tx: cervical rib and 1st rib resection, divide anterior scalene muscle
- **Subclavian vein**
  - Usually presents as **effort-induced thrombosis** of subclavian vein (Paget-von Schrötter disease; baseball pitchers) – **acutely painful, swollen, blue limb**
  - Venous thrombosis – much more common than arterial
  - Dx: **venography** is the gold standard for diagnosis, but **duplex U/S** makes the diagnosis and is quicker to get
  - 80% have associated thoracic outlet problem
  - Tx: **thrombolytics** initially; **repair at that admission** (cervical rib and 1st rib resection, divide anterior scalene muscle)
- **Subclavian artery**
  - Compression usually secondary to **anterior scalene hypertrophy** (weight lifters); least common cause of TOS
  - Symptoms – hand pain from ischemia
  - Absent radial pulse with head turned to ipsilateral side (Adson's test)
  - Dx: duplex U/S or angiogram (gold standard)
  - Tx: **surgery** → cervical rib and 1st rib resection, divide anterior scalene muscle; possible bypass graft if artery is too damaged or aneurysmal
- ■ **Motor function can remain in digits** after prolonged **hand ischemia** because motor groups are in the proximal forearm

MESENTERIC ISCHEMIA
- ■ Overall mortality 60%; usually involves the **superior mesenteric artery** (SMA)
- ■ Findings on abdominal CT that suggest intestinal ischemia – vascular occlusion, bowel wall thickening, intramural gas, portal venous gas
- ■ Most common causes of visceral ischemia:
  - **Embolic occlusion** – 50%
  - **Thrombotic occlusion** – 25%
  - **Nonocclusive** – 15%
  - **Venous thrombosis** – 5%
- ■ **SMA embolism**
  - Most commonly occurs near **origin of SMA** – heart #1 source (atrial fibrillation)
  - Pain out of proportion to exam; pain usually of sudden onset; hematochezia and peritoneal signs are late findings
  - May have a history of atrial fibrillation, endocarditis, recent MI, recent angiography
  - Dx: angiogram or abdominal CT with IV contrast
  - Tx: **embolectomy**, resect infarcted bowel if present
  - **SMA exposure** – divide ligament of Treitz, SMA is to the right of this near the base of the transverse colon mesentery
- ■ **SMA thrombosis**
  - Often history of chronic problems (food fear, weight loss)
  - Possible history of vasculitis or hypercoagulable state
  - Symptoms: similar to embolism; may have developed some collaterals
  - Dx: angiogram or abdominal CT with IV contrast

- Tx: **thrombectomy** (open or catheter directed; thrombolytics may have a role); may need **PTA with stent** or **open bypass** after the vessel is opened for any residual stenosis; resection of infarcted bowel

■ **Mesenteric vein thrombosis**
- Usually short segments of intestine involved; bloody diarrhea, crampy abdominal pain
- May have a history of vasculitis, hypercoagulable state, portal HTN
- Dx: abdominal CT scan or angiogram with venous phase
- Tx: **heparin** usual; resection of infarcted bowel if present

■ **Nonocclusive mesenteric ischemia**
- Spasm, low-flow states, hypovolemia, hemoconcentration, digoxin → final common pathway is **low cardiac output** to visceral vessels
- Risk factors: prolonged shock, CHF, prolonged cardiopulmonary bypass
- Symptoms: bloody diarrhea, pain
- **Watershed areas** (<u>Griffith's</u> - splenic flexure and <u>Sudak's</u> - upper rectum) most vulnerable
- Tx: **volume** resuscitation; catheter-directed **nitroglycerin** can ↑ visceral blood flow; also need to ↑ **cardiac output** (dobutamine); resection of infarcted bowel if present

■ **Median arcuate ligament syndrome**
- Causes **celiac artery** compression
- **Bruit near epigastrium**, chronic pain, weight loss, diarrhea
- Tx: transect **median arcuate ligament**; may need arterial reconstruction

■ **Chronic mesenteric angina**
- Weight loss secondary to **food fear** (visceral angina 30 minutes after meals)
- Get **lateral visceral vessel aortography** to see origins of **celiac** and **SMA**
- Tx: **PTA and stent**; bypass if that fails

■ **Arc of Riolan** is an important collateral between the SMA and celiac

VISCERAL AND PERIPHERAL ANEURYSMS

■ **Rupture** - most common complication of aneurysms <u>above</u> inguinal ligament
■ **Thrombosis** and **emboli** - most common complications of aneurysms <u>below</u> inguinal ligament
■ **Visceral artery aneurysms**
- Risk factors: medial fibrodysplasia, portal HTN, arterial disruption secondary to inflammatory disease (eg pancreatitis)
- **Repair all splanchnic artery aneurysms** (> 2 cm) when diagnosed (50% risk for rupture) *except* splenic
  - **Splenic artery aneurysm** - most common visceral aneurysm (more common in women; 2% risk of rupture)
    - Repair splenic artery aneurysms if **symptomatic**, if patient is **pregnant**, if occurs in **women of childbearing age**, or is > **3-4 cm**
    - High rate of pregnancy-related rupture - usually in **3rd trimester**
- Tx: **covered stent** (best); exclusion with bypass if that fails
- Splenic artery aneurysms can just be ligated if open procedure is required (have good collaterals)

■ **Renal** (> 1.5 cm) artery aneurysm - Tx: **covered stent**
■ **Iliac** (> 3.0 cm) or **femoral** (> 2.5 cm) artery aneurysms - Tx: **covered stent**
■ **Popliteal artery aneurysm**
- Most common peripheral aneurysm
- Leg exam reveals prominent popliteal pulses
- ½ are **bilateral**
- ½ have **another aneurysm elsewhere** (AAA, femoral, etc.)
- Most likely to get **thrombosis** or **emboli** with **limb ischemia**
- Can also get leg pain from compression of adjacent structures
- Dx: ultrasound

- Surgical indications: symptomatic, > 2 cm, or mycotic
- Tx: **exclusion and bypass** of all popliteal aneurysms; 25% have complication that requires amputation if not treated; *covered stent <u>not</u> recommended for these*

■ **Pseudoaneurysm**
- Collection of blood in continuity with the arterial system but <u>not</u> enclosed by all 3 layers of the arterial wall; most common location is the **femoral artery**
- Can result from percutaneous interventions or from disruption of a suture line between graft and artery
- If it occurs after **percutaneous intervention** → Tx: ultrasound-guided **compression with thrombin injection** (surgical repair if flow remains in the pseudoaneurysm after thrombin injection)
- If it occurs at a **suture line** early after surgery → *need surgical repair*
- Pseudoaneurysms that occur at suture lines late after surgery (months to years) → *suggests graft infection*

OTHER VASCULAR DISEASES

■ **Fibromuscular dysplasia**
- Young women; **HTN** if renals involved, **headaches** or **stroke** if carotids involved
- **Renal artery** most commonly involved vessel, followed by carotid and iliac
- String of beads appearance
- **Medial fibrodysplasia** most common variant (85%)
- Tx: **PTA** (*best*); bypass if that fails

■ **Buerger's disease**
- Young men, smokers
- Severe rest pain with bilateral ulceration; gangrene of digits, especially fingers
- **Corkscrew collaterals** on angiogram and severe distal disease; normal arterial tree proximal to popliteal and brachial vessels (is a <u>small vessel</u> disease)
- Tx: **stop smoking** or will require continued amputations

■ **Cystic medial necrosis syndromes**
- **Marfan's disease**
  - **Fibrillin defect** (connective tissue elastic fibers); marfanoid habitus, retinal detachment, aortic root dilatation
- **Ehlers–Danlos syndrome**
  - Many types of **collagen defects** identified
  - Easy bruising; hypermobile joints; tendency for **arterial rupture**, especially abdominal vessels
  - Get aneurysms and dissections
  - <u>No</u> angiograms → risk of laceration to vessel
  - Often too difficult to repair and need ligation of vessels to control hemorrhage

■ **Immune arteritis**
- **Temporal arteritis** (large artery)
  - Women, age > 55, headache, fever, blurred vision (risk of **blindness**)
  - Temporal artery biopsy → **giant cell** arteritis, **granulomas**
  - Inflammation of large vessels (aorta and branches)
  - Long segments of **smooth stenosis** alternating with segments of larger diameter
  - Tx: **steroids**, bypass of large vessels if needed; <u>no</u> endarterectomy
- **Polyarteritis nodosa** (medium artery)
  - Weight loss, rash, arthralgias, HTN, kidney dysfunction
  - Get **aneurysms** that thrombose or rupture
  - **Renals** most commonly involved
  - Tx: **steroids**
- **Kawasaki's disease** (medium artery)
  - Children; febrile viral illness with erythematous mucosa and epidermis
  - Get **aneurysms** of **coronary arteries** and brachiocephalic vessels

- Die from arrhythmias
- Tx: **steroids**, possible **CABG**
- **Hypersensitivity angiitis** (small artery)
  - Often secondary to drug/tumor antigens
  - Symptoms: **rash** (palpable purpura), fever, symptoms of end-organ dysfunction
  - Tx: **calcium channel blockers**, **pentoxifylline**, stop offending agent
- ■ **Radiation arteritis**
  - **Early** – sloughing and thrombosis (obliterative endarteritis)
  - **Late** (1–10 years) – fibrosis, scar, stenosis
  - **Late late** (3–30 years) – advanced atherosclerosis
- ■ **Raynaud's disease** – young women; *pallor* → *cyanosis* → *rubor*
  - Tx: **calcium channel blockers**, warmth

VENOUS DISEASE
- ■ **Greater saphenous vein** – joins femoral vein near groin; runs medially
- ■ <u>No</u> clamps on IVC → will tear
- ■ **Left renal vein** can be ligated near the IVC in emergencies because of collaterals (left gonadal vein, left adrenal vein); right renal vein does <u>not</u> have these collaterals
- ■ **Dialysis access grafts**
  - Most common failure of A-V grafts for dialysis – **venous obstruction** secondary to *intimal hyperplasia*
  - **Cimino** – radial artery to cephalic vein; wait 6 weeks to use → allows vein to mature
  - **Interposition graft** (eg brachiocephalic loop graft) – wait 6 weeks to allow fibrous scar to form
- ■ **Acquired A-V fistula** – usually secondary to trauma; can get peripheral arterial insufficiency, CHF, aneurysm, limb-length discrepancy
  - Most need repair → **lateral venous suture**; arterial side may need patch or bypass graft; try to place interposing tissue so it does not recur
- ■ **Varicose veins**
  - Smoking, obesity, low activity
  - Tx: **sclerotherapy**
- ■ **Venous ulcers**
  - Secondary to venous valve incompetence (90%)
  - Ulceration occurs above and posterior to malleoli
  - Ulcers < 3 cm often heal without surgery
  - Tx: **Unna boot** compression cures 90%
  - May need to ligate perforators or have vein stripping of greater saphenous vein (see below)
- ■ **Venous insufficiency**
  - Aching, swelling, night cramps, brawny edema, venous ulcers
  - **Edema** – secondary to incompetent perforators and/or valves
  - Elevation brings relief
  - Tx: leg wraps, ambulation with avoidance of long standing
    - Greater saphenous **vein stripping** (for saphenofemoral valve incompetence) or **removal of perforators** (if just perforator valves are incompetent; stab avulsion technique) for severe symptoms or recurrent ulceration despite medical Tx
- ■ **Superficial thrombophlebitis** – nonbacterial inflammation
  - Tx: NSAIDs, warm packs, ambulation
- ■ **Suppurative thrombophlebitis** – pus fills vein; fever, ↑ WBCs, erythema, fluctuance; usually associated with infection following a peripheral IV
  - Tx: resect entire vein
- ■ **Migrating thrombophlebitis** – pancreatic CA

■ **Normal venous Doppler ultrasound** – augmentation of flow with distal compression or release of proximal compression
■ **Sequential compression devices** (SCDs) – help prevent blood clots by ↓ venous stasis and ↑ tPA release
■ **Deep venous thrombosis** (DVT)
  • Most common in calf
  • Pain, tenderness, calf swelling
  • **Left leg 2×** more involved than right (longer left iliac vein compressed by right iliac artery)
  • Risk factors: **Virchow's triad** → venous stasis, hypercoagulability, venous wall injury
  • **Calf** DVT – minimal swelling
  • **Femoral** DVT – ankle and calf swelling
  • **Iliofemoral** DVT – leg swelling
  • **Phlegmasia alba dolens** – tenderness, pallor (whiteness), edema
    ○ Tx: heparin
  • **Phlegmasia cerulea dolens** – tenderness, cyanosis (blueness), massive edema
    ○ Tx: heparin; rarely need surgery
  • DVT Tx: **heparin, Coumadin**
  • **IVC filter indications** – contraindication to anticoagulation; PE while on Coumadin, free-floating ileofemoral thrombi; after pulmonary embolectomy
  • **Pulmonary embolism with filter in place** – comes from ovarian veins, inferior vena cava superior to filter, or from upper extremity via the superior vena cava
■ **Venous thrombosis with central line** – pull out central line if not needed, then heparin; can try to treat with systemic heparin or TPA down line if the access site is important

LYMPHATICS
■ **Do not contain a basement membrane**
■ **Not found in bone, muscle, tendon, cartilage, brain, or cornea**
■ Deep lymphatics have valves
■ **Lymphedema**
  • Occurs when lymphatics are obstructed, too few in number, or nonfunctional
  • Leads to woody edema secondary to fibrosis in subcutaneous tissue – toes, feet, ankle, leg
  • **Cellulitis** and **lymphangitis** secondary to minor trauma are big problems
  • **Strep** most common infection
  • Congenital lymphedema L > R
  • Tx: leg elevation, compression, antibiotics for infection
■ **Lymphangiosarcoma**
  • Raised blue/red coloring; early metastases to lung
  • **Stewart–Treves syndrome** – lymphangiosarcoma associated with breast axillary dissection and chronic lymphedema
■ **Lymphocele** following surgery
  • Usually after dissection in the groin (eg after femoral to popliteal bypass)
  • Leakage of **clear fluid**
  • Tx: percutaneous drainage (can try a couple of times); resection if that fails
  • Can inject **isosulfan blue dye** into foot to identify the lymphatic channels supplying the lymphocele if having trouble locating

- **Gastrin** – produced by G cells in stomach **antrum**
  - Secretion stimulated by amino acids, vagal input (acetylcholine), calcium, ETOH, antral distention, pH > 3.0
  - Secretion inhibited by pH < 3.0, somatostatin, secretin, CCK
  - Target cells – **parietal cells** and **chief cells**
  - Response – ↑ HCl, intrinsic factor, and pepsinogen secretion
  - **Omeprazole** blocks H/K ATPase of parietal cell **(final pathway for H$^+$ release)**
- **Somatostatin** – mainly produced by D (somatostatin) cells in stomach **antrum**
  - Secretion stimulated by acid in duodenum
  - Target cells – many; is the great inhibitor
  - Response – inhibits gastrin and HCl release; inhibits release of insulin, glucagon, secretin, and motilin; ↓ pancreatic and biliary output
  - **Octreotide** (somatostatin analogue) – can be used to ↓ pancreatic fistula output
- **CCK** – produced by I cells of **duodenum**
  - Secretion stimulated by amino acids and fatty acid chains
  - Response – gallbladder contraction, relaxation of sphincter of Oddi, ↑ **pancreatic enzyme secretion**
- **Secretin** – produced by S cells of **duodenum**
  - Secretion stimulated by fat, bile, pH < 4.0
  - Secretion inhibited by pH > 4.0, gastrin
  - Response – ↑ **pancreatic HCO$_3^-$ release**, inhibits gastrin release (this is reversed in patients with gastrinoma), and inhibits HCl release
    - <u>High</u> pancreatic duct output – ↑ HCO$_3^-$, ↓ Cl$^-$
    - <u>Slow</u> pancreatic duct output – ↑ Cl$^-$, ↓ HCO$_3^-$ (carbonic anhydrase in duct exchanges HCO$_3^-$ for Cl$^-$)
- **Vasoactive intestinal peptide** – produced by cells in **gut and pancreas**
  - Secretion stimulated by fat, acetylcholine
  - Response – ↑ **intestinal secretion** (water and electrolytes) and **motility**
- **Glucagon** – mainly released by alpha cells of **pancreas**
  - Secretion stimulated by ↓ glucose, ↑ amino acids, acetylcholine
  - Secretion inhibited by ↑ glucose, ↑ insulin, somatostatin
  - Response – glycogenolysis, gluconeogenesis, lipolysis, ketogenesis, ↓ gastric acid secretion, ↓ gastrointestinal motility, relaxes sphincter of Oddi
- **Insulin** – released by beta cells of the **pancreas**
  - Secretion stimulated by glucose, glucagons, CCK
  - Secretion inhibited by somatostatin
  - Response – cellular glucose uptake; promotes protein synthesis
- **Pancreatic polypeptide** – secreted by islet cells in **pancreas**
  - Secretion stimulated by food, vagal stimulation, other GI hormones
  - Response – ↓ **pancreatic** and **gallbladder secretion**
- **Motilin** – released by intestinal cells of gut
  - Secretion stimulated by duodenal acid, food, vagus input
  - Secretion inhibited by somatostatin, secretin, pancreatic polypeptide, duodenal fat
  - Response – ↑ **intestinal motility** (small bowel; phase III peristalsis) → **erythromycin** acts on this receptor
- **Bombesin** (gastrin-releasing peptide) – ↑ intestinal motor activity, ↑ pancreatic enzyme secretion, ↑ gastric acid secretion

- **Peptide YY** – released from terminal ileum following a fatty meal → inhibits acid secretion and stomach contraction; inhibits gallbladder contraction and pancreatic secretion
- **Anorexia** – mediated by hypothalamus
- **Bowel recovery**
  - Small bowel 24 hours
  - Stomach 48 hours
  - Large bowel 3–5 days

ANATOMY AND PHYSIOLOGY
■ Mucosa (squamous epithelium), submucosa, and muscularis propria (longitudinal muscle layer); _no serosa_
■ Upper ⅓ esophagus – **striated muscle**
■ Middle ⅓ and lower ⅓ esophagus – **smooth muscle**
■ Vessels directly off the aorta are the major blood supply to the thoracic esophagus

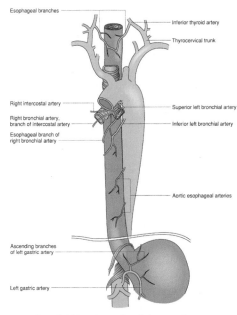

Arterial blood supply of the esophagus.

■ **Cervical esophagus** – supplied by **inferior thyroid artery**
■ **Abdominal esophagus** – supplied by **left gastric** and inferior phrenic arteries
■ **Venous drainage** – hemi-azygous and azygous veins in chest
■ **Lymphatics** – upper ⅔ drains cephalad, lower ⅓ caudad
■ **Right vagus nerve** – travels on posterior portion of stomach as it exits chest; becomes **celiac plexus**; also has the criminal nerve of Grassi → can cause persistently high acid levels postoperatively if left undivided after vagotomy
■ **Left vagus nerve** – travels on anterior portion of stomach; goes to **liver** and **biliary tree**
■ **Thoracic duct** – travels from right to left at **T4–5** as it ascends mediastinum; inserts into left subclavian vein
■ **Upper esophageal sphincter** (UES; 15 cm from incisors) – is the **cricopharyngeus muscle** (circular muscle, prevents air swallowing); recurrent laryngeal nerve innervation
  • Normal UES pressure at rest: 60 mm Hg
  • Normal UES pressure with food bolus: 15 mm Hg

- **Cricopharyngeus muscle** – most common site of esophageal perforation (usually occurs with EGD)
- **Aspiration with brainstem stroke** – failure of cricopharyngeus to relax

■ **Lower esophageal sphincter** (40 cm from incisors) – relaxation mediated by inhibitory neurons; normally contracted at resting state (prevents reflux); is an anatomic zone of high pressure, <u>not</u> an anatomic sphincter
- Normal LES pressure at rest: 15 mm Hg
- Normal LES pressure with food bolus: 0 mm Hg

■ **Anatomic areas of esophageal narrowing**
- Cricopharyngeus muscle
- Compression by the left mainstem bronchus and aortic arch
- Diaphragm

■ **Swallowing stages** – CNS initiates swallow
- **Primary peristalsis** – occurs with food bolus and swallow initiation
- **Secondary peristalsis** – occurs with incomplete emptying and esophageal distention; propagating waves
- **Tertiary peristalsis** – non-propagating, non-peristalsing (dysfunctional)
- UES and LES are normally contracted between meals

■ **Swallowing mechanism** – soft palate occludes nasopharynx, larynx rises and airway opening is blocked by epiglottis, cricopharyngeus relaxes, pharyngeal contraction moves food into esophagus; **LES relaxes** soon after initiation of swallow (**vagus** mediated)

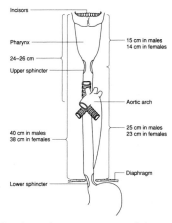

Important clinical endoscopic measurements of the esophagus in adults.

■ **Surgical approach**
- Cervical esophagus – **left**
- Upper ⅔ thoracic – **right** (avoids the aorta)
- Lower ⅓ thoracic – **left** (left-sided course in this region)

■ **Hiccoughs**
- Causes – gastric distention, temperature changes, ETOH, tobacco
- Reflex arc – vagus, phrenic, sympathetic chain T6–12

■ **Esophageal dysfunction**
- **Primary** – achalasia, diffuse esophageal spasm, nutcracker esophagus
- **Secondary** – GERD (most common), scleroderma

- **Endoscopy** – best test for **heartburn** (can visualize esophagitis)
- **Barium swallow** – best test for **dysphagia** or **odynophagia** (better at picking up masses)
- **Meat impaction** – Dx and Tx: endoscopy

PHARYNGOESOPHAGEAL DISORDERS
- Trouble in transferring food from mouth to esophagus
- Most commonly neuromuscular disease – myasthenia gravis, muscular dystrophy, stroke
- **Liquids** worse than solids
- **Plummer–Vinson syndrome** – can have upper esophageal web; Fe-deficient anemia. Tx: **dilation, Fe**; need to screen for **oral CA**

DIVERTICULA
- **Zenker's diverticulum** – caused by ↑ pressure during swallowing
  - Is a **false diverticulum** located **posteriorly**
  - Occurs between the **pharyngeal constrictors** and **cricopharyngeus**
  - Caused by **failure of the cricopharyngeus to relax**
  - Symptoms: upper esophageal dysphagia, choking, halitosis
  - Dx: **barium swallow studies**, manometry; risk for perforation with EGD and Zenker's
  - Tx: *cricopharyngeal myotomy* (key point); Zenker's itself can either be resected or suspended (removal of diverticula is not necessary)
    - Left cervical incision; leave drains in; esophagogram POD #1

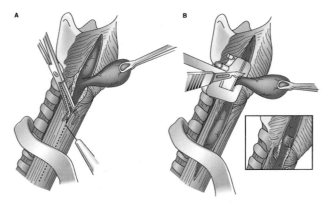

Cricopharyngomyotomy and concomitant resection of a pharyngoesophageal diverticulum. *(A)* A cricopharyngomyotomy is performed. *(B)* After completion of the cricopharyngomyotomy, the base of the pouch is crossed with a TA-30 stapler and amputated.

- **Traction diverticulum**
  - Is a **true diverticulum** – usually lies **lateral**
  - Due to inflammation, granulomatous disease, tumor
  - Usually found in the mid-esophagus
  - Symptoms: regurgitation of undigested food, dysphagia
  - Tx: excision and primary closure if symptomatic, may need palliative therapy (ie XRT) if due to invasive CA; if asymptomatic, leave alone

- **Epiphrenic diverticulum**
  - Rare; associated with **esophageal motility disorders** (eg <u>achalasia</u>)
  - Most common in the distal 10 cm of the esophagus
  - Most are asymptomatic; can have dysphagia and regurgitation
  - Dx: esophagram and esophageal manometry
  - Tx: **diverticulectomy** and **esophageal myotomy** on the side opposite the diverticulectomy if symptomatic

ACHALASIA
- **Dysphagia**, **regurgitation**, **weight loss**, respiratory symptoms
- Caused by **lack of peristalsis** and **failure of LES to relax** after food bolus
- Secondary to **neuronal degeneration** in muscle wall
- Manometry – ↑ **LES pressure, incomplete LES relaxation**, <u>no</u> **peristalsis**
- Can get tortuous dilated esophagus and epiphrenic diverticula; bird's beak appearance
- Tx: **balloon dilatation of LES** → effective in 80%; nitrates, calcium channel blocker
  - If medical Tx and dilation fail → **Heller myotomy** (left thoracotomy, **myotomy** of <u>lower</u> esophagus only; also need partial Nissen fundoplication)
- *T. cruzi* can produce similar symptoms

DIFFUSE ESOPHAGEAL SPASM
- **Chest pain**, may have dysphagia; may have psychiatric history
- Manometry – frequent **strong non-peristaltic unorganized contractions**, LES relaxes normally
- Tx: calcium channel blocker, nitrates; **Heller myotomy** if those fail (myotomy of <u>upper</u> and <u>lower</u> esophagus)
- Surgery usually less effective for diffuse esophageal spasm than for achalasia

NUTCRACKER ESOPHAGUS
- **Chest pain** and **dysphagia**
- Manometry – **high-amplitude peristaltic contractions**; LES relaxes normally
- Tx: calcium channel blocker, nitrates; **Heller myotomy** if those fail (myotomy of <u>upper</u> and <u>lower</u> esophagus)
- Surgery usually less effective for nutcracker than for achalasia

SCLERODERMA
- **Fibrous replacement** of esophageal **smooth muscle**
- Causes **dysphagia** and loss of LES tone with **massive reflux** and **strictures**
- Tx: esophagectomy usual if severe

GASTROESOPHAGEAL REFLUX DISEASE (GERD)
- **Normal anatomic protection from GERD** – need LES competence, normal esophageal body, normal gastric reservoir
- GERD caused by ↑ acid exposure to esophagus from loss of gastroesophageal barrier
- Get **heartburn** symptoms 30–60 minutes after meals; worse lying down
- Can also have asthma symptoms (cough), choking, aspiration
- Make sure patient does not have another cause for pain (check for unusual symptoms):
  - **Dysphagia/odynophagia** – need to worry about tumors
  - **Bloating** – suggests aerophagia and delayed gastric emptying (Dx: gastric emptying study)
  - **Epigastric pain** – suggests peptic ulcer, tumor

- Most treated empirically with **PPI** (omeprazole, 99% effective)
- Failure of PPI despite escalating doses (give it 3-4 weeks) → need diagnostic studies
- Dx: **pH probe** *(best test)*, **endoscopy, histology, manometry** (resting LES < 6 mm Hg)
- **Surgical indications**: failure of medical Tx, avoidance lifetime meds, young patients
- Tx: **Nissen fundoplication** → divide short gastrics, pull esophagus into abdomen, approximate crura, 270- (partial) or 360-degree **gastric fundus** wrap
  - Phrenoesophageal membrane is an extension of the **transversalis fascia**
  - Key maneuver for wrap is identification of the **left crura**
  - Complications – injury to spleen, diaphragm, esophagus, or pneumothorax
  - **Belsey** – approach is through the chest
  - **Collis gastroplasty** – when not enough esophagus exists to pull down into abdomen, can staple along stomach cardia and create a "new" esophagus (neo-esophagus)
  - Most common cause of dysphagia following Nissen – ***wrap is too tight***

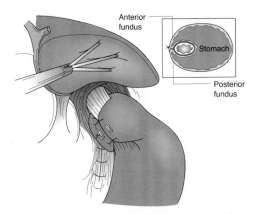

Anterior fundus

Stomach

Posterior fundus

Fixation of the fundoplication. The fundoplication is sutured in place with a single U-stitch of 2-0 Prolene pledgeted on the outside. A 60-French mercury-weighted bougie is passed through the gastroesophageal junction prior to fixation of the wrap to assure a floppy fundoplication. Inset illustrates the proper orientation of the fundic wrap.

HIATAL HERNIA
- **Type I** – sliding hernia from dilation of hiatus (most common); often associated with GERD
- **Type II** – paraesophageal; hole in the diaphragm alongside the esophagus, normal GE junction. <u>Symptoms: chest pain, dysphagia, early satiety</u>
- **Type III** – combined
- **Type IV** – entire stomach in the chest plus another organ (ie colon, spleen)
- With type II, still need **Nissen** as diaphragm repair can affect LES; also helps anchor stomach
- **Paraesophageal hernia** (type II) – usually need repair → high risk of incarceration; may want to avoid repair in the elderly and frail

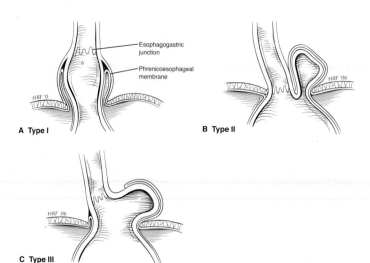

Classification of hiatal hernia. *(A)* Type 1, sliding. *(B)* Type II, pure paraesophageal. *(C)* Type III, mixed hernia. (From Critchlow J. Paraesophageal herniation. In: Fischer JE, Bland KI, et al, eds. *Mastery of Surgery.* 5th ed. Philadelphia, PA: Lippincott Williams & Wilkins; 2007, with permission.)

SCHATZKI'S RING
- Almost all patients have an associated sliding **hiatal hernia**
- Symptoms: dysphagia
- Tx: **dilatation of the ring** and **PPI** usually sufficient; *do not resect*

BARRETT'S ESOPHAGUS
- Squamous **metaplasia** to **columnar epithelium**
- Occurs with long-standing exposure to gastric reflux
- **Cancer** risk ↑ 50 times (adenocarcinoma)
- **Severe Barrett's dysplasia** is an indication for esophagectomy
- Uncomplicated Barrett's can be treated like GERD (ie PPI or Nissen) – surgery will ↓ esophagitis and further metaplasia but will **not** prevent malignancy or cause regression of the columnar lining
  - Need careful follow-up with EGD for lifetime, even after Nissen

ESOPHAGEAL CANCER
- Esophageal tumors are almost always malignant; early invasion of nodes
- Spreads quickly along **submucosal lymphatic channels**
- Symptoms: dysphagia (especially solids), weight loss
- Risk factors: ETOH, tobacco, achalasia, caustic injury, nitrosamines
- Dx: **esophagram** (best test for dysphagia)
- **Unresectability** – hoarseness (RLN invasion), Horner's syndrome (brachial plexus invasion), phrenic nerve invasion, malignant pleural effusion, malignant fistula, airway invasion, vertebral invasion
  - **Chest and abdominal CT** is the **best single test for resectability**
- **Adenocarcinoma** is the #1 esophageal cancer – **not** squamous
  - **Adenocarcinoma** – usually in **lower** ⅓ of esophagus; **liver** metastases most common
  - **Squamous cell carcinoma** – usually in **upper** ⅔ of esophagus; **lung** metastases most common

- **Nodal disease outside the area of resection** (ie supraclavicular or celiac nodes – M1 disease) – contraindication to esophagectomy
- **Pre-op chemo-XRT** may downstage tumors and make them resectable
- **Esophagectomy** – 5% mortality from surgery; curative in 20%
  - **Right gastroepiploic artery** – primary blood supply to stomach after replacing esophagus (have to divide left gastric and short gastrics)
  - **Transhiatal approach** – abdominal and neck incisions; bluntly dissect intra-thoracic esophagus; may have ↓ mortality from esophageal leaks with cervical anastomosis
  - **Ivor Lewis** – abdominal incision and right thoracotomy → exposes all of the intrathoracic esophagus; intrathoracic anastomosis
  - **3-Hole esophagectomy** – abdominal, thoracic, and cervical incisions
  - Need **pyloromyotomy** with these procedures
  - **Colonic interposition** – may be choice in young patients when you want to preserve gastric function; 3 anastomoses required; blood supply depends on colon marginal vessels
  - After esophagectomy → need contrast study on postop day 7 to rule out leak
  - **Postoperative strictures** – most can be dilated
- **Chemotherapy** – **5FU** and **cisplatin** (for node-positive disease or use pre-op to shrink tumors)
- **XRT** – may help downstage tumors
- **Malignant fistulas** – most die within 3 months due to aspiration; Tx – esophageal stent for palliation

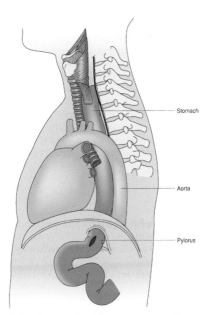

Final position of the mobilized stomach in the posterior mediastinum after transhiatal esophagectomy and cervical esophagogastric anastomosis. The gastric fundus has been suspended from the cervical prevertebral fascia, and an end-to-side cervical esophago-gastrostomy has been performed. The pylorus is now located several centimeters below the level of the diaphragmatic hiatus.

LEIOMYOMA

- Most common benign esophageal tumor; located in **muscularis propria**
- Symptoms: **dysphagia**; usually in **lower ⅔** of esophagus (<u>smooth muscle cells</u>)
- Dx: **esophagram**, endoscopic U/S (EUS), CT scan (need to rule out CA)
- **Do not biopsy** → can form scar and make subsequent resection difficult
- Tx: > **5 cm** or **symptomatic** → excision (enucleation) via thoracotomy

ESOPHAGEAL POLYPS

- Symptoms: dysphagia, hematemesis
- 2nd most common benign tumor of the esophagus; usually in the cervical esophagus
- Small lesions can be resected with endoscopy; larger lesions require cervical incision

CAUSTIC ESOPHAGEAL INJURY

- <u>No</u> NG tube. Do <u>not</u> induce vomiting. <u>Nothing</u> to drink
- **Alkali** – causes deep liquefaction necrosis, especially liquid (eg Drano)
  - Worse injury than acid; also more likely to cause cancer
- **Acid** – causes coagulation necrosis; mostly causes gastric injury
- **Chest** and **abdominal CT scan** to look for free air and signs of perforation
- **Endoscopy** to assess lesion
  - Do <u>not</u> use with suspected perforation and do <u>not</u> go past a site of severe injury
- Serial exams and plain films required
- **Degree of injury**:
  - **Primary burn** – hyperemia
    - Tx: observation and conservative therapy
    - **Conservative Tx**: IVFs, spitting, antibiotics, oral intake after 3–4 days; may need future serial dilation for strictures (usually cervical)
    - Can also get shortening of esophagus with GERD (Tx: PPI)
  - **Secondary burn** – ulcerations, exudates, and sloughing
    - Tx: prolonged observation and conservative therapy as above
    - **Indications for esophagectomy** – sepsis, peritonitis, mediastinitis, free air, mediastinal or stomach wall air, crepitance, contrast extravasation, pneumothorax, large effusion
  - **Tertiary burn** – deep ulcers, charring, and lumen narrowing
    - Tx: as above; **esophagectomy** usually necessary
    - Alimentary tract not restored until after patient recovers from the caustic injury
- Caustic esophageal perforations require esophagectomy (are <u>not</u> repaired due to extensive damage)

PERFORATIONS

- Usually the result of **EGD**
- **Cervical esophagus** near **cricopharyngeus muscle** most common site
- Symptoms: pain, dysphagia, tachycardia
- Dx: CXR initially (look for free air); **Gastrografin swallow** followed by barium swallow
- **Criteria for nonsurgical management** – contained perforation by contrast, self-draining, <u>no</u> systemic effects
  - **Conservative Tx**: IVFs, NPO, spit, broad-spectrum antibiotics
- **Non-contained perforations**:
  - If quick to diagnose it (**< 24 hours**) and area has **minimal contamination** → **primary repair** with drains
    - Need **longitudinal myotomy** to see the full extent of injury
    - Consider **muscle flaps** (eg intercostal) to cover repair

- If late to diagnose it (> **48 hours**) or area has **extensive contamination** →
  - Neck – just place **drains** *(no esophagectomy)*
  - Chest – need 1) **resection** (esophagectomy, cervical esophagostomy) or 2) **exclusion and diversion** (cervical esophagostomy, staple across distal esophagus, washout mediastinum, place chest tubes – late esophagectomy at time of gastric replacement)
  - Gastric replacement of esophagus late when patient fully recovers
- **Esophagectomy** – may be needed for any perforation (contained or non-contained) in patients with **severe intrinsic disease** (eg burned out esophagus from achalasia, esophageal CA)
■ **Boerhaave's syndrome**
  - **Forceful vomiting** followed by **chest pain** – perforation most likely to occur in the left lateral wall of esophagus, 3–5 cm above the GE junction
  - **Hartmann's sign** – mediastinal crunching on auscultation
  - *Highest mortality of all perforations* – early diagnosis and treatment improve survival
  - Dx: Gastrografin swallow
  - Tx: as above for esophageal perforations

ANATOMY AND PHYSIOLOGY

- Stomach transit time 3–4 hours
- **Peristalsis** – occurs only in distal stomach (**antrum**)
- Gastroduodenal pain sensed through afferent sympathetic fibers T5–10
- **Blood supply**
  - **Celiac trunk** – left gastric, common hepatic artery, splenic artery
    - Left gastroepiploic and short gastric are branches of splenic artery
  - **Greater curvature** – right and left gastroepiploics, short gastrics
    - Right gastroepiploic is a branch of gastroduodenal artery
  - **Lesser curvature** – right and left gastrics
    - **Right gastric** is a branch off the common hepatic artery
  - **Pylorus** – gastroduodenal artery
- Mucosa – lined with **simple columnar** epithelium

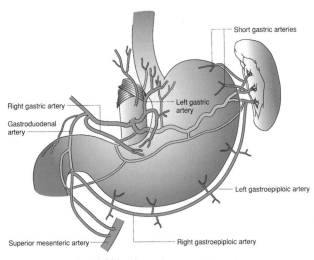

Arterial blood supply of the stomach.

- **Cardia glands** – mucus secreting
- **Fundus and body glands**
  - **Chief cells** – **pepsinogen** (1st enzyme in proteolysis)
  - **Parietal cells** – release H^+ and **intrinsic factor**
    - **Acetylcholine** (vagus nerve), **gastrin** (from G cells in antrum), and **histamine** (from mast cells) cause H^+ release
    - **Acetylcholine** and **gastrin** activate *phospholipase* (PIP → DAG + IP_3 to ↑ **Ca**); Ca-calmodulin activates **phosphorylase kinase** →↑ H^+ release
    - **Histamine** activates *adenylate cyclase* → cAMP → activates **protein kinase A** →↑ H^+ release

- **Phosphorylase kinase** and **protein kinase A** phosphorylate H^+/K^+ **ATPase** to $\uparrow H^+$ secretion and K^+ absorption
- **Omeprazole** blocks H^+/K^+ ATPase in parietal cell membrane (**final pathway for H^+** release)
- **Inhibitors of parietal cells** – somatostatin, prostaglandins (PGE_1), secretin, CCK
- **Intrinsic factor** – binds B_{12} and the complex is reabsorbed in the terminal ileum

■ **Antrum and pylorus glands**
- **Mucus** and HCO_3^- secreting glands – protect stomach
- **G cells** release **gastrin** – reason why antrectomy is helpful for ulcer disease
  - *Inhibited* by H^+ **in duodenum**
  - *Stimulated* by **amino acids, acetylcholine**
- **D cells** – secrete **somatostatin**; inhibit gastrin and acid release

■ **Brunner's glands** – in <u>duodenum</u>; secrete **alkaline mucus**
■ **Somatostatin, CCK,** and **secretin** – released with antral and duodenal acidification
■ **Rapid gastric emptying** – previous surgery (#1), ulcers
■ **Delayed gastric emptying** – diabetes, opiates, anticholinergics, hypothyroidism
■ **Trichobezoars** (hair) – hard to pull out
- Tx: EGD generally inadequate; likely need gastrostomy and removal

■ **Phytobezoars** (fiber) – often in diabetics with poor gastric emptying
- Tx: enzymes, EGD, diet changes

■ **Dieulafoy's ulcer** – vascular malformation; can bleed
■ **Ménétrièr's disease** – mucous cell hyperplasia, $\uparrow$ rugal folds

GASTRIC VOLVULUS
■ Associated with type II (paraesophageal) hernia
■ Nausea without vomiting; severe pain; usually **organoaxial volvulus**
■ Tx: reduction and Nissen

MALLORY–WEISS TEAR
■ Secondary to forceful vomiting
■ Presents as hematemesis following severe retching
■ Bleeding often stops spontaneously
■ Dx/Tx: **EGD** with **hemo-clips**; tear is usually on lesser curvature (near GE junction)
■ If continued bleeding, may need gastrostomy and oversewing of the vessel

VAGOTOMIES
■ **Vagotomy** – both truncal and proximal forms $\uparrow$ **liquid emptying** $\rightarrow$ **vagally mediated receptive relaxation is removed** (results in $\uparrow$ gastric pressure that accelerates liquid emptying)
■ **Truncal vagotomy** – divides vagal trunks at level of esophagus; $\downarrow$ **emptying of solids**
■ **Proximal vagotomy** (highly selective) – divides individual fibers, preserves "crow's foot"; **normal emptying of solids**
■ Addition of **pyloroplasty** to truncal vagotomy results in $\uparrow$ **solid emptying**
■ Other alterations caused by **truncal vagotomy**:
- **Gastric effects** – $\downarrow$ acid output by 90%, $\uparrow$ gastrin, gastrin cell hyperplasia
- **Nongastric effects** – $\downarrow$ exocrine pancreas function, $\downarrow$ postprandial bile flow, $\uparrow$ gallbladder volumes, $\downarrow$ release of vagally mediated hormones
- **Diarrhea** (40%) – most common problem following vagotomy
  - Caused by **sustained MMCs** (migrating motor complex) forcing bile acids into the colon

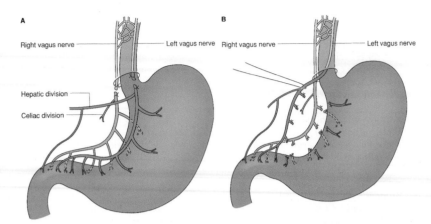

Truncal vagotomy and proximal gastric vagotomy. (*A*) With truncal vagotomy, both nerve trunks are divided at the level of the diaphragmatic hiatus. (*B*) Proximal gastric vagotomy involves division of the vagal fibers that supply the gastric fundus. Branches to the antropyloric region of the stomach are not transected, and the hepatic and celiac divisions of the vagus nerves remain intact.

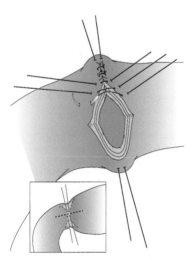

Pyloroplasty formation. A Heineke–Mikulicz pyloroplasty involves a longitudinal incision of the pyloric sphincter followed by a transverse closure.

UPPER GASTROINTESTINAL BLEEDING (UGI BLEEDING)

- **Risk factors**: previous UGI bleed, peptic ulcer disease, NSAID use, smoking, liver disease, esophageal varices, splenic vein thrombosis, sepsis, burn injuries, trauma, severe vomiting
- Dx/Tx: **EGD** (confirm bleeding is from ulcer); can potentially treat with hemo-clips, Epi injection, cautery

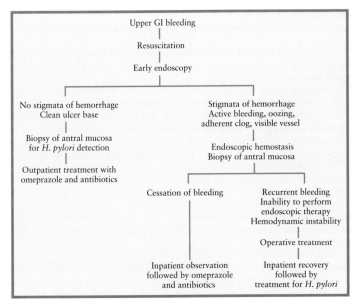

Treatment of bleeding ulceration.

- Slow bleeding and having trouble localizing source → **tagged RBC scan**
- **Biggest risk factor for rebleeding** at the time of EGD – #1 *spurting blood vessel* (60% chance of rebleed), #2 visible blood vessel (40% chance of rebleed), #3 diffuse oozing (30% chance of rebleed)
- **Highest risk factor for mortality** with non-variceal UGI bleed – *continued or re-bleeding*
- Patient with **liver failure** is likely bleeding from esophageal varices, <u>not</u> an ulcer → Tx: EGD with **variceal bands** or **sclerotherapy**; **TIPS** if that fails

DUODENAL ULCERS

- From ↑ **acid production** and ↓ **defense**
- **Most common peptic ulcer**; more common in men
- Usually in 1st part of the duodenum; **usually anterior**
  - **Anterior** ulcers <u>perforate</u>
  - **Posterior** ulcers <u>bleed</u> from <u>gastroduodenal artery</u>
- Symptoms: epigastric pain radiating to the back; abates with eating but recurs 30 minutes after
- Dx: endoscopy
- Tx: **proton pump inhibitor** (PPI; omeprazole), triple therapy for *Helicobacter pylori* → **bismuth salts**, **amoxicillin**, and **metronidazole/tetracycline** (BAM or BAT)

- Surgery for ulcer rarely indicated since **PPIs**
- Need to rule out **gastrinoma** in patients with complicated ulcer disease (Zollinger-Ellison syndrome – **gastric acid hypersecretion**, **peptic ulcers**, and **gastrinoma**)
- **Surgical indications:**
  - **Perforation**
  - **Protracted bleeding** despite EGD therapy
  - **Obstruction**
  - **Intractability** despite medical therapy
  - **Inability to rule out cancer** (ulcer remains despite treatment) → requires resection of ulcer
  - *If patient has been on a **PPI**, an **acid-reducing surgical procedure** is required in addition to surgery for any complications*
- **Surgical options** (acid-reducing surgery)
  - **Proximal vagotomy** – lowest rate of complications, no need for antral or pylorus procedure; 10%–15% ulcer recurrence; 0.1% mortality
  - **Truncal vagotomy** and **pyloroplasty** – 5%–10% ulcer recurrence, 1% mortality
  - **Truncal vagotomy** and **antrectomy** – 1%–2% ulcer recurrence (lowest rate of recurrence), 2% mortality
  - Reconstruction after antrectomy – **Roux-en-Y gastro-jejunostomy** (best)
    - Less **dumping syndrome** and **reflux gastritis** compared to Billroth I (gastro-duodenal anastomosis) and Billroth II (gastro-jejunal anastomosis)
- **Bleeding**
  - Most frequent complication of duodenal ulcers
  - Usually minor but can be life threatening
  - Major bleeding – > 6 units of blood in 24 hours or patient remains hypotensive despite transfusion
  - Tx: **EGD 1st** – hemoclips, cauterize, Epi injection
  - **Surgery** – duodenotomy and **gastroduodenal artery** (GDA) **ligation**
    - Avoid hitting common bile duct (posterior) with GDA ligation
    - If patient has been on a PPI, need acid-reducing surgery as well

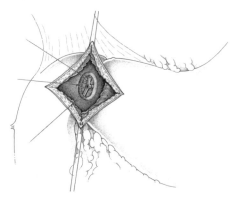

Proper suture ligation of a bleeding ulcer arising from the gastroduodenal artery requires a 3-suture ligation. The proximal and distal branches of the gastroduodenal artery are transfixed. A third suture, U type in configuration, is necessary to transfix the transverse pancreatic branch of the artery. (From Bailey RW, Martinez JM. Laparoscopic highly selective vagotomy. In: Fischer JE, Bland KI, et al, eds. *Mastery of Surgery*. 5th ed. Philadelphia, PA: Lippincott Williams & Wilkins; 2007, with permission.)

- **Obstruction**
  - **PPI** and **serial dilation** initial treatment of choice
  - Surgical options – **antrectomy** and **truncal vagotomy** (best); include ulcer in resection if it's located proximal to ampulla of Vater
  - Need to Bx area of resection to rule out CA
- **Perforation**
  - 80% will have free air
  - Patients usually have sudden sharp epigastric pain; can have generalized peritonitis
  - Pain can radiate to the pericolic gutters with dependent drainage of gastric content
  - Tx: **Graham patch** (place **omentum** over the perforation)
    - Also need acid-reducing surgery if the patient has been on a PPI

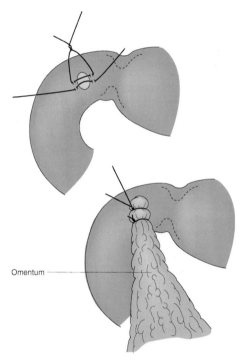

Omentum

Omental patching of perforated duodenal ulcer.

- **Intractability**
  - > 3 months without relief while on escalating doses of PPI
  - Based in EGD mucosal findings, not symptoms
  - Tx: acid-reducing surgery

GASTRIC ULCERS
- Older men; slow healing
- Risk factors: male, tobacco, ETOH, NSAIDs, *H. pylori*, uremia, stress (burns, sepsis, and trauma), steroids, chemotherapy
- 80% on lesser curvature of the stomach

- Hemorrhage is associated with higher mortality than duodenal ulcers
- Symptoms: epigastric pain radiating to the back; relieved with eating but recurs 30 minutes later; melena or guaiac-positive stools
- *Best test for H. pylori* – **histologic examination of biopsies from antrum**
- CLO test (rapid urease test) – test for *H. pylori*, detects urease released from *H. pylori*
- **Types:**
  - **Type I** – **lesser curve <u>low</u> along body of stomach**; due to ↓ <u>mucosal protection</u>
  - **Type II** – **2 ulcers** (lesser curve and duodenal); similar to duodenal ulcer with <u>high acid secretion</u>
  - **Type III** – **pre-pyloric ulcer**; similar to duodenal ulcer with <u>high acid secretion</u>
  - **Type IV** – **lesser curve <u>high</u> along cardia** of stomach; ↓ <u>mucosal protection</u>
  - **Type V** – **ulcer** associated with NSAIDs
- **Surgical indications** – perforation, bleeding not controlled with EGD, obstruction, cannot exclude malignancy, intractability (> 3 months without relief – based on mucosal findings)
- Tx: **truncal vagotomy** and **antrectomy** best for complications; try to **include the ulcer** with resection (extended antrectomy) – need **separate ulcer excision** if that is not possible (gastric ulcers are resected at time of surgery due to high risk of **gastric CA**)
  - Omental patch and ligation of bleeding vessels are <u>poor options</u> for gastric ulcers due to high recurrence of symptoms and risk of gastric CA in the ulcer

STRESS GASTRITIS
- Occurs 3–10 days after event; lesions appear in fundus first
- Tx: **PPI**
- EGD with cautery of specific bleeding point may be effective

CHRONIC GASTRITIS
- Type A (fundus) – associated with pernicious anemia, autoimmune disease
- Type B (antral) – associated with *H. pylori*
- Tx: **PPI**

GASTRIC CANCER
- **Pain** unrelieved by eating, **weight loss**
- **Antrum** has 40% of gastric cancers
- Accounts for 50% of cancer-related deaths in Japan
- Dx: EGD
- **Risk factors** – adenomatous polyps, tobacco, previous gastric operations, intestinal metaplasia, atrophic gastritis, pernicious anemia, type A blood, nitrosamines
- **Adenomatous polyps** – 15% risk of cancer. Tx: endoscopic resection
- **Krukenberg tumor** – metastases to ovaries
- **Virchow's nodes** – metastases to supraclavicular node
- **Intestinal-type gastric CA** – ↑ in high-risk populations, older men; Japan; rare in United States
  - Surgical Tx: try to perform **subtotal gastrectomy** (need 10-cm margins)
- **Diffuse gastric cancer** (linitis plastica) – in low-risk populations, women; most common type in the United States
  - Diffuse lymphatic invasion; <u>no</u> glands
  - **Less favorable prognosis** than intestinal-type gastric CA (overall 5-YS – 25%)
  - Surgical Tx: **total gastrectomy** because of diffuse nature of linitis plastica
- Chemotherapy (poor response): 5FU, doxorubicin, mitomycin C
- Metastatic disease outside area of resection → contraindication to resection unless performing surgery for palliation

- **Palliation of gastric CA**
  - **Obstruction** – proximal lesions can be **stented**; distal lesions can be bypassed with **gastrojejunostomy**
  - Low to moderate **bleeding** or **pain** – Tx: XRT
  - If these fail, consider palliative gastrectomy for obstruction or bleeding

GASTROINTESTINAL STROMAL TUMORS (GISTs)
- Most common benign gastric neoplasm, although can be malignant
- Symptoms: usually asymptomatic, but obstruction and bleeding can occur
- Hypoechoic on ultrasound; smooth edges
- Dx: biopsy – are **C-KIT–positive**
- Considered malignant if **> 5 cm** or **> 5 mitoses / 50 HPF** (high-powered field)
- Tx: **resection** with 1-cm margins
- *Chemotherapy with **imatinib*** (Gleevec; tyrosine kinase inhibitor) if malignant

MUCOSA-ASSOCIATED LYMPHOID TISSUE LYMPHOMA (MALT LYMPHOMA)
- Related to *H. pylori* infection
- Usually regresses after treatment for *H. pylori*
- Stomach most common location
- Tx: ***triple-therapy antibiotics for H. pylori*** and surveillance; if MALT does not regress, need XRT

GASTRIC LYMPHOMAS
- Have ulcer symptoms; stomach is the most common location for extra-nodal lymphoma
- Usually **non-Hodgkin's lymphoma** (B cell)
- Dx: EGD with biopsy
- Chemotherapy and XRT are primary treatment modalities; surgery for complications
- Surgery possibly indicated only for stage I disease (tumor confined to stomach mucosa) and then only partial resection is indicated
- Overall 5-year survival rate > 50%

MORBID OBESITY

Criteria for Patient Selection for Bariatric Surgery (Need All 4)
■ Body mass index > 40 kg/m² or body mass index > 35 kg/m² with coexisting comorbidities
■ Failure of nonsurgical methods of weight reduction
■ Psychological stability
■ Absence of drug and alcohol abuse

- Central obesity – worse prognosis in general population
- Operative mortality is approximately 1%
- **Gets better after surgery** – diabetes, cholesterol, sleep apnea, HTN, urinary incontinence, GERD, venous stasis ulcers, pseudotumor cerebri, joint pain, migraines, depression, polycystic ovarian syndrome, nonalcoholic fatty liver disease
- **Roux-en-Y gastric bypass**
  - Better weight loss than just banding
  - Risk of marginal ulcers, leak, necrosis, B_{12} deficiency (intrinsic factor needs acidic environment to bind B_{12}), iron-deficiency anemia (bypasses duodenum where Fe absorbed), gallstones (from rapid weight loss)

- Perform **cholecystectomy** during operation if stones present
- **UGI** on postop day 2
- **10% failure rate** due to high-carbohydrate snacking
- **Leak**
  - **Ischemia** – most common cause of leak
  - **Signs of leak** – ↑ RR, ↑ HR, abdominal pain, fever, elevated WBCs
  - Dx: **UGI**
  - Tx: **early leak** (not contained) → re-op; **late leak** (weeks out from surgery, likely contained) → percutaneous drain, antibiotics
- **Marginal ulcers** – develop in 10%. Tx: PPI
- **Stenosis** – usually responds to serial dilation
- **Dilation of excluded stomach postop** – hiccoughs, large stomach bubble
  - Dx: **AXR**; Tx: **G-tube** (gastrostomy tube)
- **Small bowel obstruction** – nausea and vomiting, intermittent abdominal pain; AXR shows dilated small bowel; this is a *surgical emergency* in patients with gastric bypass due to the high risk of **small bowel herniation**, **strangulation**, **infarction**, and subsequent **necrosis**; Tx: surgical exploration

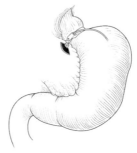

Laparoscopic adjustable gastric band. (From Jones DB, Schneider BE. Surgical management of morbid obesity. In: Fischer JE, Bland KI, et al, eds. *Mastery of Surgery*. 5th ed. Philadelphia, PA: Lippincott Williams & Wilkins; 2007, with permission.)

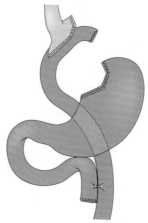

Laparoscopic proximal Roux-en-Y gastric bypass (retrocolic, retrogastric).

■ **Jejunoileal bypass**
- These operations are no longer done
- Associated with **liver cirrhosis, kidney stones,** and **osteoporosis** ($\downarrow$ Ca)
- Need to correct these patients and perform Roux-en-Y gastric bypass if ileojejunal bypasses are encountered

POSTGASTRECTOMY COMPLICATIONS
■ **Dumping syndrome**
- Can occur after gastrectomy or after vagotomy and pyloroplasty
- Occurs from rapid entering of **carbohydrates** into the small bowel
- 90% of cases resolve with medical therapy
- 2 **phases**
  - Hyperosmotic load causes **fluid shift** into bowel (hypotension, diarrhea, dizziness)
  - **Hypoglycemia** from reactive $\uparrow$ in insulin and $\downarrow$ in glucose (2nd phase rarely occurs)
- Can almost always be treated medically (and dietary changes)
- Tx: small, low-fat, low-carbohydrate, high-protein meals; no liquids with meals, no lying down after meals; **octreotide**
- **Surgical options** (rarely needed)
  - Conversion of Billroth I or Billroth II to Roux-en-Y gastrojejunostomy
  - Operations to $\uparrow$ gastric reservoir (jejunal pouch) or $\uparrow$ emptying time (reversed jejunal loop)
■ **Alkaline reflux gastritis**
- Postprandial epigastric pain associated with N/V; pain not relieved with vomiting
- Dx: evidence of **bile reflux** into stomach, histologic evidence of **gastritis**
- Tx: PPI, cholestyramine, metoclopramide
- Surgical option: conversion of Billroth I or Billroth II to Roux-en-Y gastrojejunostomy with afferent limb 60 cm distal to gastrojejunostomy
■ **Chronic gastric atony**
- Delayed gastric emptying
- Symptoms: nausea, vomiting, pain, early satiety
- Dx: gastric emptying study
- Tx: metoclopramide, prokinetics
- Surgical option: near-total gastrectomy with Roux-en-Y
■ **Small gastric remnant** (early satiety)
- Actually want this for gastric bypass patients
- Dx: EGD
- Tx: small meals
- Surgical option: jejunal pouch construction
■ **Blind-loop syndrome**
- With Billroth II or Roux-en-Y; caused by **poor motility**
- Symptoms: **pain, steatorrhea** (bacterial deconjugation of bile), B_{12} **deficiency** (bacteria use it up), malabsorption
- Caused by **bacterial overgrowth** (*E. coli*, GNRs) from stasis in afferent limb
- Dx: **EGD of afferent limb** with **aspirate and culture** for organisms
- Tx: tetracycline and Flagyl, metoclopramide to improve motility
- Surgical option: re-anastomosis with shorter (40-cm) afferent limb
■ **Afferent-loop obstruction**
- With Billroth II or Roux-en-Y; caused by **mechanical obstruction** of afferent limb
- Symptoms: RUQ pain, steatorrhea; nonbilious vomiting, pain relieved with bilious emesis
- Risk factors – long afferent limb with Billroth II or Roux-en-Y
- Dx: **CT scan**
- Tx: balloon dilation may be possible
- Surgical option: re-anastomosis with shorter (40-cm) afferent limb to relieve obstruction

- **Efferent-loop obstruction**
  - Symptoms of obstruction – nausea, vomiting, abdominal pain
  - Dx: UGI, EGD
  - Tx: balloon dilation
  - Surgical option: find site of obstruction and relieve it
- **Post-vagotomy diarrhea**
  - Secondary to non-conjugated **bile salts** in the colon (osmotic diarrhea)
  - Caused by **sustained postprandial organized MMCs**
  - Tx: cholestyramine, octreotide
  - Surgical option: reversed interposition jejunal graft
- **Duodenal stump blow-out** – place lateral duodenostomy tube and drains
- **PEG complications** – insertion into the liver or colon

ANATOMY AND PHYSIOLOGY

- ◼ **Hepatic artery variants**
  - **Right hepatic artery** off **superior mesenteric artery** (**#1 hepatic artery variant**; 20%) courses behind pancreas, posterolateral to the common bile duct
  - **Left hepatic artery** off **left gastric artery** (about 20%) – found in gastrohepatic ligament medially
- ◼ **Falciform ligament** – separates medial and lateral segments of the left lobe; attaches liver to anterior abdominal wall; extends to umbilicus and carries remnant of the umbilical vein
- ◼ **Ligamentum teres** – carries the obliterated umbilical vein to the undersurface of the liver; extends from the falciform ligament
- ◼ Line drawn from the middle of the **gallbladder fossa** to **IVC** (portal fissure or Cantlie's line) separates the right and left liver lobes

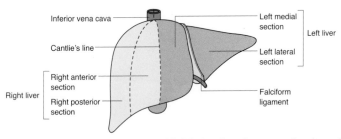

Anatomic division of the liver into right and left halves by a line extending from the gallbladder fossa posteriorly to the inferior vena cava.

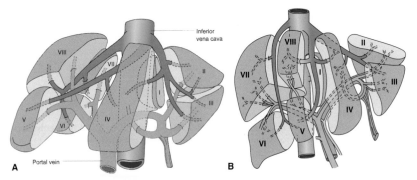

Functional divisions of the liver and liver segments according to Couinaud's nomenclature. These are both anterior views with (A) viewed slightly from the patient's left and (B) viewed slightly from the patient's right.

- ◼ **Segments**
  - I – caudate
  - II – superior left lateral segment
  - III – inferior left lateral segment
  - IV – left medial segment (quadrate lobe)

- V – inferior right anteromedial segment
- VI – inferior right posterolateral segment
- VII – superior right posterolateral segment
- VIII – superior right anteromedial segment
■ Glisson's capsule – peritoneum that covers the liver
■ Bare area – area on the posterior-superior surface of liver not covered by Glisson's capsule
■ Triangular ligaments – lateral and medial extensions of the coronary ligament on the posterior surface of the liver; made up of peritoneum
■ **Portal triad** enters **segments IV** and **V**
■ **Gallbladder** lies under **segments IV** and **V**

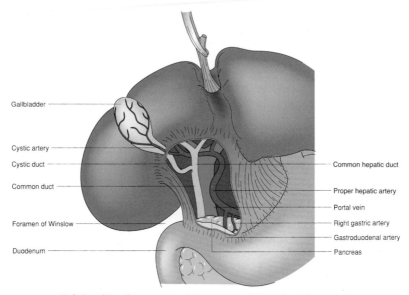

Relationship of structures within the hepatoduodenal ligament.

■ **Kupffer cells** – **liver macrophages**
■ **Portal triad** – **common bile duct** (lateral), **portal vein** (posterior), and **proper hepatic artery** (medial); come together in the **hepatoduodenal ligament** (porta hepatis)
■ **Pringle maneuver** – porta hepatis clamping; will not stop hepatic vein bleeding
■ **Foramen of Winslow** (entrance to lesser sac)
  - Anterior – portal triad
  - Posterior – IVC
  - Inferior – duodenum
  - Superior – liver
■ **Portal vein**
  - Forms from **superior mesenteric vein** joining **splenic vein** (no valves)
  - **Inferior mesenteric vein** – enters splenic vein
  - **Portal veins** – 2 in liver; ⅔ of hepatic blood flow
    - <u>Left</u> – goes to segments II, III, and IV
    - <u>Right</u> – goes to segments V, VI, VII, and VIII

■ **Arterial blood supply**
  • Right, left, and middle hepatic arteries (follows hepatic vein system below)
  • Middle hepatic artery MC a branch off the left hepatic artery
  • Most primary and secondary **liver tumors** are supplied by the <u>hepatic artery</u>
■ **Hepatic veins** – 3 hepatic veins; drain into IVC
  • <u>Left</u> – II, III, and superior IV
  • <u>Middle</u> – V and inferior IV
  • <u>Right</u> – VI, VII, and VIII
  • **Middle hepatic vein** comes off left hepatic vein in 80% before going into IVC; other 20% goes directly into IVC
  • **Accessory right hepatic veins** – drain medial aspect of right lobe directly to IVC
  • **Inferior phrenic veins** – also drain directly into the IVC
■ **Caudate lobe** – receives separate right and left portal and arterial blood flow; drains directly into IVC via separate hepatic veins
■ **Alkaline phosphatase** – normally located in <u>canalicular</u> membrane
■ **Nutrient uptake** – occurs in <u>sinusoidal</u> membrane
■ **Ketones** – usual energy source for liver; glucose is converted to glycogen and stored
  • Excess glucose converted to fat
■ **Urea** – synthesized in the liver
■ <u>**Not**</u> **made in the liver** – von Willebrand factor and factor VIII (endothelium)
■ Liver stores large amount of **fat-soluble vitamins**
■ **B$_{12}$** – the only water-soluble vitamin stored in the liver
■ **Bleeding** and **bile leak** – most common problems with hepatic resection
■ **Hepatocytes most sensitive to ischemia** – central lobular (acinar zone III)
■ 75% of normal liver can be safely resected

BILIRUBIN
■ A breakdown product of **hemoglobin** (Hgb → heme → biliverdin → bilirubin)
■ Conjugated to **glucuronic acid** (glucuronyl transferase) in the liver → improves water solubility
■ Conjugated bilirubin is actively secreted into bile
■ **Urobilinogen**
  • Breakdown of conjugated bilirubin by bacteria in the terminal ileum occurs
  • **Free bilirubin** is reabsorbed, converted to **urobilinogen**, and eventually released in the urine as **urobilin** (yellow color)
  • Excess urobilinogen turns urine dark like cola

BILE
■ Contains **bile salts** (85%), proteins, phospholipids (lecithin), cholesterol, and bilirubin
■ Final bile composition determined by active (Na/K ATPase) reabsorption of water in gallbladder
■ **Cholesterol** – used to make bile salts/acids
■ **Bile salts** are conjugated to **taurine** or **glycine** (improves water solubility)
  • <u>Primary bile acids</u> (salts) – **cholic** and **chenodeoxycholic**
  • <u>Secondary bile acids</u> (salts) – **deoxycholic** and **lithocholic** (dehydroxylated primary bile acids by bacteria in gut)
■ **Lecithin** – main biliary phospholipid
■ **Bile** solubilizes cholesterol and emulsifies fats in the intestine, forming **micelles**, which enter enterocytes by fusing with membrane

JAUNDICE
■ Occurs when total bilirubin > 2.5; 1st evident <u>under the tongue</u>
■ Maximum bilirubin is 30 unless patient had underlying renal disease, hemolysis, or bile duct–hepatic vein fistula

- Elevated **un-conjugated bilirubin** – prehepatic causes (hemolysis); hepatic deficiencies of uptake or conjugation
- Elevated **conjugated bilirubin** – secretion defects into bile ducts; excretion defects into GI tract (stones, strictures, tumor)
- **Syndromes**
  - **Gilbert's disease** – abnormal conjugation; mild defect in **glucuronyl transferase**
  - **Crigler–Najjar disease** – inability to conjugate; severe deficiency of **glucuronyl transferase**; high unconjugated bilirubin → life-threatening disease
  - **Physiologic jaundice of newborn** – immature glucuronyl transferase; high unconjugated bilirubin
  - **Rotor's syndrome** – deficiency in storage ability; high conjugated bilirubin
  - **Dubin–Johnson syndrome** – deficiency in secretion ability; high conjugated bilirubin

VIRAL HEPATITIS

- All hepatitis viral agents can cause **acute hepatitis**
- **Fulminant hepatic failure** can occur with hepatitis B, D, and E (<u>very rare</u> with A and C)
- Hepatitis B, C, and D can cause **chronic hepatitis** and **hepatoma**
- **Hepatitis A** (RNA) – serious consequences uncommon
- **Hepatitis B** (DNA)
  - Anti-HBc-IgM (c = core) is elevated in the first 6 months; IgG then takes over
  - Vaccination – have ↑ anti-HBs (s = surface) antibodies only
  - ↑ anti-HBc and ↑ anti-HBs antibodies and <u>no</u> HBs antigens (HBsAg) → patient had infection with recovery and subsequent immunity
- **Hepatitis C** (RNA) – can have long incubation period; currently most common viral hepatitis leading to liver TXP
- **Hepatitis D** (RNA) – cofactor for hepatitis B (worsens prognosis)
- **Hepatitis E** (RNA) – fulminant hepatic failure in pregnancy, most often in 3rd trimester

LIVER FAILURE

- **Most common cause of liver failure** – <u>cirrhosis</u> (palpable liver, jaundice, ascites)
- Best indicator of synthetic function in patient with cirrhosis – **prothrombin time** (PT)
- **Acute liver failure** (fulminant hepatic failure) – 80% mortality
  - Outcome determined by the course of **encephalopathy**
  - Consider **urgent liver TXP listing** if King's College criteria are met

King's College Criteria of Poor Prognostic Indicators

Acetaminophen-Induced ALF

Arterial pH < 7.3 irrespective of coma grade
OR all of the following:
INR > 6.5, creatinine > 3.4 mg/dL (300 μmol/L), grade III/IV encephalopathy

Non–Acetaminophen-Induced ALF

INR > 6.5
OR any three of the following:
Age < 10 or > 40, drug toxicity or undetermined etiology, jaundice > 7 days before encephalopathy, INR > 3.5, bilirubin > 17 mg/dL (300 μmol/L)

ALF, acute liver failure; INR, international normalized ratio.

- **Hepatic encephalopathy**
  - Liver failure leads to inability to metabolize → get buildup of ammonia, mercantanes, and false neurotransmitters
  - Causes other than liver failure for encephalopathy – GI bleeding, infection (spontaneous bacterial peritonitis [SBP]), electrolyte imbalances, drugs

- May need to embolize previous therapeutic shunts or other major collaterals
- Tx: **lactulose** – **cathartic** that gets rid of bacteria in the gut and acidifies colon (preventing NH_3 uptake by converting it to ammonium), titrate to 2–3 stools/day
  - **Limit protein intake** (< 70 g/day)
  - **Branched-chain amino acids** – metabolized by skeletal muscle, may be of some value
  - <u>No</u> antibiotics unless for a specific infection
  - **Neomycin** (gets rid of ammonia-producing bacteria from gut)
- **Cirrhosis mechanism** – hepatocyte destruction → fibrosis and scarring of liver → ↑ hepatic pressure → portal venous congestion → lymphatic overload → leakage of splanchnic and hepatic lymph into peritoneum → ascites
- **Paracentesis for ascites** – replace with albumin (1 g for every 100 cc removed)
- **Ascites** – from **hepatic/splanchnic** lymph
  - Tx: water restriction (1–1.5 L/d), ↓ NaCl (1–2 g/d), diuretics (spironolactone counteracts hyperaldosteronism seen with liver failure), paracentesis, TIPS, prophylactic antibiotics to prevent SBP (norfloxacin; used if previous SBP or current UGI bleed)
- **Aldosterone is elevated with liver failure** – secondary to impaired hepatic metabolism and impaired GFR
- **Hepatorenal syndrome** – progressive renal failure; same lab findings as prerenal azotemia; usually a sign of end-stage liver disease
  - Tx: stop diuretics, give volume; no good therapy other than liver TXP
- **Neurological changes** – asterixis; sign that liver failure is progressing
- **Postpartum liver failure with ascites** – from hepatic vein thrombosis; has an infectious component
  - Dx: SMA arteriogram with venous phase contrast
  - Tx: **heparin** and **antibiotic**

SPONTANEOUS BACTERIAL PERITONITIS
- Fever, abdominal pain, PMNs > 250 in fluid, positive cultures
- *E. coli* (#1), pneumococci, streptococci
- Most commonly mono-organism; if not, need to worry about bowel perforation
- Risk factors – prior SBP, UGI bleed (variceal hemorrhage), low-protein ascites
- Tx: 3rd-generation cephalosporins; patients usually respond within 48 hours

ESOPHAGEAL VARICES
- **Bleed** by rupture
- Tx: **banding** and **sclerotherapy** (95% effective)
  - **Vasopressin** (splanchnic artery constriction) and **octreotide** (↓ portal pressure by ↓ blood flow) can be used to temporize
  - Patients with history of CAD should receive NTG while on vasopressin
  - Sengstaken–Blakemore esophageal tube – has a balloon used to control variceal bleeding; risk of rupture of the esophagus (hardly used anymore)
- **Propranolol** – may help prevent re-bleeding; no good role acutely
- Can get later strictures from sclerotherapy; usually easily managed with dilatation
- **TIPS** is needed for refractory variceal bleeding

PORTAL HYPERTENSION
- **Pre-sinusoidal obstruction** – schistosomiasis, congenital hepatic fibrosis, portal vein thrombosis (50% of portal HTN in children)
- **Sinusoidal obstruction** – cirrhosis
- **Post-sinusoidal obstruction** – Budd–Chiari syndrome (hepatic vein occlusive disease), constrictive pericarditis, CHF
- Normal portal vein pressure < 12 mm Hg
- **Coronary veins** act as collaterals between the portal vein and the systemic venous system of the lower esophagus (azygous vein)

- Portal HTN leads to esophageal variceal hemorrhage, ascites, splenomegaly, and hepatic encephalopathy
- Shunts can decompress portal system
- **TIPS** – used for protracted bleeding, progression of coagulopathy, visceral hypoperfusion, or refractory ascites
  - Allows antegrade flow
  - Complication of TIPS – *development of* **encephalopathy**

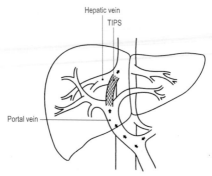

Transjugular intrahepatic portosystemic shunt (TIPS). A catheter is passed into the hepatic vein via the jugular vein. A needle, inserted through the catheter, is passed from the hepatic vein through the liver tissue into a major portal vein branch. The liver tract is dilated with an angioplasty balloon catheter, and the tract is kept open after deployment of an expandable metal stent. (From Krige JEJ, Bornman PC. Endoscopic therapy in the management of esophageal varices: injection sclerotherapy and variceal ligation. In: Fischer JE, Bland KI, et al, eds. *Mastery of Surgery.* 5th ed. Philadelphia, PA: Lippincott Williams & Wilkins; 2007, with permission.)

- **Splenorenal shunt** – low rate of encephalopathy; need to ligate left adrenal vein, left gonadal vein, inferior mesenteric vein, coronary vein, and pancreatic branches of splenic vein
  - Used only for Child's A cirrhotics who present just with bleeding (rarely used anymore)
  - Contraindicated in patients with refractory ascites, as splenorenal shunts can worsen ascites
- Child's B or C with indication for shunt → **TIPS**
- Child's A that just has bleeding as symptom → consider **splenorenal shunt** (more durable); otherwise TIPS
- **Child-Pugh Score** correlates with mortality after open shunt placement

Child-Pugh Score	1 Point	2 Points	3 Points
Albumin	> 3.5	3–3.5	< 3.0
Bilirubin	< 2.5	2.5–4	> 4
Encephalopathy	None	Minimal	Severe
Ascites	None	Treatable with meds	Refractory
INR	< 1.7	1.7–2.3	> 2.3

- Child's A (5–6 pts)   2% mortality with shunt
- Child's B (7–9 pts)   10% mortality with shunt
- Child's C (10 pts or greater)   50% mortality with shunt
- **Portal HTN in children**
  - Usually caused by **extra-hepatic portal vein thrombosis**
  - Most common cause of **massive hematemesis** in children

BUDD–CHIARI SYNDROME
- Occlusion of hepatic veins or IVC
- RUQ pain, hepatosplenomegaly, ascites, fulminant hepatic failure, muscle wasting, variceal bleeding
- Dx: angiogram with venous phase, CT angiogram; liver biopsy shows sinusoidal dilatation, congestion, centrilobular congestion
- Tx: **porta-caval shunt** (needs to connect to the IVC above the obstruction)

SPLENIC VEIN THROMBOSIS
- Can lead to **isolated gastric varices** without elevation of pressure in the rest of the portal system
- These gastric varices can **bleed**
- Splenic vein thrombosis is most often caused by **pancreatitis**
- Tx: **splenectomy** if symptomatic

LIVER ABSCESSES
- **Amebic**
  - ↑ LFTs; ↑ in **right lobe** of liver, usually single
  - Primary infection occurs in the colon → **amebic colitis**
  - Risk factors – travel to Mexico, ETOH; fecal–oral transmission
  - Positive serology for *Entamoeba histolytica* – 90% have infection
  - Symptoms: fever, chills, RUQ pain, ↑ WBCs, jaundice, hepatomegaly
  - Reaches liver via **portal vein**
  - Cultures of abscess often sterile → protozoa exist only in peripheral rim
  - Can usually diagnose based on CT characteristics
  - Tx: **Flagyl**; aspiration *only* if refractory; surgery *only* if free rupture
- *Echinococcus*
  - Forms cyst (hydatid cyst)
  - Positive **Casoni skin test**, positive **serology**
  - **Sheep** – carriers; **dogs** – human exposure; ↑ in **right lobe** of the liver
  - *Do not aspirate → can leak out and cause **anaphylactic shock***
  - Abdominal CT shows ectocyst (calcified) and endocyst (double-walled cyst)
  - Pre-op ERCP for jaundice, ↑ LFTs, or cholangitis to check for communication with the biliary system
  - Tx: **pre-op albendazole** (2 weeks) and **surgical removal** (intra-op can inject cyst with alcohol to kill organisms, then aspirate out); need to get all of cyst wall
  - Do not spill cyst contents – can cause anaphylactic shock
- **Schistosomiasis**
  - Maculopapular rash, ↑ eosinophils
  - Sigmoid colon – primary infection; fine granulation tissue, petechiae, ulcers
  - Can cause variceal bleeding
  - Tx: **praziquantel** and control of variceal bleeding
- **Pyogenic abscess**
  - Account for 80% of all abscesses
  - Symptoms: fever, chills, weight loss, RUQ pain, ↑ LFTs, ↑ WBCs, sepsis
  - ↑ in right lobe; 15% mortality with sepsis
  - GNRs – #1 organism (***E. coli***)
  - Most commonly secondary to **contiguous infection** from **biliary tract**
  - Can occur following **bacteremia** from other types of infections (diverticulitis, appendicitis)
  - Dx: aspiration
  - Tx: **CT-guided drainage** and **antibiotics**; surgical drainage for unstable condition and continued signs of sepsis

BENIGN LIVER TUMORS

- **Hepatic adenomas**
  - Women, steroid use, OCPs
  - 80% are symptomatic; 20% risk of significant bleeding (rupture)
  - Can become malignant
  - More common in **right lobe**
  - Symptoms: pain, ↑ LFTs, ↓ BP (from rupture), palpable mass
  - Dx: no Kupffer cells in adenomas, thus **no uptake on sulfur colloid scan** (cold)
    - MRI demonstrates a hypervascular tumor
  - Tx:
    - Asymptomatic – stop OCPs; if regression, no further therapy is needed; if no regression, patient needs resection of the tumor
    - Symptomatic – tumor resection for bleeding and malignancy risk; embolization if multiple and unresectable
- **Focal nodular hyperplasia**
  - Has **central stellate scar** that may look like cancer
  - No malignancy risk; very unlikely to rupture
  - Dx: abdominal CT; has Kupffer cells, so **will take up sulfur colloid on liver scan**
  - MRI/CT scan demonstrates a hypervascular tumor
  - Tx: conservative therapy (*no resection*)
- **Hemangiomas**
  - Most common benign hepatic tumor
  - Rupture rare; most asymptomatic; more common in women
  - Avoid biopsy → risk of hemorrhage
  - Dx: MRI and CT scan show **peripheral to central enhancement**
    - Appears as a **hypervascular** lesion
  - Tx: conservative unless symptomatic, then **surgery ± pre-op embolization**; steroids (possible XRT) for unresectable disease
  - **Rare complications of hemangioma** – consumptive **coagulopathy** (Kasabach–Merritt syndrome) and **CHF**; these complications are usually seen in children
- **Solitary cysts**
  - Congenital; women, right lobe; walls have a characteristic blue hue
  - Complications from these cysts are rare; most can be left alone

MALIGNANT LIVER TUMORS

- **Metastases:primary ratio** is **20:1**
- **Hepatocellular CA** (hepatoma)
  - **Most common cancer worldwide**
  - Risk factors – HepB (#1 cause worldwide), HepC, ETOH, hemochromatosis, alpha-1-antitrypsin deficiency, primary sclerosing cholangitis, aflatoxins, hepatic adenoma, steroids, pesticides
  - **Not** risk factors – primary biliary cirrhosis, Wilson's disease
  - **Clear cell, lymphocyte infiltrative**, and **fibrolamellar types** (adolescents and young adults) have the best prognosis
  - **AFP level** correlates with tumor size
  - 30% 5-year survival rate with resection
  - Few hepatic tumors are resectable secondary to cirrhosis, portohepatic involvement, or metastases
  - Need 1-cm margin
  - Tumor recurrence most likely in the liver after resection
- **Hepatic sarcoma**
  - Risk factors – PVC, Thorotrast, arsenic → rapidly fatal
- **Isolated colon CA metastases to liver** – can resect if you leave enough liver for the patient to survive; 35% 5-year survival rate after resection for cure
- **Primary liver tumors** – hypervascular
- **Metastatic liver tumors** – hypovascular

ANATOMY AND PHYSIOLOGY

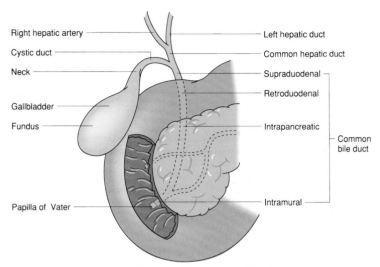

Anatomic divisions of the common bile duct.

- Gallbladder lies beneath **segments IV** and **V**
- **Cystic artery** branches off right hepatic artery
  - Is found in the **triangle of Calot** (**cystic duct** [lateral], **common bile duct** [medial], **liver** [superior])
- **Right hepatic** (lateral) and retroduodenal branches of the **gastroduodenal artery** (medial) supply the hepatic and common bile duct (9- and 3-o'clock positions when performing endoscopic retrograde cholangiopancreatography [ERCP]); considered longitudinal blood supply
- **Cystic veins** drain into the **right branch of the portal vein**
- **Lymphatics** are on the **right side** of the common bile duct
- Parasympathetic fibers come from **left** (anterior) **trunk of the vagus**
- Sympathetic fibers from T7–10 (**splanchnic and celiac ganglions**)
- Gallbladder has **no submucosa**; mucosa is **columnar** epithelium
- Common bile duct and common hepatic duct **do not have peristalsis**
- Gallbladder normally fills by **contraction of sphincter of Oddi** at the ampulla of Vater
  - **Morphine** – contracts the sphincter of Oddi
  - **Glucagon** – relaxes the sphincter of Oddi
- **Normal sizes**: common bile duct (CBD) < 8 mm (< 10 mm after cholecystectomy), gallbladder wall < 4 mm, pancreatic duct < 4 mm
- After cholecystectomy, total bile salt pools ↓
- Highest concentration of **CCK** and **secretin cells** are in the **duodenum**
- **Rokitansky–Aschoff sinuses** – epithelial invaginations in the gallbladder wall; formed from ↑ gallbladder pressure
- **Ducts of Luschka** – biliary ducts that can leak after a cholecystectomy; lie in the gallbladder fossa

- **Bile excretion regulation**
  - ↑ **bile excretion** – CCK, secretin, and vagal input
  - ↓ **bile excretion** – somatostatin, sympathetic stimulation
  - **Gallbladder contraction** – CCK causes constant, steady, tonic contraction
- **Essential functions of bile**:
  - Fat-soluble vitamin absorption
  - Essential fat absorption
  - Bilirubin and cholesterol excretion
- **Gallbladder** – forms concentrated bile by **active resorption of NaCl and water**

	Na (mEq/L)	Cl (mEq/L)	Bile Salts (mEq/dL)	Cholesterol (mEq/dL)
Hepatic bile	140–170	50–120	1–50	50–150
Gallbladder bile	225–350	1–10	250–350	300–700

- Active resorption of **conjugated bile salts** occurs in the **terminal ileum** (50%)
- Passive resorption of **nonconjugated bile salts** can occur in the **small intestine** (45%) and **colon** (5%)
- Postprandial gallbladder emptying is maximum at 2 hours (80%)
- Bile secreted by **hepatocytes** (80%) and **bile canalicular cells** (20%)
- Color of bile is mostly due to **conjugated bilirubin**
- **Stercobilin** – breakdown product of conjugated bilirubin in gut; gives stool brown color
- **Urobilinogen** – conjugated bilirubin is broken down in the gut and reabsorbed; gets converted to urobilinogen and eventually urobilin, which is released in the urine (yellow color)

CHOLESTEROL AND BILE ACID SYNTHESIS
- HMG CoA → (**HMG CoA reductase**) → cholesterol → (**7-alpha-hydroxylase**) → bile salts (acids)
- **HMG CoA reductase** – rate-limiting step in cholesterol synthesis

GALLSTONES
- Occur in 10% of the population; vast majority are asymptomatic
- Only 10% of gallstones are radiopaque
- **Nonpigmented stones**
  - **Cholesterol stones** – caused by **stasis, calcium nucleation**, and ↑ **water reabsorption** from gallbladder
  - Also caused by ↓ **lecithin** and **bile salts**
  - Found almost exclusively in the gallbladder
  - Most common type of stone found in the United States (75%)
- **Pigmented stones** – most common worldwide
  - **Calcium bilirubinate stones** – caused by solubilization of unconjugated bilirubin with precipitation
  - Dissolution agents (monooctanoin) do <u>not</u> work on pigmented stones
  - **Black stones**
    - Can be caused by **hemolytic disorders, cirrhosis, ileal resection** (loss of bile salts), **chronic TPN**
    - Factors for development – ↑ bilirubin load, ↓ hepatic function, and bile stasis → get **calcium bilirubinate stones**
    - Almost always form in gallbladder
    - Tx: **cholecystectomy** if symptomatic

- **Brown stones** (primary CBD stones, formed in ducts, Asians)
  - **Infection** causing deconjugation of bilirubin
  - **E. coli** most common – produces beta-glucuronidase, which deconjugates bilirubin with formation of **calcium bilirubinate**
  - Need to check for ampullary stenosis, duodenal diverticula, abnormal sphincter of Oddi
  - Most commonly **form in the bile ducts** (are *primary common bile duct stones*)
  - Tx: almost all patients with primary stones need a biliary drainage procedure – **sphincteroplasty** (90% successful)
- <u>Cholesterol</u> stones and <u>black</u> stones found in the CBD are considered *secondary common bile duct stones*

CHOLECYSTITIS
- Caused by obstruction of the **cystic duct** by a gallstone
- Results in gallbladder wall distention and wall inflammation
- Symptoms: RUQ pain, referred pain to the right shoulder and scapula, nausea and vomiting, loss of appetite
  - Attacks frequently occur after a fatty meal; pain is persistent (unlike biliary colic)
- Murphy's sign – patient resists deep inspiration with deep palpation to the RUQ secondary to pain
- **Alkaline phosphatase** and **WBCs** are frequently elevated
- **Suppurative cholecystitis** associated with frank purulence in the gallbladder → can be associated with sepsis and shock
- Most common organisms in cholecystitis – **E. coli (#1)**, *Klebsiella*, *Enterococcus*
- **Stone risk factors** – age > 40, female, obesity, pregnancy, rapid weight loss, vagotomy, TPN (pigmented stones), ileal resection (pigmented stones)
- **Ultrasound** – 95% sensitive for picking up stones → hyperechoic focus, posterior shadowing, movement of focus with changes in position
  - Best initial evaluation test for **jaundice** or **RUQ pain**
  - Findings suggestive of **acute cholecystitis** – gallstones, gallbladder wall thickening (> 4 mm), pericholecystic fluid
  - Dilated CBD (> 8 mm) suggests CBD stone and obstruction
- **HIDA scan** – technetium taken up by liver and excreted in the biliary tract
- **CCK-CS test** (cholecystokinin cholescintigraphy)
  - Most sensitive test for cholecystitis (also uses HIDA above)
  - Indications for **cholecystectomy** after CCK-CS test:
    - If **gallbladder not seen** (the cystic duct likely has a stone in it)
    - Takes > **60 minutes to empty** (chronic cholecystitis)
    - **Ejection fraction < 40%** (biliary dyskinesia)
- **Indications for <u>immediate</u> ERCP** (signs that a common bile duct stone is present) – jaundice, cholangitis, U/S shows stone in CBD
- **Indications for <u>pre-op</u> ERCP** (any of following needs to be persistently high for > 24 hours to justify pre-op ERCP) – **AST** or **ALT** (> 200), **bilirubin** (> 4), or **amylase** or **lipase** (> 1,000)
  - **< 5%** of patients undergoing cholecystectomy will have a retained CBD stone → 95% of these are cleared with ERCP
- **Tx for cholecystitis** – cholecystectomy; cholecystostomy tube can be placed in patients who are very ill and cannot tolerate surgery
- **ERCP** – best treatment for late common bile duct stone
  - Sphincterotomy allows for removal of stone
  - Risks: bleeding, pancreatitis, perforation
- **Biliary colic** – transient cystic duct obstruction caused by passage of a gallstone
  - Resolves within 4-6 hours

- **Air in the biliary system** most commonly occurs with previous ERCP and sphincterotomy
  - Can also occur with cholangitis or erosion of the biliary system into the duodenum (ie gallstone ileus)
- **Bacterial infection of bile** – dissemination from **portal system** is the most common route (<u>not</u> retrograde through sphincter of Oddi)
- **Highest incidence of positive bile cultures** occurs with **postoperative strictures** (usually *E. coli*, often polymicrobial)

ACALCULOUS CHOLECYSTITIS
- Thickened wall, RUQ pain, ↑ WBCs, <u>no</u> stones
- Occurs most commonly after severe burns, prolonged TPN, trauma, or major surgery
- Primary pathology is **bile stasis** (narcotics, fasting), leading to distention and ischemia
- Also have ↑ **viscosity** secondary to **dehydration**, **ileus**, **transfusions**
- Ultrasound shows **sludge**, gallbladder wall thickening, and pericholecystic fluid
- HIDA scan is positive
- Tx: cholecystectomy; percutaneous drainage if patient too unstable

EMPHYSEMATOUS GALLBLADDER DISEASE
- Gas in the gallbladder wall – can see on plain film
- ↑ in diabetics; usually secondary to *Clostridium perfringens*
- Symptoms: severe, rapid-onset abdominal pain, nausea, vomiting, and sepsis
- Perforation more common in these patients
- Tx: **emergent cholecystectomy**; percutaneous drainage if patient is too unstable

GALLSTONE ILEUS
- **Fistula** between **gallbladder** and **duodenum** that releases stone, causing small bowel obstruction; elderly
  - Can see **pneumobilia** (air in the biliary system) on plain film
- **Terminal ileum** – most common site of obstruction
- Tx: remove stone through enterotomy proximal to obstruction
  - Perform cholecystectomy and fistula resection if patient can tolerate it (if old and frail, just leave the fistula)

COMMON BILE DUCT INJURIES
- Most commonly occur after laparoscopic cholecystectomy
- **Intraoperative CBD injury** – if < 50% the circumference of the common bile duct, can probably perform primary repair; in all other cases, will likely need hepaticojejunostomy (or choledochojejunostomy)
- Persistent **nausea and vomiting** or **jaundice** following **laparoscopic cholecystectomy** → get **U/S** to look for fluid collection
  - If **fluid collection is present**, may be bile leak → percutaneous drain into the collection
    - If fluid is bilious, get ERCP → sphincterotomy and stent if due to cystic duct remnant leak, small injuries to the hepatic or common bile duct, or a leak from a duct of Luschka
    - Larger lesions (ie complete duct transection) will require hepaticojejunostomy or choledochojejunostomy (see below for timing)
  - If **fluid collection not present** and the hepatic ducts are dilated, likely have a completely transected common bile duct (PTC tube initially, then hepaticojejunostomy or choledochojejunostomy)
    - For lesions that cause <u>early symptoms (≤ 7 days)</u> – **hepaticojejunostomy**
    - For lesions that cause <u>late symptoms (> 7 days)</u> – **hepaticojejunostomy** 6–8 weeks after injury (tissue too friable for surgery after 7 days)

- **Sepsis** following **laparoscopic cholecystectomy** → fluid resuscitation and stabilize
  - May be due to complete transection of the CBD and cholangitis → get U/S to look for dilated intrahepatic ducts or fluid collections (pathway same as above)
- **Anastomotic leaks** following transplantation or hepaticojejunostomy → usually handled with percutaneous drainage of fluid collection followed by **ERCP with temporary stent** (leak will heal)

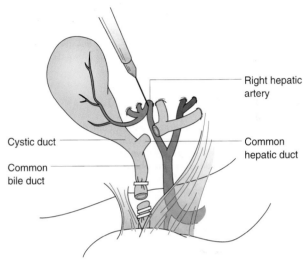

Cystic duct

Common bile duct

Right hepatic artery

Common hepatic duct

Classic laparoscopic bile duct injury. The common bile duct is mistaken for the cystic duct and transected. A variable extent of the extrahepatic biliary tree is resected with the gallbladder. The right hepatic artery, in background, is also often injured.

BILE DUCT STRICTURES
- **Ischemia** following **laparoscopic cholecystectomy** – most important cause of late postoperative biliary strictures
- Other causes – **chronic pancreatitis, gallbladder CA, bile duct CA**
- Symptoms: sepsis, cholangitis, jaundice
- Bile duct strictures without a history of pancreatitis or biliary surgery is CA until proven otherwise
- Dx: **MRCP** (magnetic resonance cholangiopancreatography) defines anatomy, looks for mass → if CA not ruled out with MRCP, need ERCP with brush biopsies
- Tx: if due to **ischemia** or **chronic pancreatitis** → *choledochojejunostomy* (best long-term solution)
  - If due to CA, follow appropriate workup

HEMOBILIA
- Fistula between **bile duct** and **hepatic arterial system** (most commonly)
- Patients classically present with UGI bleed, jaundice, and RUQ pain
- Most commonly occurs with **trauma** or **percutaneous instrumentation** to liver (eg PTC tube)
- Dx: angiogram
- Tx: **angioembolization**; operation if that fails

GALLBLADDER ADENOCARCINOMA
- Rare although most common CA of the biliary tract
- Four times more common than bile duct CA; most have stones
- **Liver** – most common site of metastasis
- **Porcelain gallbladder** – risk of gallbladder CA (15%) → these patients need cholecystectomy
- 1st spreads to **segments IV** and **V**; 1st nodes are the cystic duct nodes (right side)
- Symptoms: **jaundice** 1st (bile duct invasion with obstruction) then **RUQ pain**
- Tx: if muscle <u>not</u> involved – **cholecystectomy** sufficient
  - If **in muscle** but not beyond – need **wedge resection** of **segments IVb** and **V**
  - If **beyond muscle** and **still resectable** – need **formal resection** of **segments IVb and V**
- High incidence of **tumor implants** in trocar sites when discovered after laparoscopic cholecystectomy (laparoscopic approach *contraindicated* for gallbladder CA)
- Overall 5-year survival – 5%

BILE DUCT CANCER (CHOLANGIOCARCINOMA)
- Occurs in elderly; males
- Risk factors: *C. sinensis* infection, ulcerative colitis, choledochal cysts, primary sclerosing cholangitis, chronic bile duct infection
- Symptoms: <u>early</u> – **painless jaundice**; <u>late</u> – **weight loss**, pruritus
- Persistent ↑ in **bilirubin** and **alkaline phosphatase**
- Dx: **MRCP** (defines anatomy, looks for mass)
- Invades contiguous structures early
- Discovery of a **focal bile duct stenosis** in patients without a history of biliary surgery or pancreatitis is highly suggestive of bile duct CA
- Tx (consider surgery if no distant metastases and tumor is resectable):
  - **Upper ⅓** (Klatskin tumors)
    - Most common type, worst prognosis, usually unresectable
    - Tx: can try <u>lobectomy</u> and stenting of contralateral bile duct if localized to either the right or left lobe
  - **Middle ⅓** – <u>hepaticojejunostomy</u>
  - **Lower ⅓** – <u>Whipple</u>
- Palliative stenting for unresectable disease
- Overall 5-year survival rate – 20%

CHOLEDOCHAL CYSTS
- Female gender; Asians; 90% are extrahepatic; 15% CA risk (cholangiocarcinoma)
- Older patients have episodic pain, fever, jaundice, cholangitis
- Infants can have symptoms similar to biliary atresia
- Most are type I – fusiform or saccular dilatation of extrahepatic ducts (very dilated)
- Caused by **abnormal reflux of pancreatic enzymes** during uterine development
- Tx: **cyst excision** with **hepaticojejunostomy** and **cholecystectomy** usual
- **Type IV** cysts are partially intrahepatic, and **type V** (Caroli's disease) are totally intrahepatic → will need **partial liver resection** or **liver TXP**

PRIMARY SCLEROSING CHOLANGITIS
- Men in 4th–5th decade
- Can be associated with ulcerative colitis, pancreatitis, diabetes
- Symptoms: jaundice, fatigue, pruritus (from bile acids), weight loss, RUQ pain
- Get **multiple strictures** throughout the hepatic ducts
- Leads to **portal HTN** and **hepatic failure** (progressive fibrosis of intrahepatic and extrahepatic ducts)

- Does <u>not</u> get better after colon resection for ulcerative colitis
- Complications – cirrhosis, cholangiocarcinoma
- Tx: **liver TXP** needed long term for most; PTC tube drainage, choledochojejunostomy or balloon dilatation of dominant strictures may provide some symptomatic relief
  - **Cholestyramine** – can ↓ pruritus symptoms (↓ bile acids)
  - **UDCA** (ursodeoxycholic acid) – can ↓ symptoms (↓ bile acids) and improve liver enzymes

PRIMARY BILIARY CIRRHOSIS
- Women; medium-sized hepatic ducts
- Cholestasis → cirrhosis → portal hypertension
- Symptoms: jaundice, fatigue, pruritus, xanthomas
- Have **antimitochondrial antibodies**
- <u>No</u> increased risk for cancer
- Tx: **liver TXP**

CHOLANGITIS
- Usually caused by **obstruction of the bile duct** (most commonly due to gallstones)
- Can also be caused by **indwelling tubes** (eg PTC tube)
- **Charcot's triad** – RUQ pain, fever, jaundice
- **Reynolds' pentad** – Charcot's triad plus mental status changes and shock (suggests sepsis)
- **E. coli** (#1) and **Klebsiella** – most common organisms
- **Colovenous reflux** occurs at > 200 mm Hg pressure → **systemic bacteremia**
- Dx: ↑ AST/ALT, bilirubin, alkaline phosphatase, and WBCs
  - U/S – dilated CBD (> 8 mm, > 10 mm after cholecystectomy) if due to obstruction of the biliary system
- Stricture and hepatic abscess are late complications of cholangitis
- Renal failure – #1 serious complication; related to **sepsis**
- Other causes – biliary strictures, neoplasm, choledochal cysts, duodenal diverticula
- Tx: *fluid resuscitation and antibiotics* initially
  - **Emergent ERCP** with **sphincterotomy** and **stone extraction**; if ERCP fails, place PTC tube to decompress the biliary system
  - If the patient has cholangitis due to infected PTC tube, **change the PTC tube**

SHOCK FOLLOWING LAPAROSCOPIC CHOLECYSTECTOMY
- **Early** (1st 24 hours) – hemorrhagic shock from clip that fell off cystic artery
- **Late** (after 1st 24 hours) – septic shock from accidental clip on CBD with subsequent cholangitis

OTHER CONDITIONS
- **Adenomyomatosis** – thickened nodule of mucosa and muscle associated with Rokitansky–Aschoff sinus
  - Not premalignant; does not cause stones, can cause RUQ pain
  - Tx: cholecystectomy
- **Granular cell myoblastoma** – benign neuroectoderm tumor of gallbladder
  - Can occur in biliary tract with signs of cholecystitis
  - Tx: cholecystectomy
- **Cholesterolosis** – speckled cholesterol deposits on the gallbladder wall
- **Gallbladder polyps** – if > 1 cm, need to worry about malignancy
  - Polyps in patients > 60 years more likely malignant
  - Tx: cholecystectomy

- **Delta bilirubin** – bound to albumin covalently, half-life of 18 days; may take a while to clear after long-standing jaundice
- **Mirizzi syndrome** – compression of the common hepatic duct by 1) a stone in the gallbladder infundibulum or 2) inflammation arising from the gallbladder or cystic duct extending to the contiguous hepatic duct, causing common hepatic duct stricture; Tx: cholecystectomy; may need hepaticojejunostomy for hepatic duct stricture
- **Ceftriaxone** – can cause gallbladder sludging and cholestatic jaundice
- **Indications for asymptomatic cholecystectomy** – in patients undergoing liver TXP or gastric bypass procedure (if stones are present)

CHAPTER 33. PANCREAS

ANATOMY AND PHYSIOLOGY

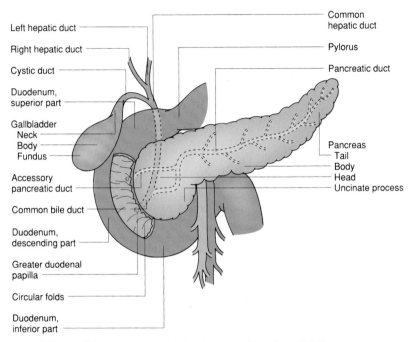

Relation of the pancreas to the duodenum and extrahepatic biliary system.

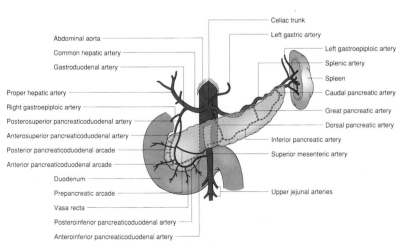

Arterial supply to the pancreas.

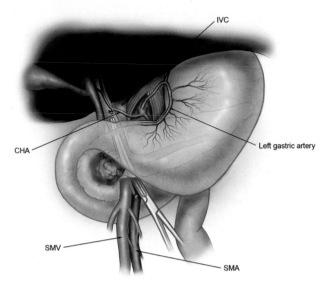

Relationship between the superior mesenteric vein and superior mesenteric artery. (Modified from Evans DB, Lee JE, Tamm EP, et al. Pancreaticoduodenectomy [Whipple operation] and total pancreatectomy for cancer. In: Fischer JE, Bland KI, et al, eds. *Mastery of Surgery*. 5th ed. Philadelphia, PA: Lippincott Williams & Wilkins; 2007, with permission.)

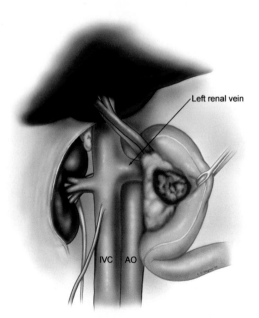

Kocher maneuver and relationship between the aorta and inferior vena cava. (Modified from Evans DB, Lee JE, Tamm EP, et al. Pancreaticoduodenectomy [Whipple operation] and total pancreatectomy for cancer. In: Fischer JE, Bland KI, et al, eds. *Mastery of Surgery*. 5th ed. Philadelphia, PA: Lippincott Williams & Wilkins; 2007, with permission.)

- **Head** (including uncinate), **neck, body**, and **tail**
- **Uncinate process** – rests on aorta, behind SMV
- **SMV** and **SMA** – lay behind neck of pancreas
- **Portal vein** – forms behind the neck (SMV and splenic vein)
- **Blood supply**
  - **Head** – **superior** (off GDA) and **inferior** (off SMA) **pancreaticoduodenal arteries** (anterior and posterior branches for each)
  - **Body** – great, inferior, and caudal pancreatic arteries (all off **splenic artery**)
  - **Tail** – splenic, gastroepiploic, and dorsal pancreatic arteries
- **Venous drainage** into the **portal system**
- **Lymphatics** – celiac and SMA nodes
- **Ductal cells** – secrete **HCO_3^- solution** (have carbonic anhydrase)
- **Acinar cells** – secrete **digestive enzymes**
- **Exocrine function of the pancreas** – amylase, lipase, trypsinogen, chymotrypsinogen, carboxypeptidase; HCO_3^-
  - **Amylase** – only pancreatic enzyme secreted in active form; hydrolyzes alpha 1–4 linkages of glucose chains
- **Endocrine function of the pancreas**
  - **Alpha cells** – glucagon
  - **Beta cells** (at center of islets) – insulin
  - **Delta cells** – somatostatin
  - **PP or F cells** – pancreatic polypeptide
  - **Islet cells** – also produce vasoactive intestinal peptide (VIP), serotonin
- **Islet cells** receive **majority of blood supply** related to size
  - After islets, blood goes to acinar cells
- **Enterokinase** – released by the duodenum, activates trypsinogen to trypsin
  - Trypsin activates other pancreatic enzymes including trypsinogen
- **Hormonal control of pancreatic excretion**
  - **Secretin** – ↑ HCO_3^- mostly
  - **CCK** – ↑ pancreatic enzymes mostly
  - **Acetylcholine** – ↑ HCO^- and enzymes
  - **Somatostatin** and **glucagons** – ↓ exocrine function
  - **CCK** and **secretin** – most released by cells in the duodenum
- **Ventral pancreatic bud**
  - Connected to duct of Wirsung; migrates posteriorly, to the right, and clockwise to fuse with the dorsal bud
  - Forms uncinate and inferior portion of the head
- **Dorsal pancreatic bud** – body, tail, and superior aspect of the pancreatic head; has duct of Santorini
- **Duct of Wirsung** – major pancreatic duct that merges with CBD before entering duodenum
- **Duct of Santorini** – small accessory pancreatic duct that drains directly into duodenum

ANNULAR PANCREAS
- 2nd portion of duodenum trapped in pancreatic band; can see double bubble on abdominal x-ray; get **duodenal obstruction** (N/V, abdominal pain)
- Associated with Down syndrome; forms from the ventral pancreatic bud from failure of clockwise rotation
- Tx: **duodenojejunostomy** or **duodenoduodenostomy**; possible sphincteroplasty
  - Pancreas not resected

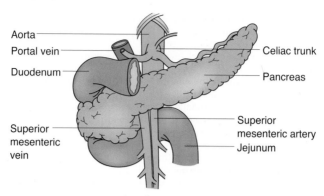

Annular pancreas.

PANCREAS DIVISUM
- Failed fusion of the pancreatic ducts; can result in pancreatitis from duct of Santorini (accessory duct) stenosis
- Most are asymptomatic; some get pancreatitis
- Dx: ERCP – **minor papilla** will show long and large duct of Santorini; **major papilla** will show short duct of Wirsung
- Tx: **ERCP with sphincteroplasty**; open sphincteroplasty if that fails

HETEROTOPIC PANCREAS
- Most commonly found in **duodenum**
- Usually asymptomatic
- Surgical resection if symptomatic

ACUTE PANCREATITIS
- **Gallstones** and **ETOH** most common etiologies in the United States
  - Other etiologies – ERCP, trauma, hyperlipidemia, hypercalcemia, viral infection, medications (azathioprine, furosemide, steroids, cimetidine)
  - **Gallstones** – can obstruct the ampulla of Vater, causing impaired extrusion of zymogen granules and activation of degradation enzymes → leads to pancreatic auto-digestion
  - **ETOH** – can cause auto-activation of pancreatic enzymes while still in the pancreas
- Symptoms: **abdominal pain** radiating to the back, **nausea**, **vomiting**, **anorexia**
  - Can also get **jaundice**, left **pleural effusion**, **ascites**, or **sentinel loop** (dilated small bowel near the pancreas as a result of the inflammation)
- Mortality rate 10%; hemorrhagic pancreatitis mortality 50%
- Pancreatitis without obvious cause → need to worry about malignancy
- **Ranson's criteria**
  - On admission → age > 55, WBC > 16, glucose > 200, AST > 250, LDH > 350
  - After 48 hours: Hct ↓ 10%, BUN ↑ of 5, Ca < 8, PaO_2 < 60, base deficit > 4, fluid sequestration > 6 L
  - 8 Ranson criteria met → mortality rate near 100%
- Labs: ↑ **amylase**, **lipase**, and **WBCs**
- **Ultrasound** – needed to check for gallstones and possible CBD dilatation
- **Abdominal CT** – to check for complications (**necrotic pancreas** will <u>not</u> uptake contrast)
- Tx: **NPO**, aggressive **fluid resuscitation**
  - **ERCP** is needed in patients with **gallstone pancreatitis** and **retained CBD stones** → perform sphincterotomy and stone extraction
  - Antibiotics for stones, severe pancreatitis, failure to improve, or suspected infection

- **TPN** may be necessary during recovery period
- Patients with gallstone pancreatitis should undergo **cholecystectomy** when recovered from pancreatitis (same hospital admission)
- Morphine should be avoided as it can contract the sphincter of Oddi and worsen attack
- **Bleeding**
  - **Grey Turner sign** – flank ecchymosis
  - **Cullen's sign** – periumbilical ecchymosis
  - **Fox's sign** – inguinal ecchymosis
- **15% get pancreatic necrosis** – leave sterile necrosis <u>alone</u>
  - **Infected necrosis** (fever, sepsis, positive blood cultures; may need to sample necrotic pancreatic fluid with CT-guided aspiration to get diagnosis) → Tx: need *surgical debridement*
  - **Pancreatic abscesses** → Tx: need *surgical debridement*
  - CT-guided drainage of infected pancreatic necrosis or pancreatic abscess is generally <u>not</u> effective
  - **Gas** in necrotic pancreas = infected necrosis or abscess (need **open debridement**)
- **Infection** – leading cause of death with pancreatitis; usually GNRs
- Surgery only for infected pancreatitis or pancreatic abscess
- **Obesity** – most important risk factor for necrotizing pancreatitis
- **ARDS** – related to release of phospholipases
- **Coagulopathy** – related to release of proteases
- **Pancreatic fat necrosis** – related to release of phospholipases
- **Mild ↑ amylase** and **lipase** can be seen with cholecystitis, perforated ulcer, sialoadenitis, small bowel obstruction (SBO), and intestinal infarction

PANCREATIC PSEUDOCYSTS
- Most common in patients with **chronic pancreatitis**
  - Cysts <u>not</u> associated with pancreatitis – **need to R/O CA** (eg mucinous cystadenocarcinoma)
- Symptoms: pain, fever, weight loss, bowel obstruction from compression
- Often occurs in the **head** of the pancreas; is a non-epithelialized sac
- Most **resolve spontaneously** (especially if < 5 cm)
- Tx: *expectant management for __3 months__* – (*most **resolve on their own**; also allows pseudocyst to mature if cystogastrostomy is required)
  - May need to place these patients on **TPN** if unable to eat
  - *Surgery only for* **continued symptoms** (Tx: **cystogastrostomy**, open or percutaneous) or pseudocysts that are **growing** (Tx: **resection** to R/O CA)
- **Complications of pancreatic pseudocyst** – infection of cyst, portal or splenic vein thrombosis
- **Incidental cysts** <u>not</u> associated with pancreatitis should be *resected* (worry about **intraductal papillary-mucinous neoplasms [IPMNs]** or **mucinous cystadenocarcinoma**) <u>unless</u> the cyst is purely serous and non-complex
- **Non-complex, purely serous cystadenomas** have an extremely low malignancy risk (< 1%) and can be followed

PANCREATIC FISTULAS
- Most **close spontaneously** (especially if low output < 200 cc/day)
- Tx: allow drainage, NPO, TPN, **octreotide**
  - If failure to resolve with medical management, can try **ERCP**, **sphincterotomy**, and **pancreatic stent** placement (fistula will usually close, then remove stent)

PANCREATITIS-ASSOCIATED PLEURAL EFFUSION (OR ASCITES)
- Caused by retroperitoneal leakage of pancreatic fluid from the pancreatic duct or a pseudocyst (is <u>not</u> a pancreatic–pleural fistula); majority close on their own

- Tx: **thoracentesis** (or paracentesis) followed by conservative Tx (**NPO**, **TPN**, and **octreotide** – follow pancreatic fistula pathway above)
  - **Amylase** will be elevated in the fluid

CHRONIC PANCREATITIS
- Corresponds to irreversible **parenchymal fibrosis**
- **ETOH** most common cause; idiopathic 2nd most common
- **Pain** most common problem; anorexia, weight loss, malabsorption, steatorrhea, recurrent acute pancreatitis
- <u>Endocrine</u> function usually **preserved** (Islet cell preserved); <u>exocrine</u> function **decreased**
- Can cause **malabsorption of fat-soluble vitamins** (Tx: pancrelipase)
- Dx: **abdominal CT** will show **shrunken pancreas** with **calcifications**
  - **Ultrasound** – shows pancreatic ducts > 4 mm, cysts, and atrophy

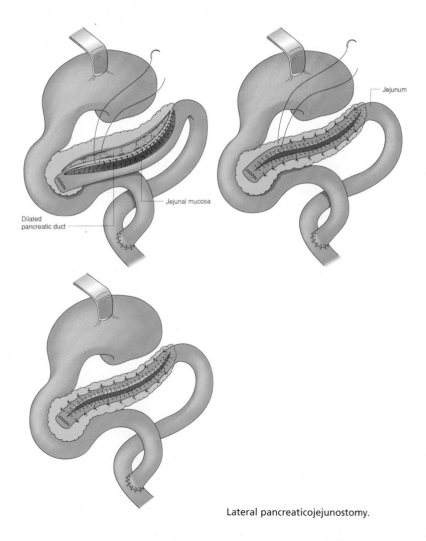

Lateral pancreaticojejunostomy.

- **ERCP** – very sensitive at diagnosing chronic pancreatitis
- Advanced disease – **chain of lakes** → alternating segments of dilation and stenosis in pancreatic duct
- Tx: supportive, including **pain control** and nutritional support (**pancrelipase**)
- **Surgical indications** – pain that interferes with quality of life, nutrition abnormalities, addiction to narcotics, failure to rule out CA, biliary obstruction
- **Surgical options**
    - **Puestow procedure** – pancreaticojejunostomy, for enlarged ducts > 8 mm (most patients improve) → open along main pancreatic duct and drain into jejunum
    - **Distal pancreatic resection** – for normal or small ducts and only distal portion of the gland is affected
    - **Whipple** – for normal or small ducts with isolated pancreatic head disease
    - **Beger-Frey** (duodenal preserving head "core-out") – for normal or small ducts with isolated pancreatic head enlargement
    - **Bilateral thoracoscopic splanchnicectomy** or **celiac ganglionectomy** may be used for **pain control**
    - **Common bile duct** (CBD) **stricture** – causes CBD dilation; Tx: **hepaticojejunostomy or choledochojejunostomy** for pain, jaundice, progressive cirrhosis, or cholangitis (make sure the stricture is not pancreatic CA)
- **Splenic vein thrombosis** – <u>chronic pancreatitis</u> most common cause
    - Can get bleeding from isolated **gastric varices** that form as collaterals
    - Tx: **splenectomy** for isolated bleeding gastric varices

PANCREATIC INSUFFICIENCY
- Usually the result of long-standing pancreatitis or occurs after total pancreatectomy (over 90% of the function must be lost)
- Generally refers to exocrine function
- Symptoms: **malabsorption** and **steatorrhea**
- Dx: **fecal fat testing**
- Tx: high-carbohydrate, high-protein, low-fat diet; **pancreatic enzymes** (Pancrease)

JAUNDICE WORKUP
- **Ultrasound 1st**
    - **Positive CBD stones, no mass** → ERCP (allows extraction of stones)
    - **No CBD stones, no mass** → MRCP
    - **Positive mass** → MRCP

PANCREATIC ADENOCARCINOMA
- Male predominance; usually 6th–7th decades of life
- Symptoms: **weight loss** (most common symptom), **jaundice, pain**
- **20% 5-year survival rate with resection**
- Risk factors – **tobacco #1**
- **CA 19-9** – serum marker for pancreatic CA
- 95% have **p16 mutation** (tumor suppressor, binds **cyclin** complexes)
- Lymphatic spread 1st
- **70%** are in the **head**
    - 50% invade portal vein, SMV, or retroperitoneum at time of diagnosis (unresectable disease)
    - Metastases to peritoneum, omentum, or liver – indicate unresectable disease
    - Metastases to celiac or SMA nodal system (nodal systems outside area of resection) – indicate unresectable disease
    - Most cures in patients with pancreatic head disease
- **90%** are **ductal adenocarcinoma**
    - Others (more favorable prognosis) – papillary or mucinous cyst-adenocarcinoma

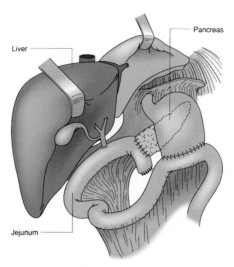

Reconstruction after standard pancreaticoduodenectomy (Whipple; the gallbladder is usually resected with the procedure).

- Labs: typically show ↑ conjugated **bilirubin** and **alkaline phosphatase**
- Patients with a **resectable mass** (and no signs of metastatic disease) in the pancreas do **not** need a biopsy because you are taking it out regardless. If the patient appears to have metastatic disease, a biopsy is warranted to direct therapy
- **MRCP** good at differentiating dilated ducts secondary to chronic pancreatitis versus CA
  - **Signs of CA on MRCP** – duct with irregular narrowing, displacement, destruction; can also detect vessel involvement
- **Abdominal CT** – may show the lesion and double-duct sign for pancreatic head tumors (dilation of both the pancreatic duct and CBD)
- For **unresectable disease**, consider **palliation** with **biliary stents** or **hepaticojejunostomy** (for biliary obstruction), **gastrojejunostomy** (for duodenal obstruction), and **celiac plexus ablation** (for pain)
- Complications from Whipple – **delayed gastric emptying** #1 (Tx – metoclopramide), **fistula** (Tx: conservative therapy), **leak** (place drains and Tx like a fistula), **marginal ulceration** (Tx: PPI)
- **Bleeding** after Whipple or other pancreatic surgery – go to **angio for** *embolization* (the tissue planes are very friable early after surgery, and bleeding is hard to control operatively)
- Chemo-XRT usual postop (**gemcitabine**)
- Prognosis for non-metastatic disease related to nodal invasion and ability to get a clear margin

NON-FUNCTIONAL ENDOCRINE TUMORS
- Represent ⅓ of pancreatic endocrine neoplasms
- 90% of the nonfunctional tumors are **malignant**
- Tend to have a more **indolent and protracted course** compared with pancreatic adenocarcinoma
- Resect these lesions: metastatic disease precludes resection
- **5FU** and **streptozocin** may be effective
- Liver metastases most common

FUNCTIONAL ENDOCRINE PANCREATIC TUMORS

- Represents ⅔ of pancreatic endocrine neoplasms
- **Octreotide** – effective for insulinoma, glucagonoma, gastrinoma, VIPoma
- **Most common in pancreatic head** – gastrinoma, somatostatinoma
- All tumors can respond to debulking
- **Liver** metastatic spread – 1st for all
- **Insulinoma**
  - **Most common islet cell tumor of the pancreas**
  - Symptoms: **Whipple's triad** → fasting **hypoglycemia** ($<$ 50), **symptoms** of hypoglycemia (palpitations, ↑ HR, and diaphoresis), and **relief with glucose**
  - **90%** are **benign** and evenly distributed throughout pancreas
  - Dx: insulin to glucose ratio $>$ 0.4 after fasting; ↑ C peptide and proinsulin (→ if not elevated, suspect **Munchausen's syndrome**)
  - Tx: enucleate if $<$ 2 cm; formal resection if $>$ 2 cm
    - For metastatic disease → **5-FU** and **streptozocin**; octreotide
- **Gastrinoma** (Zollinger–Ellison syndrome [ZES])
  - Most common pancreatic islet cell tumor in **MEN-1 patients**
  - 50% **malignant** and 50% **multiple**
  - 75% **spontaneous** and 25% **MEN-1**
  - Majority in **gastrinoma triangle** – common bile duct, neck of pancreas, third portion of the duodenum

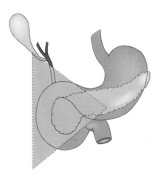

Most gastrinomas are found within the gastrinoma triangle.

- Symptoms: **refractory** or **complicated ulcer disease** and **diarrhea** (improved with PPI)
- **Serum gastrin** usually $>$ 200; 1,000s is diagnostic
- **Secretin stimulation test** – ZES patients: ↑ gastrin ($>$ 200); normal patients: ↓ gastrin
- Tx: enucleation if $<$ 2 cm; formal resection if $>$ 2 cm
  - Malignant disease → excise suspicious nodes
  - Cannot find tumor → perform duodenostomy and look inside duodenum for tumor (15% of microgastrinomas there)
  - **Duodenal tumor** – resection with primary closure; may need Whipple if extensive; be sure to check pancreas for primary
  - **Debulking** – can improve symptoms
  - **Octreotide scan** – single best study for localizing tumor

- **Glucagonoma**
  - Symptoms: **diabetes**, stomatitis, **dermatitis** (**rash** – necrolytic migratory erythema), weight loss
  - Diagnosis: fasting glucagon level
  - Most **malignant**; most in **distal pancreas**
  - Zinc, amino acids, or fatty acids may treat skin rash
- **VIPoma** (Verner–Morrison syndrome)
  - Symptoms: **watery diarrhea, hypokalemia**, and achlorhydria (WDHA)
  - Hypokalemia from diarrhea
  - Dx: exclude other causes of diarrhea; ↑ VIP levels
  - Most **malignant**; most in **distal pancreas**, 10% extrapancreatic (retroperitoneal, thorax)
- **Somatostatinoma**
  - **Very rare**
  - Symptoms: diabetes, gallstones, steatorrhea, hypochlorhydria
  - Diagnosis: fasting somatostatin level
  - Most **malignant**; most in **head of pancreas**
  - Perform cholecystectomy with resection

ANATOMY AND PHYSIOLOGY

- Short gastrics and splenic artery are end arteries
- Splenic vein is posterior and inferior to the splenic artery
- Spleen serves as an **antigen-processing center** for macrophages
- Is the largest producer of **IgM**
- **85% red pulp** – acts as a filter for aged or damaged RBCs
  - **Pitting** – removal of abnormalities in RBC membrane
    - Howell–Jolly bodies – nuclear remnants
    - Heinz bodies – hemoglobin
  - **Culling** – removal of less deformable RBCs
- **15% white pulp** – immunologic function; contains lymphocytes and macrophages
  - Major site of **bacterial clearance that lacks preexisting antibodies**
  - Site of removal of **poorly opsonized bacteria, particles,** and **cellular debris**
  - Antigen processing occurs with interaction between **macrophages** and **helper T cells**

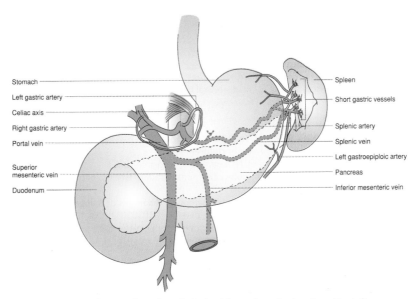

Stomach
Left gastric artery
Celiac axis
Right gastric artery
Portal vein
Superior mesenteric vein
Duodenum

Spleen
Short gastric vessels
Splenic artery
Splenic vein
Left gastroepiploic artery
Pancreas
Inferior mesenteric vein

The arterial blood flow to the spleen is derived from the splenic artery, the left gastroepiploic artery, and the short gastric arteries (vasa brevia). The venous drainage into this portal vein is also shown.

- **Tuftsin** – an opsonin; facilitates phagocytosis → produced in spleen
- **Properdin** – activates alternate complement pathway → produced in spleen
- **Hematopoiesis** – occurs in spleen before birth and in conditions such as myeloid dysplasia
- Spleen serves as a **reservoir for platelets**
- **Accessory spleen** (20%) – most commonly found at *splenic hilum*

- **Indication for splenectomy** – idiopathic thrombocytopenic purpura (ITP) far greater than for thrombotic thrombocytopenic purpura (TTP)
- ITP most common nontraumatic condition requiring splenectomy

IDIOPATHIC THROMBOCYTOPENIC PURPURA (ITP)
- This can occur from many etiologies – drugs, viruses, etc.
- Caused by **anti-platelet antibodies** (IgG) – bind platelets; results in **decreased platelets**
- Petechiae, gingival bleeding, bruising, soft tissue ecchymosis
- **Spleen is normal**
- In children < 10 years, ITP usually resolves spontaneously (avoid splenectomy in children)
- Tx: *steroids* (primary therapy); **gammaglobulin** if steroid resistant
- Splenectomy indicated for those who <u>fail steroids</u> → removes IgG production and source of phagocytosis; 80% respond after splenectomy
- Give platelets 1 hour before surgery

THROMBOTIC THROMBOCYTOPENIC PURPURA (TTP)
- Associated with medical reactions, infections, inflammation, autoimmune disease
- **Loss of platelet inhibition** – leads to thrombosis and infarction, profound thrombocytopenia
- Purpura, fever, mental status changes, renal dysfunction, hematuria, hemolytic anemia
- 80% respond to medical therapy
- Tx: *plasmapheresis* (primary); immunosuppression
- Death most commonly due to **intracerebral hemorrhage** or acute renal failure
- Splenectomy *rarely* indicated

POST-SPLENECTOMY SEPSIS SYNDROME (PSSS)
- 0.1% risk after splenectomy; ↑ risk in **children**
- *S. pneumoniae* (#1), *H. influenzae*, *N. meningitidis* – most common
- Secondary to specific lack of immunity (immunoglobulin, IgM) to capsulated bacteria
- Highest in patients with splenectomy for **hemolytic disorders** or **malignancy**
- Children also have ↑ risk of mortality after developing PSSS
- Try to wait until at least **5 years old** before performing splenectomy → allows antibody formation; child can get fully immunized
- Most episodes occur within 2 years of splenectomy
- Children < 10 years should be given prophylactic antibiotics for 6 months (controversial)
- **Vaccines needed <u>*before*</u> splenectomy** – *Pneumococcus, Meningococcus, H. influenzae*

Definition of Hypersplenism

Decrease in circulating cell count of erythrocytes and/or platelets and/or leukocytes
and
Normal compensatory hematopoietic responses present in bone marrow
and
Correction of cytopenia by splenectomy
with or without
Splenomegaly

HEMOLYTIC ANEMIAS – MEMBRANE PROTEIN DEFECTS

- **Spherocytosis**
  - **Most common congenital hemolytic anemia requiring splenectomy**
  - **Spectrin** deficit (**membrane protein**) deforms RBCs and leads to splenic sequestration (**hypersplenism**)
  - Causes pigmented stones, anemia, reticulocytosis, jaundice, splenomegaly
  - Try to perform splenectomy after age 5; give immunizations first
  - Tx: **splenectomy** and **cholecystectomy**
  - Splenectomy curative
- **Elliptocytosis**
  - Symptoms and mechanism similar to spherocytosis; less common
  - Spectrin and protein 4.1 deficit (**membrane protein**)

HEMOLYTIC ANEMIAS: NON–MEMBRANE PROTEIN DEFECTS

- **Pyruvate kinase deficiency**
  - Results in congenital hemolytic anemia
  - Causes altered glucose metabolism; RBC survival enhanced by splenectomy
  - Is the most common congenital hemolytic anemia <u>not</u> involving a membrane protein that requires splenectomy
- **G6PD deficiency**
  - Precipitated by infection, certain drugs, fava beans
  - Splenectomy usually <u>not</u> required
- **Warm antibody–type acquired immune hemolytic anemia** – indication for splenectomy
- **Sickle cell anemia** – HgbA replaced with HgbS
  - Spleen usually autoinfarcts and splenectomy <u>not</u> required
- **Beta thalassemia**
  - Most common thalassemia; due to persistent HgbF
  - Major – both chains affected; minor – 1 chain, asymptomatic
  - Symptoms: pallor, retarded body growth, head enlargement
  - **Splenectomy** (if patient has splenomegaly) may ↓ hemolysis and symptoms
  - Most die in teens secondary to hemosiderosis
  - Medical Tx: blood transfusions and iron chelators (deferoxamine, deferiprone)

HODGKIN'S DISEASE

- A – asymptomatic
- B – symptomatic (night sweats, fever, weight loss) → unfavorable prognosis
- Stage I – 1 area or 2 contiguous areas on the same side of diaphragm
- Stage II – 2 non-contiguous areas on the same side of diaphragm
- Stage III – involved on each side of diaphragm
- Stage IV – liver, bone, lung, or any other non-lymphoid tissue except spleen
- See **Reed–Sternberg cells**
- **Lymphocyte predominant** – best prognosis
- **Lymphocyte depleted** – worst prognosis
- **Nodular sclerosing** – most common
- Tx: chemo
- **MCC of chylous ascites** – *lymphoma*

NON-HODGKIN'S LYMPHOMA

- Worse prognosis than Hodgkin's; 90% are **B-cell** lymphomas
- Generally systemic disease by the time the diagnosis is made
- Tx: chemo

OTHER CONDITIONS

- **Hairy cell leukemia** – Tx: rarely need splenectomy
- **Spontaneous splenic rupture** – mononucleosis, malaria, sepsis, sarcoid, leukemia, polycythemia vera
- **Splenosis** – splenic implants; usually related to trauma
- **Hyposplenism** – see Howell–Jolly bodies
- **Pancreatitis** – most common cause of splenic artery or splenic vein thrombosis
- **Postsplenectomy changes** – ↑ RBCs, ↑ WBCs, ↑ platelets; if platelets $> 1 \times 10^6$, give ASA
- **Hemangioma** – #1 splenic tumor overall; #1 benign splenic tumor; Tx: splenectomy if symptomatic
- **Non-Hodgkin's lymphoma** – #1 malignant splenic tumor
- **Splenic cysts** – surgery if symptomatic or > 10 cm
- **Sarcoidosis of spleen** – anemia, ↓ platelets; Tx: splenectomy for symptomatic splenomegaly
- **Felty's syndrome** – rheumatoid arthritis, hepatomegaly, splenomegaly; Tx: splenectomy for symptomatic splenomegaly
- **Splenic abscess** – Tx: splenectomy usual (bleeding risk with percutaneous drainage)
- **Echinococcal splenic cyst** – Tx: splenectomy

Results of Splenectomy/Hyposplenic Condition

ERYTHROCYTES
- Howell–Jolly bodies (nuclear fragments)
- Heinz bodies (hemoglobin deposits)
- Pappenheimer bodies (iron deposits)
- Target cells
- Spur cells (acanthocytes)

PLATELETS
- Transient thrombocytosis

LEUKOCYTES
- Transient leukocytosis
- Persistent lymphocytosis
- Persistent monocytosis

Guidelines for Prevention of Postsplenic Sepsis

- Vaccinate with polyvalent pneumococcal vaccine at least 10–14 days prior to splenectomy, if possible
- If splenectomy is urgent, wait until at least 14 days postprocedure to vaccinate
- For high-risk patients (immunosuppressed, children < 10 years of age), meningococcal vaccine and *Haemophilus influenza* vaccine
- Antibiotic prophylaxis for children < 5 years of age
- Early antibiotic treatment for initial signs of infection
- MedicAlert bracelet

ANATOMY AND PHYSIOLOGY
- **Small intestine** – nutrient and water absorption
- **Large intestine** – water absorption
- **Duodenum**
  - **Bulb** (1st portion) – 90% of ulcers here
  - **Descending** (2nd) – contains ampulla of Vater (duct of Wirsung) and duct of Santorini
  - **Transverse** (3rd)
  - **Ascending** (4th)
  - Descending and transverse portions are **retroperitoneal**
  - 3rd and 4th portions – transition point at the acute angle between the aorta (posterior) and **SMA** (anterior)
  - Vascular supply is **superior** (off gastroduodenal artery) and **inferior** (off SMA) **pancreaticoduodenal arteries**
    - Both have anterior and posterior branches
    - Many communications between these arteries

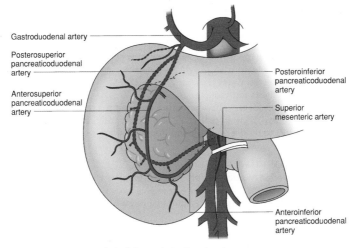

Arterial supply to the duodenum.

- **Jejunum**
  - 100 cm long; long vasa recta, circular muscle folds
  - Is the **maximum site of all absorption** except for B_{12} (terminal ileum), bile acids (ileum – non-conjugated; terminal ileum – conjugated), iron (duodenum), and folate (terminal ileum)
  - 95% of NaCl absorbed and 90% of water absorbed in jejunum
  - Vascular supply – SMA
- **Ileum** – 150 cm long; short vasa recta, flat
  - Vascular supply – SMA
- **Intestinal brush border** – maltase, sucrase, limit dextrinase, lactase
- **Normal sizes** – small bowel/transverse colon/cecum → **3/6/9 cm**

217

- SMA eventually branches into the **ileocolic artery**
- **Cell types**
  - **Absorptive cells**
  - **Goblet cells** (mucin secretion)
  - **Paneth cells** (secretory granules, enzymes)
  - **Enterochromaffin cells** (APUD, 5-hydroxytryptamine release, carcinoid precursor)
  - **Brunner's glands** (alkaline solution)
  - **Peyer's patches** (lymphoid tissue); increased in the ileum
  - **M cells** – antigen-presenting cells in intestinal wall
- **IgA** – released into gut; also in mother's milk
- **Fe** – small bowel has both heme and Fe transporters
- **Migrating motor complex** (gut motility)
  - Phase I – rest
  - Phase II – acceleration and gallbladder contraction
  - Phase III – peristalsis
  - Phase IV – deceleration
  - **Motilin** is most important hormone in migrating motor complex (acts on **phase III**)
- **Bile salts** (acids)
  - **95% of bile salts are reabsorbed**
    - 50% passive absorption (non-conjugated bile salts) – 45% ileum, 5% colon
    - 50% active resorption (conjugated bile salts) in **terminal ileum** (Na/K ATPase); conjugated bile salts are absorbed only in the terminal ileum
  - Gallstones form after terminal ileum resection from malabsorption of bile salts

SHORT-GUT SYNDROME
- Diagnosis is made on symptoms, not length of bowel
- Symptoms: diarrhea, steatorrhea, weight loss, nutritional deficiency
- Lose fat, B_{12}, electrolytes, water
- **Sudan red stain** – checks for fecal fat
- **Schilling test** – checks for B_{12} absorption (radiolabeled B_{12} in urine)
- Probably need at least 75 cm to survive off TPN; 50 cm with competent ileocecal valve
- Tx: **restrict fat**, **PPI** to reduce acid, **Lomotil** (diphenoxylate and atropine)

CAUSES OF STEATORRHEA
- **Gastric hypersecretion of acid** $\rightarrow \downarrow$ pH $\rightarrow \uparrow$ intestinal motility; interferes with fat absorption
- **Interruption of bile salt resorption** (eg terminal ileum resection) interferes with micelle formation and fat absorption
- Tx: control diarrhea (Lomotil); $\downarrow$ oral intake, especially fats; **Pancrease, PPI**

NONHEALING FISTULA
- **"FRIENDS"** – mnemonic for causes of nonhealing fistula: **f**oreign body, **r**adiation, **i**nflammatory bowel disease, **e**pithelialization, **n**eoplasm, **d**istal obstruction, **s**epsis/infection
- High-output fistulas are more likely with proximal bowel (duodenum or proximal jejunum) and are less likely to close with conservative management
- Colonic fistulas are more likely to close than those in small bowel
- Patients with **persistent fever** – need to check for **abscess** (fistulogram, abdominal CT, upper GI with small bowel follow-through)
- Most fistulas are **iatrogenic** and treated conservatively 1st $\rightarrow$ NPO, TPN, skin protection (stoma appliance), octreotide
- Majority close spontaneously without surgery
- Surgical options: resect bowel segment containing fistula and perform primary anastomosis

OBSTRUCTION
- **Without previous surgery** (most common)
  - Small bowel – <u>hernia</u>
  - Large bowel – <u>cancer</u>
- **With previous surgery** (most common)
  - Small bowel – <u>adhesions</u>
  - Large bowel – <u>cancer</u>

Symptoms and Signs of Bowel Obstruction

Symptom or Sign	Proximal Small Bowel (Open Loop)	Distal Small Bowel (Open Loop)	Small Bowel (Closed Loop)	Colon and Rectum
Pain	Intermittent, intense, colicky; often relieved by vomiting	Intermittent to constant	Progressive, intermittent constant; rapidly worsens	Continuous
Vomiting	Large volumes; bilious and frequent	Low volume and frequency; progressively feculent with time	May be prominent (reflex)	Intermittent, not prominent; feculent when present
Tenderness	Epigastric or periumbilical; quite mild unless strangulation is present	Diffuse and progressive	Diffuse, progressive	Diffuse
Distention	Absent	Moderate to marked	Often absent	Marked
Obstipation	May not be present	Present	May not be present	Present

Adapted from Schuffler MD, Sinanan MN. Intestinal obstruction and pseudo-obstruction. In: Sleisenger MH, Fordtran JS, eds. *Gastrointestinal Disease.* 5th ed. Philadelphia, PA: WB Saunders; 1993:898.

- Symptoms: nausea and vomiting, crampy abdominal pain, failure to pass gas or stool
- Abdominal x-ray: air–fluid level, distended loops of small bowel, distal decompression

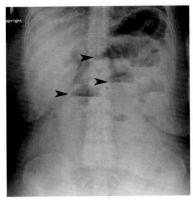

Plain upright abdominal film of a patient with small intestinal obstruction. Note the air–fluid levels in the stomach and multiple dilated loops of small intestine (*black arrows*) and absence of air in the colon or rectum.

- 3rd spacing of fluid into bowel lumen occurs – need **aggressive fluid resuscitation**
- Air with bowel obstruction – from **swallowed nitrogen**
- Tx: bowel rest, NG tube, IV fluids $\rightarrow$ cures 80% of partial SBO, 40% of complete SBO
- Surgical indications: **progressing pain**, **peritoneal signs**, **fever**, **increasing WBCs**, (all signs of strangulation or perforation), or **failure to resolve**

GALLSTONE ILEUS
- Small bowel obstruction from **gallstone** usually in the **terminal ileum**
- Classically see **air in the biliary tree** in a patient with small bowel obstruction
- Caused by a **fistula** between the **gallbladder** and **second portion of duodenum**
- Tx: remove stone from terminal ileum
  - Can leave gallbladder and fistula if patient too sick
  - If not too sick, perform cholecystectomy and close duodenum

MECKEL'S DIVERTICULUM
- 2 ft from ileocecal valve; 2% of population; usually presents in 1st 2 years of life with bleeding; is a true diverticulum
- Caused by failure of closure of the **omphalomesenteric duct**
- Accounts for 50% of all **painless lower GI bleeds in children < 2 years**
- **Pancreas tissue** – most common tissue found in Meckel's (can cause **diverticulitis**)
- **Gastric mucosa** – most likely to be symptomatic (**bleeding** most common)
- **Obstruction** – most common presentation in adults
- **Incidental** $\rightarrow$ usually not removed unless gastric mucosa suspected (diverticulum feels thick) or has a very narrow neck
- Dx: can get a **Meckel's scan** (^{99}Tc) if having trouble localizing (mucosa lights up)
- Tx: **diverticulectomy** for uncomplicated diverticulitis or bleeding
  - Need **segmental resection** for **complicated** diverticulitis (eg perforation), **neck > ⅓ the diameter** of the normal bowel lumen, or if **diverticulitis involves the base**

DUODENAL DIVERTICULA
- Need to rule out gallbladder-duodenal fistula
- Observe unless perforated, bleeding, causing obstruction, or highly symptomatic
- Frequency of diverticula: duodenal > jejunal > ileal
- Tx: **segmental resection** if symptomatic
  - If **juxta-ampullary** usually can't get resection and need **choledochojejunostomy** for biliary or **ERCP with stent** for pancreatitis symptoms (_avoid_ Whipple here)

CROHN'S DISEASE
- Inflammatory bowel disease causing intermittent **abdominal pain**, **diarrhea**, and **weight loss**; can also cause bowel obstructions and fistulas
- 15–35 years old at 1st presentation; $\uparrow$ in Ashkenazi Jews
- Extraintestinal manifestations – arthritis, arthralgias, pyoderma gangrenosum, erythema nodosum, ocular diseases, growth failure, megaloblastic anemia from folate and vitamin B_{12} malabsorption
- Can occur anywhere from mouth to anus; usually **spares rectum**
- **Terminal ileum** – most commonly involved bowel segment
- **Anal/perianal disease** – 1st presentation in 5%
  - Tx: Flagyl
  - **Anal disease most common symptom** – large skin tags

■ **Most common sites for initial presentation**
  • **Terminal ileum** and cecum – 40%
  • Colon only – 35%
  • Small bowel only – 20%
  • Perianal – 5%
■ Dx: colonoscopy with biopsies and enteroclysis can help make the diagnosis

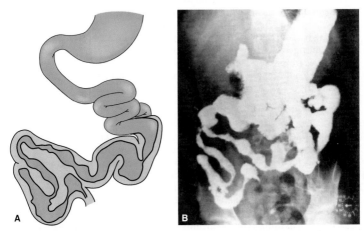

Typical radiographic appearance of extensive jejunoileal Crohn's disease.

■ **Pathology** – transmural involvement, segmental disease (skip lesions), cobblestoning, narrow deep ulcers, creeping fat, fistulas
■ Medical Tx: **5-ASA** and **loperamide** for maintenance; **steroids** for acute flares
  • **Remicade** (infliximab; TNF-α inhibitor) – for fistulas or steroid-resistant disease
  • <u>No</u> agents affect the natural course of disease
  • **TPN** – may induce remission and fistula closure with small bowel Crohn's disease
■ **90%** eventually need an **operation**
■ **Surgical indications** – unlike ulcerative colitis, surgery is <u>not</u> curative
  • **Obstruction** – often partial and can be initially treated conservatively
  • **Abscess** – usually treated with percutaneous drainage
  • **Megacolon** – perforation occurs in 15%; usually contained
  • **Hemorrhage** – unusual in Crohn's but can occur
  • **Blind loop obstruction** – need resection
  • **Fissures** – <u>no</u> lateral internal sphincteroplasty in patients with Crohn's disease
  • **Enterocutaneous fistula** – can usually be treated conservatively
  • **Perineal fistula** – unroof and rule out abscess; let heal on its own
  • **Anorectovaginal fistulas** – may need <u>rectal advancement flap</u>; possible colostomy
  • Do not need clear margins; just get 2 cm away from gross disease with surgery
■ **Patients with diffuse disease of colon** – proctocolectomy and ileostomy the procedures of choice (<u>no</u> pouches or ilio-anal anastomosis with Crohn's)
■ **Incidental finding of inflammatory bowel disease** in patient with presumed appendicitis who has normal appendix – Tx: **remove appendix** if cecum not involved (avoids future confounding diagnosis)

- **Stricturoplasty** (longitudinal incision through stricture, close transversely)
  - Consider if patient has multiple bowel strictures to save small bowel length
  - Probably not good for patient's 1st operation as it leaves disease behind
  - 10% leakage/abscess/fistula rate with stricturoplasty (all of which can usually be treated conservatively)
- 50% recurrence rate requiring surgery for Crohn's disease after resection
- **Complications from removal of terminal ileum**
  - ↓ **B$_{12}$ uptake** can result in **megaloblastic anemia**
  - ↓ **bile salt uptake** causes osmotic **diarrhea** (bile salts) and **steatorrhea** (fat) in colon
  - ↓ **oxalate binding to calcium secondary to** ↑ **intraluminal fat** (fat binds Ca) → oxalate then gets absorbed in colon → released in urine → **Ca oxalate kidney stones** (hyperoxaluria)
  - **Gallstones** can form after terminal ileum resection from malabsorption of bile salts

CARCINOID
- **Serotonin** is produced by **Kulchitsky cells** (enterochromaffin cell or argentaffin cell)
  - Part of amine precursor uptake decarboxylase system **(APUD)**
  - **5-HIAA** is a breakdown product of serotonin – can measure this in urine
- **Bradykinin** – also released by carcinoid tumors
- **Carcinoid syndrome** – caused by bulky **liver metastases**
  - Intermittent **flushing** (kallikrein) and **diarrhea** (serotonin) – hallmark symptoms
  - Can also get **asthma-type symptoms** (bradykinin) and **right heart valve lesions**
  - If patient has carcinoid syndrome with small bowel carcinoid primary, it **indicates metastasis to liver** (liver usually clears serotonin)
  - If resection of liver metastases is performed, perform cholecystectomy in case of future embolization
  - **Octreotide scan** – best for *localizing* tumor not seen on CT scan
  - **Chromogranin A level** – highest sensitivity for *detecting* a carcinoid tumor
- **Appendix carcinoid** – most common site for carcinoid tumor (50% of carcinoids arise here; ileum and rectum next most common)
- **Small bowel carcinoid** – patients at ↑ risk for **multiple primaries** and **second unrelated malignancies**
- **Carcinoid Tx:**
  - **Carcinoid in appendix** – < 2 cm → appendectomy; ≥ 2 cm or involving base → right hemicolectomy
  - **Carcinoid anywhere else in GI tract** → treat like cancer (segmental resection with lymphadenectomy)
  - **Chemotherapy** – **streptozocin** and **5FU**; usually just for **unresectable disease**
  - **Octreotide** – useful for carcinoid syndrome palliation
  - **Bronchospasm** – Tx: **aprotinin**
  - **Flushing** – Tx: **α-blockers** (phenothiazine)
  - **False 5-HIAA** – fruits
  - **Crohn's pancolitis** – same **colon CA** risk as ulcerative colitis

INTUSSUSCEPTION IN ADULTS
- Can occur from small bowel or cecal tumors
- Most common presentation is obstruction
- Worrisome in adults as it often has a **malignant lead point** (ie cecal CA)
- Tx: resection

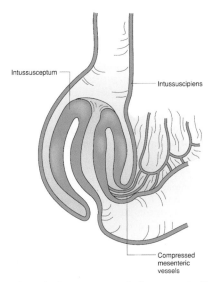

Intussusceptum

Intussuscipiens

Compressed
mesenteric
vessels

Anatomy of intussusception. The intussusceptum is the segment of bowel that invaginates into the intussuscipiens.

BENIGN SMALL BOWEL TUMORS
- **Adenomas** – most found in duodenum; present with bleeding, obstruction
  - Need resection when identified (often done with endoscope)
- **Peutz–Jeghers syndrome** (autosomal dominant) – **hamartomas** throughout GI tract (small and large bowel); mucocutaneous melanotic skin pigmentation; patients have ↑ extraintestinal malignancies (most common – **breast CA**) and a small risk of GI malignancies; _**no prophylactic colectomy**_

MALIGNANT SMALL BOWEL TUMORS
- **Adenocarcinoma** (rare) – most common malignant small bowel tumor
  - High proportion is in the **duodenum**
  - Symptoms: obstruction, jaundice
  - Tx: resection and adenectomy; **Whipple** if in **2nd portion of duodenum**
- **Duodenal CA risk factors**: FAP, Gardner's, polyps, adenomas, von Recklinghausen's
- **Leiomyosarcoma**
  - Usually in **jejunum** and **ileum**; most extraluminal
  - Hard to differentiate compared with leiomyoma (> 5 mitoses/HPF, atypia, necrosis)
  - Make sure it is not a GIST (check for C-Kit)
  - Tx: resection; <u>no</u> adenectomy required
- **Lymphoma**
  - Usually in **ileum**; associated with Wegener's, SLE, AIDS, Crohn's, celiac sprue
  - Usually **NHL B cell** type
  - Post-transplantation – ↑ **risk of bleeding** and **perforation**
  - Dx: abdominal CT, node sampling
  - Tx: **wide en bloc resection** (include nodes) unless 1st or 2nd portion of the duodenum (chemo-XRT, <u>no</u> Whipple)
  - 40% 5-year survival rate

STOMAS
- **Parastomal hernias** – highest incidence with colostomies; generally well tolerated and do not need repair unless symptomatic
- *Candida* – most common stomal infection
- **Diversion colitis** (Hartmann's pouch) – secondary to lack of short-chain fatty acids
  • Tx: short-chain fatty acid enemas
- **Ischemia** – most common cause of stenosis of stoma
  • Tx: dilation if mild
- **Crohn's disease** – most common cause of fistula near stoma site
- **Abscesses** – underneath stoma site, often caused by irrigation device
- **Gallstones** and **uric acid kidney stones** – increased in patients with ileostomy

APPENDICITIS
- **Appendicitis** – 1st: anorexia; 2nd: abdominal pain (periumbilical); 3rd: vomiting
- Pain gradually migrates to the RLQ as peritonitis sets in
- Most commonly occurs in patients 20–35 years
- Patients can have normal WBC count
- **CT scan** - <u>diameter > 7 mm</u> or <u>wall thickness > 2 mm</u> (looks like a bull's eye), fat stranding, no contrast in appendiceal lumen; try to give rectal contrast
- **Midpoint of anti-mesenteric border** – area most likely to **perforate**
- **Hyperplasia** – most common cause in children; can follow a viral illness
- **Fecalith** – most common cause in adults
- Luminal obstruction is followed by distention of the appendix, venous congestion and thrombosis, ischemia, gangrene necrosis, and finally rupture
- **Nonoperative situation** – CT scan shows walled-off perforated appendix (usually in **elderly**)
  • Tx: **percutaneous drainage** and **interval appendectomy** at later date as long as symptoms are improving
  • Consider follow-up barium enema or colonoscopy to rule out perforated cecal colon CA
- **Children** and **elderly** have higher propensity to rupture secondary to <u>delayed diagnosis</u>
  • Children often have **higher fever** and more **vomiting and diarrhea**
  • **Elderly** – signs and symptoms can be minimal; may need right hemicolectomy if cancer suspected
- **Appendicitis is infrequent in infants**
- **Perforation** – patient generally more ill; can have evidence of sepsis
- **Appendicitis during pregnancy**
  • **Most common cause** of **acute abdominal pain** in the **1st trimester**
  • More likely to **occur** in the **2nd trimester** but is not the most common cause of abdominal pain
  • More likely to **perforate** in the **3rd trimester** – confused with contractions
  • **Need to make the incision where the patient is having pain** – the appendix is *displaced superiorly (cephalad)*
  • May have symptoms of RUQ pain in the 3rd trimester
  • 35% fetal mortality with rupture
  • Women with suspected appendicitis need beta-HCG drawn and abdominal ultrasound to rule out OB/GYN causes of abdominal pain

OTHER APPENDIX
- **Appendix mucocele** – can be benign or malignant mucous papillary tumor; needs resection (**should open** for these so you don't spill tumor contents)
  • Need right hemicolectomy if malignant
  • Can get **pseudomyxoma peritonei** with rupture (spread of tumor implants throughout the peritoneum)
  • **MCC of death** - **small bowel obstruction** from peritoneal tumor spread

- **Regional ileitis** – can mimic appendicitis; 10% go on to Crohn's disease
- **Gastroenteritis** – nausea, vomiting, diarrhea
- **Presumed appendicitis** but find ruptured ovarian cyst, thrombosed ovarian vein, or regional enteritis not involving cecum → **still perform appendectomy** (prevents future confounding diagnosis)

ILEUS
- Causes include surgery (most common), electrolyte abnormalities (↓ K), peritonitis, ischemia, trauma, drugs
- **Ileus** – dilatation is uniform throughout the stomach, small bowel, colon, and rectum *without* decompression
- **Obstruction** – there is <u>bowel decompression</u> distal to the obstruction

TYPHOID ENTERITIS (SALMONELLA)
- Children; get RLQ pain, diarrhea, fever, headaches, maculopapular rash, leukopenia; rare bleeding/perforation
- Tx: **Bactrim**

ANATOMY AND PHYSIOLOGY

■ Colon secretes **K** and reabsorbs **Na and water** (mostly in right colon and cecum)
■ **4 layers** – mucosa (columnar epithelium) → submucosa → muscularis propria → serosa
  • **Muscularis mucosa** – small interwoven inner muscle layer just below mucosa but above basement membrane
  • **Muscularis propria** – circular layer of muscle
■ Ascending, descending, and sigmoid colon are all **retroperitoneal**
  • Peritoneum covers anterior upper and middle ⅓ of the rectum
■ **Plicae semilunares** – transverse bands that form haustra
■ **Taenia coli** – 3 bands that run longitudinally along colon. At rectosigmoid junction, the taeniae become broad and completely encircle the bowel.

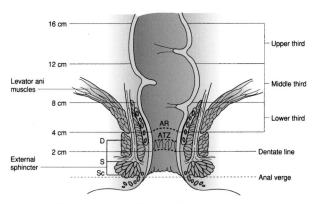

Anorectal anatomy with important landmarks. Approximate measurements are relative to the anal verge. D, deep; S, superficial; Sc, subcutaneous; AR, anorectal ring; ATZ, anal transition zone.

■ **Vascular supply**
  • **Ascending** and ⅔ **of transverse colon** supplied by **SMA** (ileocolic, right and middle colic arteries)
  • ⅓ **transverse**, **descending colon**, **sigmoid colon**, and **upper portion of the rectum** supplied by **IMA** (left colic, sigmoid branches, superior rectal artery)
  • **Marginal artery** – runs along colon margin, connecting SMA to IMA (provides collateral flow)
  • **Arc of Riolan** – short direct connection between SMA and IMA
  • 80% of blood flow goes to mucosa and submucosa
■ **Venous drainage** follows arterial except IMV, which goes to the splenic vein
  • Splenic vein joins the SMV to form the portal vein behind the pancreas
■ **Superior rectal artery** – branch of **IMA**
■ **Middle rectal artery** – branch of **internal iliac** (the lateral stalks during low anterior resection [LAR] or abdominoperineal resection [APR] contain the middle rectal arteries)
■ **Inferior rectal artery** – branch of <u>internal pudendal</u> (which is a branch of **internal iliac**)
■ Superior and middle rectal veins drain into the IMV and eventually the portal vein
■ Inferior rectal veins drain into the internal iliac veins and eventually the caval system

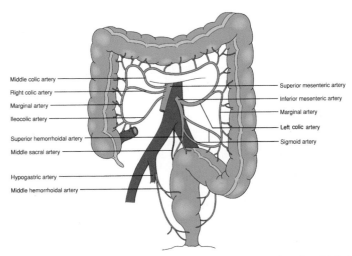

Arterial blood supply of the colon. The superior mesenteric artery (SMA) and inferior mesenteric artery (IMA) are the major blood supplies to the colon.

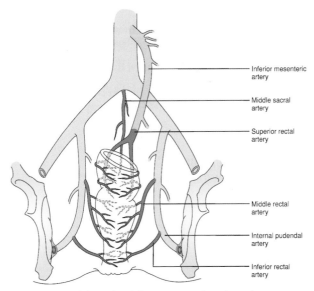

Arterial supply of the rectum and anal canal.

- ■ **Superior** and **middle rectum** – drain to IMA nodal lymphatics
- ■ **Lower rectum** – drains primarily to IMA nodes, also to internal iliac nodes
- ■ Bowel wall contains mucosal and submucosal lymphatics
- ■ **Watershed areas**
  - • Splenic flexure (Griffith's point) – SMA and IMA junction
  - • Rectum (Sudak's point) – superior rectal and middle rectal junction
  - • Colon more sensitive to ischemia than small bowel secondary to ↓ collaterals

- **External sphincter** (puborectalis muscle) – under CNS (voluntary) control
  - Inferior rectal branch of **internal pudendal nerve**
  - Is the continuation of the **levator ani muscle** (striated muscle)
- **Internal sphincter** – involuntary control
  - Is the continuation of the **muscularis propria** (smooth muscle)
  - Is normally contracted
- **Meissner's plexus** – inner nerve plexus
- **Auerbach's plexus** – outer nerve plexus
- **Pelvic splanchnic nerves** – parasympathetic
- **Lumbar** and **sacral plexus** – sympathetic
- **From anal verge** – anal canal 0–5 cm, rectum 5–15 cm, rectosigmoid junction 15–18 cm
- **Levator ani** – marks the transition between anal canal and rectum
- **Crypts of Lieberkühn** – mucus-secreting goblet cells
- **Colonic inertia** – slow transit time; patients may need subtotal colectomy
- **Short-chain fatty acids** – main nutrient of colonocytes
- **Stump pouchitis** (diversion or disuse proctitis) – Tx: short-chain fatty acids
- **Infectious pouchitis** – Tx: metronidazole (Flagyl)
- **Denonvilliers fascia** (anterior) – rectovesicular fascia in men; rectovaginal fascia in women
- **Waldeyer's fascia** (posterior) – rectosacral fascia

POLYPS
- **Hyperplastic polyps** – most common polyp; no cancer risk
- **Tubular adenoma** – most common (75%) intestinal neoplastic polyp
  - These are generally pedunculated
- **Villous adenoma** – most likely to produce symptoms
  - These are generally sessile and larger than tubular adenomas
  - 50% of villous adenomas have **cancer**
- **> 2 cm**, **sessile**, or **villous** lesions have ↑ cancer risk
- Polyps have left-side predominance
- Most **pedunculated polyps** can be removed endoscopically
- If not able to get all of the polyp (which usually occurs with **sessile polyps**) → need **segmental resection**

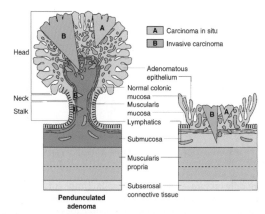

Diagrammatic representation of cancer-containing polyps. Pedunculated adenoma is described on the left and a sessile adenoma on the right. In carcinoma in situ, malignant cells are confined to the mucosa. These lesions are adequately treated by endoscopic polypectomy. Polypectomy is adequate treatment for invasive carcinoma only if the margin is sufficient (2 mm), the carcinoma is not poorly differentiated, and no evidence of venous or lymphatic invasion is found.

- **High-grade dysplasia** – basement membrane is intact (carcinoma in situ)
- **Intramucosal cancer** – into muscularis mucosa (carcinoma in situ → still has not gone through basement membrane)
- **Invasive cancer** – into submucosa (T1)
- **Screening** – at **50** for **normal risk**, at **40** (or 10 years before youngest case) for **intermediate risk** (eg family history of colon CA)
- **Screening options** – 1) **colonoscopy** every 10 years; *or* 2) **high-sensitivity fecal occult blood testing** every 3 years and **flexible sigmoidoscopy** every 5 years; *or* 3) **high-sensitivity fecal occult blood testing** annually
  - **Double contrast barium enema** or **CT colonography** every 5 years may be alternatives to above
  - **False-positive guaiac** – beef, vitamin C, iron, cimetidine
  - **No colonoscopy with** recent MI, splenomegaly, pregnancy (if fluoroscopy planned)
- **Polypectomy shows T1 lesion** – polypectomy is adequate if margins are clear (2 mm), is well differentiated, and has no vascular/lymphatic invasion; otherwise, need formal colon resection
- **Extensive low rectal villous adenomas with atypia** – Tx: transanal excision (can try mucosectomy) as much of the polyp as possible
  - **No** APR unless cancer is present
- **Pathology shows T1 lesion after transanal excision of rectal polyp** → transanal excision is adequate if margins are clear (2 mm), it is well differentiated, and it has no vascular/lymphatic invasion
- **Pathology shows T2 lesion after transanal excision of rectal polyp** → patient needs APR or LAR

COLORECTAL CANCER
- **2nd leading cause of CA death**
- Symptoms: **anemia**, **constipation**, and **bleeding**
- Red meat and **fat** → O_2 radicals are thought to have a role
- Colon CA has had an association with *Clostridium septicum* infection
- **Colon CA** – main gene mutations are **APC**, **DCC**, **p53**, and **k-ras**
- **Sigmoid colon** – most common site of primary
- **Disease spread**
  - Spreads to **nodes** first
  - **Nodal status** – most important prognostic factor
  - **Liver** – #1 site of metastases; lung – #2 site of metastases
    - Portal vein → **liver metastases**; iliac vein → **lung metastases**
    - **Liver metastases** – if resectable and leaves adequate liver function, patients have 35% 5-year survival (5-YS) rate
    - **Lung metastases** – 25% 5-YS rate in selected patients after resection
    - **Isolated liver** or **lung metastases** should be **resected**
  - 5% get drop metastases to **ovaries**
  - **Rectal CA** – can metastasize to **spine directly via Batson's plexus** (venous)
  - **Colon CA** typically does not go to bone
  - Colorectal CA growing into adjacent organs can be resected en bloc with a portion of the adjacent organ (ie partial bladder resection)
- **Lymphocytic penetration** – patients have an improved prognosis
- **Mucoepidermoid** – worst prognosis
- **Rectal ultrasound** – good at assessing depth of invasion (sphincter involvement), recurrence, and presence of enlarged nodes
- Need **total colonoscopy** to rule out **synchronous** lesions in patients with colorectal CA
- **Goals of resection**
  - En bloc resection, adequate margins, and regional adenectomy
  - **Most right-sided colon CAs** can be treated with primary anastomosis without ostomy
  - **Rectal pain with rectal CA** – patient needs APR
  - Generally need **2-cm margins**

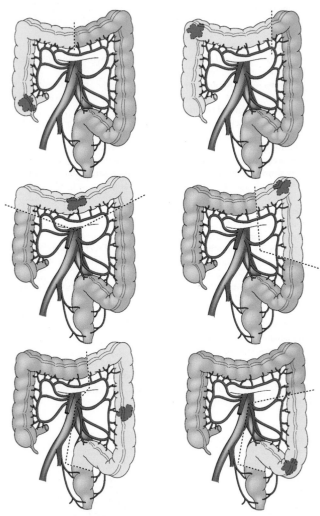

Segmental resections for cancers of the colon and upper third of the rectum. Note the blood supply taken with each form of resection.

- ■ **Intraoperative ultrasound** (U/S) – best method of picking up intrahepatic metastases
  - • Conventional U/S resolution: 10 mm
  - • Abdominal CT: 5–10 mm
  - • Abdominal MRI: 5–10 mm (better resolution than CT)
  - • Intraoperative U/S: 3–5 mm
- ■ **Abdominoperineal resection** (APR)
  - • Permanent colostomy; anal canal is excised along with the rectum
  - • Can have impotence and bladder dysfunction (injured pudendal nerves)
  - • Indicated for malignant lesions only (not benign tumors) that are not amenable to LAR
  - • Need at least a 2-cm margin (2 cm from levator ani muscles) for LAR, otherwise will need APR
  - • Risk of local recurrence higher with rectal CA than with colon CA in general

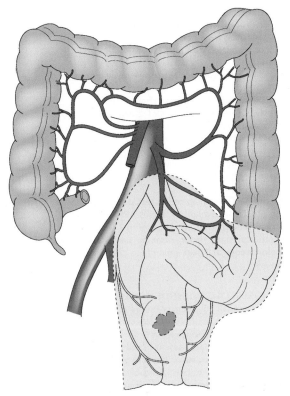

Extent of surgery in abdominoperineal resection.

- **Preoperative chemo-XRT** – produces complete response in some patients with rectal CA; preserves sphincter function in some

---

TNM STAGING SYSTEM FOR COLORECTAL CANCER
- **T1**: into submucosa. **T2**: into muscularis propria. **T3**: into serosa or through muscularis propria if no serosa is present. **T4**: through serosa into free peritoneal cavity or into adjacent organs/structures if no serosa is present
- **N0**: nodes negative. **N1**: 1–3 nodes positive, **N2**: ≥ 4 nodes positive, **N3**: central nodes positive
- **M1**: distant metastases

Stage	TNM Status
0	Tis, N0, M0
I	T1–2, N0, M0
IIA	T3, N0, M0
IIB	T4, N0, M0
IIIA	T1–2, N1, M0
IIIB	T3–4, N1, M0
IIIC	Any T, N2, M0
IV	Any T, Any N, M1

- **Low rectal T1** (limited to submucosa) – can be excised transanally if < 4 cm, has negative margins (need 1 cm), is well differentiated, and there is no neurologic or vascular invasion; otherwise, patient needs APR or LAR
- **Low rectal T2 or higher** – Tx: APR or LAR
- **Chemotherapy**
  - **Stage III** and **IV colon CA** (nodes positive or distant metastases) → **postop chemo,** no XRT
  - **Stage II** and **III rectal CA** → **pre-op chemo-XRT**
  - **Stage IV rectal CA** → **chemo and XRT ± surgery** (possibly just colostomy, may want to avoid APR in patients with metastatic disease)
  - **Chemo** – *5FU*, *leucovorin*, and *oxaliplatin* (FOLFOX)
- **XRT**
  - ↓ local recurrence and ↑ survival when combined with chemotherapy
  - **XRT damage** – rectum most common site of injury → vasculitis, thrombosis, ulcers, strictures
  - **Pre-op chemo-XRT** may help shrink **rectal tumors**, allowing down-staging of the tumor and possibly allowing LAR versus APR
- **20% have a recurrence** (usually occurs within 1 year)
  - 5% get another primary – ***main reason for surveillance colonoscopy***
- **Follow-up colonoscopy at 1 year** – mainly to check for **new primary colon CA** (metachronous)

FAMILIAL ADENOMATOUS POLYPOSIS (FAP)
- Autosomal dominant; all have cancer by age 40
- **APC gene** – chromosome 5
- 20% of FAP syndromes are spontaneous
- Polyps <u>not</u> present at birth; are present in **puberty**
- Do <u>not</u> need colonoscopy for surveillance in patients with suspected FAP → just need flexible sigmoidoscopy to check for polyps
- All need **total colectomy prophylactically** at **age 20**
- **Also get duodenal polyps** → need to check duodenum with endoscopy every 2 years
- **Surgery** – **proctocolectomy, rectal mucosectomy,** and **ileoanal pouch** (J-pouch)
  - Need lifetime surveillance of residual rectal mucosa
  - **Total proctocolectomy with end ileostomy** is also an option
  - Following colectomy, most common cause of death in FAP patients is **periampullary tumors of duodenum**
- **Gardner's syndrome** – patients get colon CA (associated with APC gene) and desmoid tumors/osteomas
- **Turcot's syndrome** – patients get colon CA (associated with APC gene) and brain tumors

LYNCH SYNDROMES (HEREDITARY NONPOLYPOSIS COLON CANCER)
- 5% of population, autosomal dominant
- Associated with **DNA mismatch repair gene**
- Predilection for right-sided and multiple cancers
- **Lynch I** – just colon CA risk
- **Lynch II** – patients <u>*also*</u> have ↑ risk of ovarian, endometrial, bladder, and stomach cancer
- **Amsterdam criteria** for **Lynch syndrome** – "3, 2, 1" → at least **3** first-degree relatives, over **2** generations, **1** with cancer before age 50
- Need surveillance colonoscopy starting at age 25 or 10 years before primary relative got cancer (also need surveillance program for the other CA types in the family)
- 50% get metachronous lesions within 10 years; often have multiple primaries
- Need **total proctocolectomy** with first cancer operation

SIGMOID VOLVULUS
- More common with high-fiber diets (Iran, Iraq)
- Occurs in debilitated psychiatric patients, neurologic dysfunction, laxative abuse
- Symptoms: pain, distention, and obstipation
- Causes closed-loop obstruction – **sigmoid colon twists on itself**
- Abdominal x-ray – bent inner tube sign; Gastrografin enema may show bird's beak sign (tapered colon)
- Do not attempt decompression with gangrenous bowel or peritoneal signs → go to OR for sigmoidectomy
- Tx: **decompress with colonoscopy** (80% reduce, 50% will recur), give bowel prep, and perform sigmoid colectomy during same admission

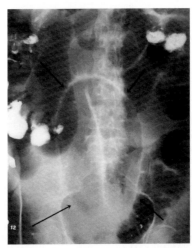

Plain supine abdominal film of a patient with sigmoid volvulus. The centrally located sigmoid loop is outlined by trapped air. The proximal small intestine is dilated as well, suggesting that the volvulus has been present for sufficient time to cause accumulation of air and fluid proximally. (Courtesy of John Braver, M.D., Department of Radiology, Brigham and Women's Hospital, Harvard Medical School, Boston, MA.)

CECAL VOLVULUS
- Less common than sigmoid volvulus; occurs in 20s–30s
- Can appear as an SBO, with dilated cecum in the RLQ
- Can try to decompress with colonoscopy but unlikely to succeed (only 20%)
- Tx: **OR → right hemicolectomy** probably best treatment; can try cecopexy if colon is viable and patient is frail

ULCERATIVE COLITIS
- Symptoms: **bloody diarrhea, abdominal pain, fever,** and **weight loss**
- Involves the **mucosa** and **submucosa**
- Strictures and fistulae unusual with ulcerative colitis
- **Spares anus** – unlike Crohn's disease
  - Usually starts distally in **rectum** and is contiguous (<u>no</u> skip areas like Crohn's)
  - **Bleeding** is universal and has mucosal friability with <u>pseudopolyps and collar button ulcers</u>
  - Always need to rule out infectious etiology
  - Backwash ileitis can occur with proximal disease

Clinicopathologic Features of Ulcerative Colitis Versus Crohn Disease

Manifestation	Ulcerative Colitis	Crohn Disease
Transmural inflammation	Seldom	Common
Granulomas	Seldom	> 50%
Fissuring	Rare	Common
Fibrosis	Rare	Common
Submucosal inflammation	Rare	Common
Crypt abscesses	Common	Uncommon
Small-bowel involvement	Rare (backwash ileitis)	Common
Anatomic location	Continuous	Skip
Rectal involvement	Common	May be spared
Bleeding	Common	Absent
Fistulas	Rare	Common
Perianal disease	Rare	Common
Ulcers	Rare	Common
Surrounding mucosa	Pseudopolyps	Relatively normal
Cobblestoning of mucosa	None	Long-standing disease
Mucosal friability	Common	Uncommon
Vascular pattern	Absent	Normal
Fat wrapping	Rare	Common

- **Barium enema** – with chronic disease see loss of haustra, narrow caliber, short colon, and loss of redundancy
- **Medical Tx: sulfasalazine** (or 5-ASA) and **loperamide** for maintenance therapy
  - **Steroids** for acute flares
  - 5-ASA and sulfasalazine can maintain remission in ulcerative colitis
  - Consider cyclosporine or infliximab for steroid-resistant disease
- **Toxic colitis** and **toxic megacolon**
  - <u>Toxic colitis</u>: > 6 bloody stools/d, fever, ↑ HR, drop in Hgb, leukocytosis
  - <u>Toxic megacolon</u>: above plus distension, abdominal pain and tenderness
  - <u>Initial Tx</u>: **NG tube, fluids, steroids, bowel rest**, and **antibiotics** (ciprofloxacin and Flagyl) will treat 50% adequately; other 50% require surgery
  - Follow clinical response and abdominal radiographs
  - *Avoid* barium enemas, narcotics, anti-diarrheal agents, and anti-cholinergics

Indications for Surgery with Toxic Colitis and Toxic Megacolon

Absolute	Relative
Pneumoperitoneum	Inability to promptly control sepsis
Diffuse peritonitis	Increasing megacolon
Localized peritonitis with increasing abdominal pain and/or colonic distension > 10 cm	Failure to improve within 24–48 h
	Increasing toxicity or other signs of clinical deterioration
Uncontrolled sepsis	Continued transfusion requirements
Major hemorrhage	

Modified from Rothenberger DA, Bullard KM. Surgery for toxic megacolon. In: Fischer JE, Bland KI, et al, eds. *Mastery of Surgery*. 5th ed. Philadelphia, PA: Lippincott Williams & Wilkins; 2007, with permission.

- **Perforation with ulcerative colitis** – <u>transverse colon</u> more common
- **Perforation with Crohn's** – <u>distal ileum</u> most common
- **Surgical indications for ulcerative colitis**: massive hemorrhage, refractory toxic mega-colon, acute fulminant ulcerative colitis (occurs in 15%), obstruction, <u>any</u> dysplasia, cancer, intractability, systemic complications, failure to thrive, and long-standing disease (> 10 years) as prophylaxis against colon CA (some controversy here)

- **Emergent/urgent resections** – total proctocolectomy and bring up ileostomy
  - Perform definitive hook-up later
- **Elective resections**
  - **Ileoanal anastomosis** – rectal mucosectomy, J-pouch, and ileoanal (low rectal) anastomosis; <u>not</u> used with Crohn's disease
    - Can protect bladder and sexual function
    - Need lifetime surveillance of residual rectal area
    - Many ileoanal anastomoses need resection secondary to cancer, dysplastic changes, refractory pouchitis, or pouch failure (incontinence)
    - Need temporary diverting ileostomy (6–8 weeks) while pouch heals
    - **Leak** (most common major morbidity) – can lead to sepsis (Tx: drainage, antibiotics)
    - **Infectious pouchitis** – Tx: Flagyl
  - **APR with ileostomy** – can also be performed
- **Cancer risk** is **1% per year** starting **10 years after initial diagnosis** for patients with **pancolitis**
  - Cancer more evenly distributed throughout colon
  - Need yearly colonoscopy starting 8–10 years after diagnosis
- **Extraintestinal manifestations of ulcerative colitis**
  - Most common extraintestinal manifestation requiring total colectomy – **failure to thrive in children**
  - **Do <u>not</u> get better with colectomy** → primary sclerosing cholangitis, ankylosing spondylitis
  - **Get better with colectomy** → most ocular problems, arthritis, and anemia
  - **50% get better** → pyoderma gangrenosum
  - **HLA B27** – sacroiliitis, ankylosing spondylitis, ulcerative colitis
  - Can get **thromboembolic disease**
  - **Pyoderma gangrenosum** – Tx: steroids

CARCINOID OF THE COLON AND RECTUM

- Represents 15% of all carcinoids; infrequent cause of carcinoid syndrome
- Metastases related to size of tumor
- ⅔ of colon carcinoids have either local or systemic spread
- **Low rectal carcinoids**
  - **< 2 cm** → wide local excision with negative margins
  - **> 2 cm or invasion of muscularis propria** → APR
- **Colon or high rectal carcinoids** → formal resection with adenectomy

COLONIC OBSTRUCTION

- **Colon perforation with obstruction** – most likely to occur in **cecum**
  - Law of LaPlace: tension = pressure × diameter
- **Closed-loop obstructions** – can be worrisome; can have rapid progression and perforation with minimal distention
  - Competent ileocecal valve can lead to closed-loop obstruction
- **Colonic obstruction** – #1 cancer; #2 diverticulitis
- **Pneumatosis intestinalis** – air on the bowel wall, associated with ischemia and dissection of air through areas of bowel wall
- **Air in the portal system** – usually indicates significant infection or necrosis of the large or small bowel; often an ominous sign

OGILVIE'S SYNDROME

- Pseudoobstruction of colon
- Associated with opiate use; bedridden or older patients; recent surgery, infection, or trauma
- Get a **massively dilated colon**, which can **perforate**

■ Tx: check and replace electrolytes (especially K); discontinue drugs that slow the gut (eg morphine); NGT
  • If **colon > 10 cm** (high risk of perforation) → **decompression** with colonoscopy and **neostigmine**; cecostomy if that fails

AMOEBIC COLITIS
■ ***Entamoeba histolytica***; from contaminated food and water with feces that contain cysts
■ **Primary infection** – occurs in colon; **secondary infection** – occurs in liver
■ Risk factors – travel to Mexico, ETOH; fecal–oral transmission
■ Symptoms: similar to ulcerative colitis (dysentery); chronic more common form (3–4 bowel movements/day, cramping, and fever)
■ Dx: endoscopy → ulceration, trophozoites; 90% have anti-amebic antibodies
■ Tx: **Flagyl**, diiodohydroxyquin

ACTINOMYCES
■ Can present as a mass, abscess, fistula, or induration; suppurative and granulomatous
■ Cecum most common location; can be confused with CA
■ Pathology shows **yellow-white sulfur granules**
■ Tx: **penicillin** or tetracycline, drainage of any abscess

DIVERTICULA
■ Herniation of mucosa through the colon wall at sites where arteries enter the muscular wall
■ Circular muscle thickens adjacent to diverticulum with luminal narrowing
■ Caused by **straining** (↑ intraluminal pressure)
■ Most diverticula occur on **left side** (80%) in the sigmoid colon
  • **Bleeding** is more likely with right-sided diverticula (50% of bleeds occur on right)
  • **Diverticulitis** is more likely to present on the left side
■ Present in 35% of the population

LOWER GI BLEEDING
■ Stool guaiac can stay positive up to 3 weeks after bleed
■ **Hematemesis** – bleeding anywhere from pharynx to ligament of Treitz
■ **Melena** – passage of tarry stools; need as little as 50 cc

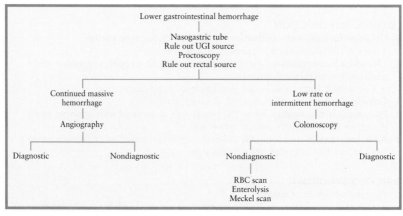

Diagnostic steps in the evaluation of acute lower gastrointestinal hemorrhage. UGI, upper gastrointestinal; RBC, red blood cell.

- **Azotemia after GI bleed** – caused by production of urea from bacterial action on intraluminal blood ($\uparrow$ BUN; also get elevated total bilirubin)
- **Arteriography** – bleeding must be $\geq$ 0.5 cc/min
- **Tagged RBC scan** – bleeding must be $\geq$ 0.1 cc/min

DIVERTICULITIS
- Result of mucosal perforations in the diverticulum with adjacent fecal contamination
- Denotes infection and inflammation of the colonic wall as well as surrounding tissue
- LLQ pain, tenderness, fever, $\uparrow$ WBCs
- Dx: CT scan is needed only if worried about complications of disease
- Need **follow-up colonoscopy** after an episode of diverticulitis to rule out **colorectal cancer**
- Most common complication – **abscess formation**; can usually **percutaneously drain**
  - **Signs of complication** – obstruction symptoms, fluctuant mass, peritoneal signs, temperature > 39, and WBCs > 20
- **Uncomplicated diverticulitis** – Tx: **levofloxacin** and **Flagyl**; bowel rest for 3–4 days (mild cases can be treated as an outpatient)
- **Surgery** – for **significant complications** (total obstruction not resolved with medical therapy, perforation, or abscess formation not amenable to percutaneous drainage) or **inability to exclude cancer**
  - Need to resect all of the **sigmoid colon** down to the superior rectum (distal margin should be **normal rectum**)
- **Right-sided diverticulitis** – 80% discovered at the time of incision for appendectomy
  - Tx: right hemicolectomy
- **Colovesicular fistula** – fecaluria, pneumouria
  - Occurs in men; women are more likely to get **colovaginal fistula**
  - **Cystoscopy** is the best diagnostic test
  - Tx: close bladder opening, resect involved segment of colon, and perform reanastomosis, diverting ileostomy; interpose omentum between the bladder and colon

DIVERTICULOSIS BLEEDING
- Most common cause of lower GI bleed
- Usually causes significant bleeding
- 75% stops spontaneously; recurs in 25%
- Caused by disrupted **vasa rectum**; creates **arterial bleeding**
- Dx: **NG tube** to rule out upper GI source
  - **Colonoscopy** usually as a 1st step $\rightarrow$ can be therapeutic (hemo-clips best) and can localize bleeding should surgery be required
  - **Angio** 1st if **massive bleed** (hypotension, tachycardia) – want to localize area for surgery; may be able to treat at angio with highly selective coil embolization
  - **Go to operating room** if hypotensive and not responding to resuscitation $\rightarrow$ colectomy at site of bleeding if identified or subtotal colectomy if bleeding source has not been localized
  - **Tagged RBC scan** for intermittent bleeds that are hard to localize
- Tx: **colonoscopy** can ligate bleeder
  - With arteriography, can use vasopressin (to temporize) or **highly selective coil embolization**; also demonstrates where the bleed is should surgery be required
  - May need segmental colectomy or possible subtotal colectomy if bleeding is not localized and not controlled
- Patients with recurrent diverticular bleeds should have resection of the area

ANGIODYSPLASIA BLEEDING
- ↑ on right side of colon
- Bleeds are usually less severe than diverticular bleeds but are more likely to recur (80%)
- Causes **venous bleeding**
- Soft signs of angiodysplasia on angiogram – **tufts, slow emptying**
- 20% of patients with angiodysplasia have **aortic stenosis** (usually gets better after valve replacement)

ISCHEMIC COLITIS
- Symptoms: abdominal pain, bright red bleeding
- Can be caused by a low-flow state (eg recent MI, CHF), ligation of the IMA at surgery (eg AAA repair), embolus or thrombosis of the IMA, sepsis
- **Splenic flexure** and **upper rectum** most vulnerable to low-flow state
- **Griffith's point** (splenic flexure) – SMA and IMA junction
- **Sudeck's point** – superior rectal and middle rectal artery junction
- Dx: CT scan or endoscopy → cyanotic edematous mucosa covered with exudates
  - Lower ⅔ of the rectum is spared → supplied by the middle and inferior rectal arteries (off internal iliacs)
  - If gangrenous colitis is suspected (peritonitis), no colonoscopy and go to OR → sigmoid resection or left hemicolectomy usual

PSEUDOMEMBRANOUS COLITIS (*C. DIFFICILE* COLITIS)
- Symptoms: watery, green, mucoid diarrhea; pain and cramping
- Can occur up to 3 weeks after antibiotics; increased in postop, elderly, and ICU patients
- Carrier state not eradicated; 15% recurrence
- Key finding – **PMN inflammation of mucosa** and **submucosa**
  - Pseudomembranes, plaques, and ringlike lesions
- Most common in the distal colon
- Dx: *C. difficile* **toxin**
- Tx: oral – vancomycin or Flagyl; IV – Flagyl
  - Lactobacillus can also help; stop other antibiotics or change them

NEUTROPENIC TYPHLITIS (ENTEROCOLITIS)
- Follows chemotherapy when WBCs are low (nadir)
- Can mimic surgical disease
- Can often see pneumatosis intestinalis (not a surgical indication here)
- Tx: **antibiotics**; patients will improve when WBCs ↑; surgery only for free perforation

OTHER COLON DISEASES
- Other causes of colitis – *Salmonella, Shigella, Campylobacter*, CMV, *Yersinia* (can mimic appendicitis in children), other viral infections, *Giardia*
- *Yersinia* – can mimic appendicitis; comes from contaminated food (feces/urine)
  - Tx: tetracycline or Bactrim
- **Megacolon** – propensity for volvulus; enlargement is proximal to non-peristalsing bowel
  - **Hirschsprung's disease** – rectosigmoid most common. Dx: rectal biopsy
  - *Trypanosoma cruzi* – most common acquired cause, secondary to destruction of nerves

Arterial supply to the anus – inferior rectal artery
Venous drainage – above the dentate is **internal hemorrhoid plexus** and below the dentate is **external hemorrhoid plexus**

HEMORRHOIDS

- Left lateral, right anterior, and right posterior hemorrhoidal plexuses
- **External hemorrhoids** cause pain when they thrombose
  - Distal to the dentate line, covered by sensate squamous epithelium; can cause pain, swelling, and itching
- **Internal hemorrhoids** cause bleeding or prolapse
  - **Primary** – slides below dentate with strain
  - **Secondary** – prolapse that reduces spontaneously
  - **Tertiary** – prolapse that has to be manually reduced
  - **Quaternary** – not able to reduce
- Tx: **fiber** and **stool softeners** (prevent straining); sitz baths
- **Thrombosed external hemorrhoid** → lance open (if > 72 hours) or elliptical excision (if < 72 hours) to relieve pain
- **Surgical indications**: recurrence, thrombosis multiple times, large external component
- External hemorrhoids can be resected with **elliptical excision**
- Can **band primary** and **secondary** internal hemorrhoids
  - Do not band external hemorrhoids (painful)
- **Surgery** for **tertiary** and **quaternary** internal hemorrhoids – 3 quadrant resection
  - Need to resect down to the **internal anal sphincter** (do not go through it)
  - Postop – sitz baths, stool softener, high-fiber diet

RECTAL PROLAPSE

- Starts 6–7 cm from anal verge
- Secondary to pudendal neuropathy and laxity of the anal sphincters
- ↑ with female gender, straining, chronic diarrhea, previous pregnancy, and redundant sigmoid colons
- Prolapse involves all layers of the rectum
- **Medical Tx**: high-fiber diet
- **Surgical Tx**:
  - **Perineal rectosigmoid resection** (Altemeier) transanally if patient is older and frail
  - **Low anterior resection** and **pexy** of residual colon if good condition patient

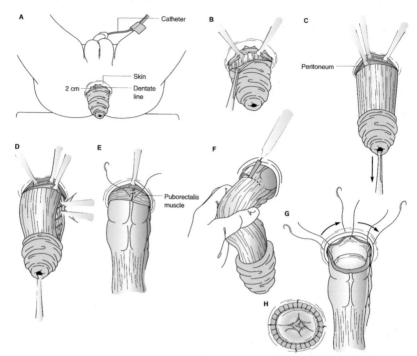

Perineal rectosigmoidectomy. The patient is placed in the lithotomy position with both legs in gynecologic stirrups. *(A and B)* A circular incision is made on the prolapsed rectum 2 cm proximal to the dentate line. *(C)* The peritoneal attachment is dissected from the anterior rectal wall, thus opening into the peritoneal cavity. *(D)* The mesorectum or mesosigmoid is clamped and divided laterally and posteriorly. *(E)* The previously opened peritoneum is sutured to the anterior wall of the rectum or sigmoid colon as high as possible. This is followed by approximation of the puborectalis (optional). *(F)* The anterior wall of the protruding rectum is cut 1 cm distal to the anal verge. *(G)* Stay sutures of 3-0 synthetic absorbable material are placed in four quadrants. *(H)* Anastomosis with running stitches.

CONDYLOMATA ACUMINATA
- Cauliflower mass; papillomavirus (HPV)
- Tx: laser surgery

ANAL FISSURE
- Caused by a split in the anoderm
- 90% in **posterior midline**
- Causes pain and bleeding after defecation; chronic ones will see a **sentinel pile**
- Medical Tx: **sitz baths**, **bulk**, **lidocaine jelly**, and **stool softeners** (90% heal)
- Surgical Tx: **lateral subcutaneous internal sphincterotomy**
- Fecal incontinence is the most serious complication of surgery
- Do <u>not</u> perform surgery if secondary to Crohn's disease or ulcerative colitis
- **Lateral or recurrent fissures** – worry about inflammatory bowel disease

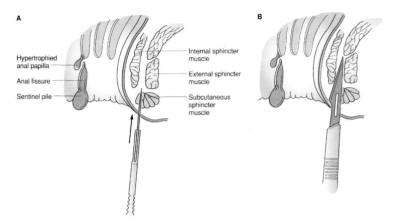

Lateral internal sphincterotomy (closed technique). *(A)* Triad of fissure, sentinel pile, and hypertrophied anal papilla. With an anal speculum used for exposure of the lateral quadrant, a no. 11 scalpel blade stabs into the subcutaneous tissue from the anal verge to the dentate line, with the knife in the horizontal position. *(B)* The knife is turned 90 degrees, and the internal sphincter muscle is cut while the anal canal is stretched open.

ANORECTAL ABSCESS
- Can cause severe pain
- **Perianal**, **intersphincteric**, and **ischiorectal abscesses** can be drained through the skin (all are below the levator muscles)
  - **Intersphincteric** and **ischiorectal abscesses** can form horseshoe abscess
- **Supralevator abscesses** need to be drained transrectally
- Antibiotics cellulitis, DM, immunosuppressed, or prosthetic hardware

PILONIDAL CYSTS
- Sinus or abscess formation over the sacrococcygeal junction; ↑ in men
- Tx: drainage and packing; follow-up surgical resection of cyst

FISTULA-IN-ANO
- Do <u>not</u> need to excise the tract
- Often occurs after anorectal abscess formation
- **Goodsall's rule**
  - Anterior fistulas connect with anus/rectum in a straight line
  - Posterior fistulas go toward a midline internal opening in the anus/rectum
- Tx: **lower ⅓** of the external anal sphincter → **fistulotomy** (open tract up, curettage out, let it heal by secondary intention)
  - **Upper ⅔** of the external anal sphincter → **rectal advancement flap**
  - Most worrisome complication here is **risk of incontinence** – you want to avoid damage to the external anal sphincter so fistulotomy is not used for fistulas above the lower ⅓ of the external anal sphincter

RECTOVAGINAL FISTULAS

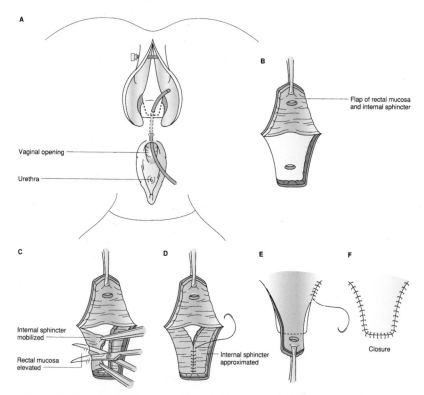

A

Vaginal opening

Urethra

B

Flap of rectal mucosa
and internal sphincter

C

Internal sphincter
mobilized

Rectal mucosa
elevated

D

Internal sphincter
approximated

E

F

Closure

Endorectal advancement of anorectal flap. *(A)* Exposure is gained by an anal speculum, and the fistula is identified. Outline of endorectal flap, extending proximally to
7 cm from the anal verge. *(B)* The full-thickness flap is created to include the internal
sphincter muscle. *(C)* Lateral mobilization is made on each side in the submucosal plane.
(D) Anorectal wall on each side is approximated. *(E and F)* The endorectal flap is pulled
down to cover the wound and sutured. The fistula is excised. The aperture in the vagina
is not sutured but is left open for drainage.

- ■ **Simple** – low to mid-vagina
  - • Tx: trans-anal **rectal mucosa advancement flap**
  - • Many obstetrical fistulas heal spontaneously
- ■ **Complex** – high in vagina
  - • Tx: **abdominal** or combined **abdominal and perineal approach** usual; resection
    and re-anastomosis of rectum, close hole in vagina, interpose omentum, tempo-
    rary ileostomy

ANAL INCONTINENCE
- ■ **Neurogenic** (gaping hole) – no good treatment
- ■ **Abdominoperineal descent** – chronic damage to levator ani muscle and pudendal
  nerves (obesity, multiparous women) and anus falls below levators; Tx: high-fiber
  diet, limit to 1 bowel movement a day; hard to treat
- ■ **Obstetrical trauma** – Tx: **anterior anal sphincteroplasty**

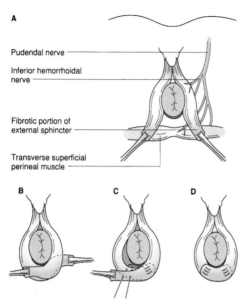

Overlapping anal sphincteroplasty.

AIDS ANORECTAL PROBLEMS
- **Kaposi's sarcoma** – see nodule with ulceration; most common cancer in patients with AIDS
- **CMV** – see shallow ulcers; similar presentation as appendicitis. Tx: ganciclovir
- **HSV** – #1 rectal ulcer
- **B cell lymphoma** – can look like abscess or ulcer
- Need biopsies of these ulcers to rule out cancer and figure out above

ANAL CANCER
- Association with **HPV and XRT**
- Anal canal – above dentate line
- Anal margin – below dentate line
- **Anal canal lesions** *(above dentate line)*
  - **Squamous cell CA** (eg epidermoid CA, mucoepidermoid CA, cloacogenic CA, basaloid CA)
    - **Symptoms**: pruritus, bleeding, and palpable mass
    - Tx: **Nigro protocol** *(chemo-XRT with **5FU** and **mitomycin**)*, **not** surgery
    - Cures 80%
    - APR for treatment failures or recurrent cancer
  - **Adenocarcinoma**
    - Tx: APR usual; WLE if < 3 cm, < ⅓ circumference, limited to submucosa (T1 tumors, 2–3 mm margin needed), well differentiated, and no vascular/lymphatic invasion; needs about 1 cm margin
    - Postoperative chemo/XRT same as rectal CA
  - **Melanoma**
    - 3rd most common site for melanoma (skin and eyes #1 and #2)
    - ⅓ has spread to mesenteric lymph nodes

- Hematogenous spread to the liver and the lung is early and accounts for most deaths
- Symptomatic disease is often associated with significant metastatic disease
- Most common symptom – **rectal bleeding**
- Most tumors are lightly pigmented or not pigmented at all
- Tx: APR usual; margin dictated by depth of lesion standard for melanoma

■ **Anal margin lesions** *(below dentate line)* – have better prognosis than anal canal lesions
- **Squamous cell CA**
  - Ulcerating, slow growing; men with better prognosis
  - Metastases – go to **inguinal nodes**
  - **WLE** for lesions **< 5 cm** (need 0.5 cm margin)
  - **Chemo-XRT** (**5-FU** and **cisplatin**) primary Tx for lesions **> 5 cm**, if involving sphincter or if positive nodes (trying to preserve the sphincter here and avoid APR)
  - Need inguinal node dissection if clinically positive
- **Basal cell CA** – central ulcer, raised edges, rare metastases
  - Tx: WLE usually sufficient, only need 3-mm margins; rare need for APR unless sphincter involved

NODAL METASTASES
■ **Superior and middle rectum** – IMA nodes
■ **Lower rectum** – primarily IMA nodes, also to internal iliac nodes
■ **Upper ⅔ of anal canal** – internal iliac nodes
■ **Lower ⅓ of anal canal** – inguinal nodes

INGUINAL HERNIAS

- **External abdominal oblique fascia** – forms the <u>inguinal ligament</u> (shelving edge) at inferior portion of the inguinal canal
- **Internal abdominal oblique** – forms <u>cremasteric muscles</u>
- **Transversalis muscle** – along with the conjoined tendon, forms inguinal canal <u>floor</u>
- **Conjoined tendon** – composed of the aponeurosis of the internal abdominal oblique and transversalis muscles
- **Inguinal ligament** (Poupart's ligament) – from external abdominal oblique fascia, runs from anterior superior iliac spine to the pubis; anterior to the femoral vessels
  - **Lacunar ligament** – where the inguinal ligament splays out to insert in the pubis
- **Cooper's ligament** – <u>pectineal ligament</u>; posterior to the femoral vessels; lies against bone
- **Vas deferens** – runs medial to cord structures
- **Hesselbach's triangle** – rectus muscle, inferior inguinal ligament, and inferior epigastrics
  - **Direct hernias** are inferior/medial to the epigastric vessels
  - **Indirect hernias** are superior/lateral to the epigastric vessels
- **Indirect hernias** – most common; from persistently patent processus vaginalis
- **Direct hernias** – lower risk of incarceration; rare in females, higher recurrence than indirect
- **Pantaloon hernia** – direct and indirect components

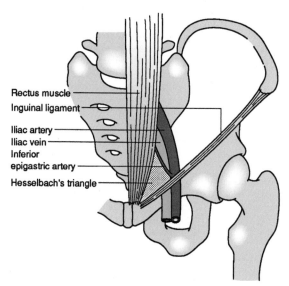

The inguinal (Hesselbach's) triangle.

- **Risk factors for inguinal hernia in adults**: age, obesity, heavy lifting, COPD (coughing), chronic constipation, straining (BPH), ascites, pregnancy, peritoneal dialysis
- **Incarcerated hernia** – can lead to bowel strangulation; should be repaired emergently

- **Sliding hernias** – retroperitoneal organ makes up part of the hernia sac
  - **Females** – ovaries or fallopian tubes most common
  - **Males** – cecum or sigmoid most common
  - Bladder can also be involved
- **Females with ovary in canal**
  - Ligate the round ligament
  - Return ovary to peritoneum
  - Perform biopsy if looks abnormal
- **Hernias in infants and children**
  - Just perform high ligation (nearly always indirect)
  - Open sac prior to ligation
- **Lichtenstein repair** = mesh; recurrence ↓ with use of **mesh** (↓ tension)
- **Bassini repair** – approximation of the conjoined tendon and transversalis fascia (superior) to the free edge of the inguinal ligament (shelving edge, inferior)
- **Cooper's ligament repair** – approximation of the conjoined tendon and transversalis fascia (superior) to Cooper's ligament (pectineal ligament, inferior)
  - Needs a relaxing incision in the external abdominal oblique fascia
  - Can use this for femoral hernia repair
- **Laparoscopic hernia repair** – indicated for bilateral or recurrent inguinal hernia
- **Urinary retention** – most common early complication following hernia repair
- **Wound infection** – 1%
- **Recurrence rate** – 2%
- **Testicular atrophy** – usually secondary to dissection of the distal component of the hernia sac causing vessel disruption
  - Thrombosis of **spermatic cord veins**
  - Usually occurs with indirect hernias
- **Pain after hernia** – usually compression of **ilioinguinal nerve**
  - Tx: local infiltration can be diagnostic and therapeutic
- **Ilioinguinal nerve injury** – loss of cremasteric reflex; numbness on ipsilateral penis, scrotum, and thigh
  - Nerve is usually injured at the external ring; nerve runs on top of cord
- **Genitofemoral nerve injury** – usually injured with laparoscopic hernia repair
  - Genital branch – cremaster (motor) and scrotum (sensory)
  - Femoral branch – upper lateral thigh (sensory)
- **Cord lipomas** – should be removed

FEMORAL HERNIA
- Most common in males, although incidence is increased in females compared to inguinal hernias
- Femoral canal boundaries – Cooper's ligament (posterior), inguinal ligament (anterior), femoral vein (lateral), and Poupart's ligament (medial)
- **Femoral hernia** is medial to the femoral vein and lateral to the lymphatics (in empty space)
- High risk of incarceration → may need to **divide the inguinal ligament** to reduce the bowel
- Hernia passes under the inguinal ligament
- Characteristic **bulge on the anterior–medial thigh** below the ligament
- Hernia is usually repaired through an inguinal approach with Cooper's ligament repair

OTHER HERNIAS
- **Umbilical hernia**
  - ↑ incidence in African Americans; often close on their own
  - Delay repair until age 5 years
  - Risk of incarceration in adults, not children

- **Spigelian hernia**
  - Lateral border of rectus muscle, adjacent to the **linea semilunaris**
  - Almost always inferior to the semicircularis
  - Occurs between the muscle fibers of the internal abdominal oblique muscle and insertion of the external abdominal oblique aponeurosis into the rectus sheath
- **Obturator hernia** (anterior pelvis)
  - Can present as tender medial thigh mass or as small bowel obstruction
  - **Howship–Romberg sign** – inner thigh pain with internal rotation
  - Elderly women, previous pregnancy, bowel gas below superior pubic ramus
  - Tx: operative reduction, may need mesh; check other side for similar defect
- **Sciatic hernia** (posterior pelvis)
  - Herniation through the greater sciatic foramen; high rate of strangulation
- **Incisional hernia** – most likely to recur; inadequate closure is the most common cause

RECTUS SHEATH

- Anterior – complete
- Posterior – absent below semicircularis (below umbilicus)
- The posterior aponeurosis of the internal abdominal oblique and transversalis aponeurosis move anterior below the umbilicus
- **Rectus sheath hematomas**
  - Most common after trauma; epigastric vessel injury
  - Painful abdominal wall mass
  - Mass more prominent and painful with flexion of the rectus muscle (Fothergill's sign)
  - Tx: nonoperative usual, surgery if expanding

DESMOID TUMORS

- Women, benign but locally invasive; ↑ recurrences
- Gardner's syndrome
- Painless mass
- Tx: wide local excision if possible; if involving significant small bowel mesentery, excision may not be indicated → often not completely resectable
  - Medical Tx: **sulindac** and **tamoxifen**

RETROPERITONEAL FIBROSIS

- Can occur with hypersensitivity to methysergide
- **IVP** most sensitive test (constricted ureters)
- Symptoms usually related to **trapped ureters** and **lymphatic obstruction**
- Tx: steroids, nephrostomy if infection is present, and surgery if renal function becomes compromised (free up ureters and wrap in **omentum**)

MESENTERIC TUMORS

- Of the primary tumors, most are cystic
  - **Malignant tumors** – closer to the **root** of the mesentery
  - **Benign tumors** – more **peripheral**
- Malignant – **liposarcoma** (#1), leiomyosarcoma
- Dx: abdominal CT
- Tx: resection

RETROPERITONEAL TUMORS

- 15% in children, others in 5th–6th decade
- Malignant > benign

- Most common malignant retroperitoneal tumor – #1 **lymphoma**, #2 liposarcoma
- Symptoms: vague abdominal and back pain
- **Retroperitoneal sarcomas**
  - < 25% resectable; local recurrence in 40%; 10% 5-year survival rate
  - Have pseudocapsule but cannot shell out → would leave residual tumor
  - Metastases go to the lung

OMENTAL TUMORS
- Most common omental solid tumor is **metastatic disease**
- Omentectomy for metastatic cancer has a role for some cancers (eg ovarian CA)
- Omental cysts are usually asymptomatic, can undergo torsion
- Primary solid omental tumors are rare; ⅓ are malignant
  - <u>No</u> biopsy → can bleed
  - Tx: resection

PERITONEAL MEMBRANE
- Blood is absorbed through fenestrated lymphatic channels in the peritoneum
- Most drugs are not removed with peritoneal dialysis
- NH_3, Ca, Fe, and lead are removed
- Movement of fluid into the peritoneal cavity can occur with hypertonic intra-peritoneal saline load (mechanism of peritoneal dialysis); can cause hypotension

CO_2 PNEUMOPERITONEUM
- Cardiopulmonary dysfunction can occur with intra-abdominal pressure > 20
- *Increased*: mean arterial pressure, pulmonary artery pressure, HR, systemic vascular resistance, central venous pressure, mean airway pressure, peak inspiratory pressure, and CO_2
- *Decreased*: pH, venous return (IVC compression), cardiac output, renal flow secondary to decreased cardiac output
- Hypovolemia lowers pressure necessary to cause compromise
- PEEP worsens effects of pneumoperitoneum
- CO_2 can cause some ↓ in myocardial contractility
- **CO_2 embolus** – Tx: head down, turn patient to the left (sudden rise in $ETCO_2$ and hypotension); can try to aspirate CO2 through central line; prolonged CPR

SURGICAL TECHNOLOGY
- **Harmonic scalpel**
  - Cost-effective for medium vessels (short gastrics)
  - Disrupts protein H-bonds, causes coagulation
- **Ultrasound**
  - **B-mode** used most commonly (B = brightness; assesses relative density of structures)
  - **Shadowing** – dark area posterior to object indicates mass
  - **Enhancement** – brighter area posterior to object indicates fluid-filled cyst
  - **Duplex**
    - **Lower frequencies** – deep structures
    - **Higher frequencies** – superficial structures
- **Argon beam** – energy transferred across argon gas
  - Depth of necrosis related to power setting (2 mm); causes superficial coagulation
  - Is non-contact – good for hemostasis of the liver and spleen; smokeless

- **Laser** – return of electrons to ground state releases energy as heat → coagulates and vaporizes
  - Used for condylomata acuminata (wear mask)
- **Nd:YAG laser** – good for deep tissue penetration; good for bronchial lesions
  - 1–2 mm cuts, 3–10 mm vaporizes, and 1–2 cm coagulates
- **Gore-Tex** (PTFE) – cannot get fibroblast ingrowth
- **Dacron** (polypropylene) – allows fibroblast ingrowth
- **Incidence of vascular or bowel injury with Veress needle or trocar** – 0.1%

ANATOMY AND PHYSIOLOGY

■ **Gerota's fascia** – around kidney
■ **Anterior to posterior** – renal vein, renal artery, and renal pelvis
   • **Right renal artery** crosses posterior to the IVC
■ **Ureters** cross **over iliac vessels**
■ **Left renal vein** – can be ligated from IVC secondary to increased collaterals (left adrenal vein, left gonadal vein, and left ascending lumbar vein); right renal vein lacks collaterals
   • **Left renal vein** usually crosses anterior aorta
■ **Epididymis** – connects to vas deferens
■ **Hypotension** – most common cause of acute renal insufficiency following surgery

KIDNEY STONES

■ **Symptoms**: severe colicky pain, restlessness
■ **Urinalysis** – blood or stones
■ **Abdominal CT** – can demonstrate stones and associated hydronephrosis
■ **Calcium oxalate** stones – most common (75%); radiopaque; ↑ in patients with terminal ileum resection due to ↑ oxalate absorption in colon
■ **Struvite** stones (magnesium ammonium phosphate; radiopaque) – occur with infections (*Proteus mirabilis*) that are <u>urease</u> producing; cause <u>staghorn calculi</u> (fill renal pelvis)
■ **Uric acid** stones (radiolucent) – ↑ in patients with ileostomies, gout, and myeloproliferative disorders
■ **Cysteine stones** (radiolucent) – associated with congenital disorders in the reabsorption of cysteine (cystinuria)
■ **Surgery indications** for kidney stones:
   • Intractable pain or infection
   • Progressive obstruction
   • Progressive renal damage
   • Solitary kidney
■ 90% of kidney stones opaque; > 6 mm not likely to pass
■ Tx: **ESWL** (extra-corporeal shock wave lithotripsy); other options – ureteroscopy with stone extraction or placement of stent past obstruction, percutaneous nephrostomy tube, open nephrolithotomy

TESTICULAR CANCER

■ **#1 cancer killer** in men 25–35
■ Symptom: **painless hard mass**
■ **Testicular mass** – patient needs an **orchiectomy** through an **inguinal incision** (<u>not</u> a trans-scrotal incision → do not want to disrupt lymphatics)
   • The testicle and attached mass constitute the biopsy specimen
■ Most testicular masses are **malignant**
■ **Ultrasound** can help with diagnosis
■ Chest and abdominal CT – to check for retroperitoneal and chest metastases
■ **LDH** correlates with tumor bulk
■ Check **B-HCG** and **AFP level**
■ 90% are **germ cell** – seminoma or nonseminoma
■ **Undescended testicles** (cryptorchidism) – ↑ risk of testicular CA
   • Most likely to get seminoma

- ■ **Seminoma**
  - #1 testicular tumor
  - 10% of seminomatous tumors have beta-HCG elevation
  - Should <u>not</u> have AFP elevation (if elevated, need to treat like non-seminomatous)
  - **Seminoma** is **extremely sensitive to XRT**
  - Tx: all stages get *orchiectomy and retroperitoneal XRT*
    - Chemo reserved for **metastatic disease** or **bulky retroperitoneal disease** (cisplatin, bleomycin, VP-16)
    - Surgical resection of residual disease after above
- ■ **Nonseminomatous testicular CA**
  - **Types** – embryonal, teratoma, choriocarcinoma, yolk sac
  - **Alpha fetoprotein** and **beta-HCG** – 90% have these markers
  - Classically, tumors with ↑ teratoma components are more likely to metastasize to the retroperitoneum
  - Tx: all stages get *orchiectomy and retroperitoneal node dissection*
    - *Stage II or greater* – also give chemo *(cisplatin, bleomycin, VP-16)*
    - Surgical resection of residual disease after above

PROSTATE CANCER
- ■ **Posterior lobe** – most common site
- ■ **Bone** – most common site of metastases
  - **Osteoblastic**; x-ray demonstrates **hyperdense areas**
- ■ Many patients become impotent after resection; can get incontinence
- ■ Can also get urethral strictures
- ■ Dx: transrectal Bx, chest/abd pelvic CT, PSA, alkaline phosphatase; possible bone scan
- ■ **Intracapsular tumors** and no metastases (T1 and T2) → options:
  - XRT <u>or</u>
  - Radical prostatectomy + pelvic lymph node dissection (if life span > 10 years) <u>or</u>
  - Nothing (depending on age and health)
- ■ **Extracapsular invasion** or **metastatic disease**
  - Tx: **XRT** and **androgen ablation** (leuprolide [LH–RH blocker], flutamide [testosterone blocker], or bilateral orchiectomy)
- ■ **Stage IA disease found with TURP** – Tx: nothing
- ■ **With prostatectomy, PSA should go to 0 after 3 weeks** → if not, get bone scan to check for metastases
- ■ **A normal PSA is < 4** in a patient who has a prostate gland
  - **PSA** can be ↑ with prostatitis, BPH, and chronic catheterization
- ■ ↑ **alkaline phosphatase** in a patient with prostate CA → worrisome for metastases or extracapsular disease

RENAL CELL CARCINOMA (RCC, HYPERNEPHROMA)
- ■ #1 primary tumor of kidney (15% calcified)
- ■ Risk factor: **smoking**
- ■ **Abdominal pain**, **mass**, and **hematuria**
- ■ ⅓ have metastatic disease at the time of diagnosis → can perform **wedge resection** of **isolated lung** or **colon metastases**
- ■ **Lung** – most common location for RCC metastases
- ■ **Erythrocytosis** can occur secondary to ↑ erythropoietin (HTN)
- ■ Tx: **radical nephrectomy** with regional nodes; XRT, chemotherapy
  - Radical nephrectomy takes kidney, adrenal, fat, Gerota's fascia, and regional nodes
  - Predilection for growth in the IVC; can still resect even if going up IVC → can pull the tumor thrombus out of the IVC
  - Partial nephrectomies should be considered only for patients who would require dialysis after nephrectomy

- Most common tumor in kidney – **metastasis from the breast CA**
- **RCC paraneoplastic syndromes** – erythropoietin, PTHrp, ACTH, insulin
- **Transitional cell CA of renal pelvis** – Tx: radical nephroureterectomy
- **Oncocytomas** – benign
- **Angiomyolipomas** – hamartomas; can occur with tuberous sclerosis; **benign**
- **Von Hippel–Lindau syndrome** – multifocal and recurrent RCC, renal cysts, CNS tumors, and pheochromocytomas

BLADDER CANCER
- Usually **transitional cell CA**
- **Painless hematuria**
- Males; prognosis based on stage and grade
- Risk factors: smoking, aniline dyes, and cyclophosphamide
- Dx: cystoscopy
- Tx: **intravesical BCG** or **transurethral resection if muscle is not involved (T1)**
  - **If muscle wall is invaded** (T2 or greater) → cystectomy with ileal conduit, chemotherapy (MVAC: methotrexate, vinblastine, Adriamycin [doxorubicin], and cisplatin), and XRT
  - Metastatic disease – chemotherapy
- **Ileal conduit is standard reconstruction option** – avoid stasis as this predisposes to infection, stones (calcium resorption), and ureteral reflux
- **Reservoirs or neobladders** may also be options
- **Squamous cell CA of bladder** – schistosomiasis infection

TESTICULAR TORSION
- Peaks in 15-year-olds
- Torsion is usually toward the midline
- Tx: **bilateral orchiopexy**
  - If testicle not viable, resection and orchiopexy of contralateral testis

URETERAL TRAUMA
- If going to repair end-to-end →
  - Spatulate ends
  - Use **absorbable suture** to avoid stone formation
  - **Stent the ureter** to avoid stenosis
  - **Place drains** to identify and potentially help treat leaks
- Avoid stripping the soft tissue on the ureter, as it will compromise blood supply

BENIGN PROSTATIC HYPERTROPHY (BPH)
- Arises in **transitional zone**
- **Symptoms**: nocturia, frequency, dysuria, weak stream, and urinary retention
- **Initial therapy**
  - **Alpha blockers** – terazosin, doxazosin (relax smooth muscle)
  - **5-alpha-reductase inhibitors** – finasteride (inhibits the conversion of testosterone to dihydrotestosterone → inhibits prostate hypertrophy)
- **Surgery** (trans-urethral resection of prostate; TURP): for recurrent UTIs, gross hematuria, stones, renal insufficiency, or failure of medical therapy
  - **Post-TURP syndrome** – hyponatremia secondary to irrigation with water; can precipitate **seizures** from cerebral edema
  - Tx: careful correction of Na with diuresis
- Most patients with TURP have retrograde ejaculation

NEUROGENIC BLADDER
- Most commonly secondary to spinal compression
- Patient urinates all the time
- Nerve injury above T-12
- Tx: surgery to improve bladder resistance

NEUROGENIC OBSTRUCTIVE UROPATHY
- Incomplete emptying
- Nerve injury below T-12; can occur with APR
- Tx: intermittent catheterization

INCONTINENCE
- **Stress incontinence** (cough, sneeze)
  - Because of hypermobile urethra or loss of sphincter mechanism; women
  - Tx: Kegel exercises, alpha-adrenergic agents, surgery for urethral suspension or pubovaginal sling
- **Overflow incontinence**
  - Incomplete emptying of an enlarged bladder
  - Obstruction (BPH) leads to the distention and leakage
  - Tx: TURP

OTHER UROLOGIC DISEASES
- **Ureteropelvic obstruction** – Tx: pyeloplasty
- **Vesicoureteral reflux** – Tx: reimplantation with long bladder portion
- **Ureteral duplication** – most common urinary tract abnormality; Tx: reimplantation if obstruction occurs
- **Ureterocele** – Tx: resect and reimplant if symptomatic
- **Hypospadias** – ventral urethral opening; Tx: repair at 6 months with penile skin
- **Epispadias** – dorsal urethral opening; Tx: surgery
- **Horseshoe kidney** – usually joined at lower poles
  - Complications: UTI, urolithiasis, and hydronephrosis
  - Tx: may need pyeloplasty
- **Polycystic kidney disease** – resection only if symptomatic
- **Failure of closure of urachus** – connection between umbilicus and bladder; occurs in patients with bladder outlet obstructive disease (wet umbilicus)
  - Tx: resection of sinus/cyst and closure of the bladder; relieve bladder outlet obstruction
- **Epididymitis** – sterile epididymitis can occur from ↑ abdominal straining
- **Varicocele** – worrisome for <u>renal cell CA</u> (left gonadal vein inserts into left renal vein; obstruction by renal tumor causes varicocele); could also be caused by another retroperitoneal malignancy
- **Spermatocele** – fluid-filled cystic structure separate from and superior to the testis along the epididymis; Tx: surgical removal if symptomatic
- **Hydrocele in adult** – if acute, suspect tumor elsewhere (pelvic, abdominal); translucent
- **Pneumaturia** – most common cause is diverticulitis and subsequent formation of colovesical fistula; Dx – cystoscopy
- **WBC casts** – pyelonephritis, glomerulonephritis
- **RBC casts** – glomerulonephritis
- **Interstitial nephritis** – fever, rash, arthralgias, eosinophils
- **Vasectomy** – 50% pregnancy rate after repair of vasectomy

- **Priapism** – Tx: aspiration of the corpus cavernosum with dilute epinephrine or phenylephrine
  - May need to create a communication through the glans with scalpel
  - Risk factors: sickle-cell anemia, hypercoagulable states, trauma, intracorporeal injections for impotence
- **SCC of penis** – penectomy with 2-cm margin
- **Indigo carmine or methylene blue** – used to check for urine leak
- **Phimosis found at time of laparotomy** – Tx: dorsal slit
- **Erythropoietin** – ↓ production in patients with renal failure

CHAPTER 40. GYNECOLOGY

LIGAMENTS
- **Round ligament** – allows anteversion of the uterus
- **Broad ligament** – contains uterine vessels
- **Infundibular ligament** – contains ovarian artery, nerve, and vein
- **Cardinal ligament** – holds cervix and vagina

ULTRASOUND
- Very good at diagnosing disorders of the female genital tract

PREGNANCY
- Can see most pregnancies on ultrasound at 6 weeks
- **Gestational sac** is seen with beta-HCG of 1,500
- **Fetal pole** usually is seen with beta-HCG of 6,000

ABORTIONS
- **Missed** – 1st-trimester bleeding, closed os, positive sac on ultrasound, and no heartbeat
- **Threatened** – 1st-trimester bleeding, positive heartbeat
- **Incomplete** – tissue protrudes through os
- **Ectopic pregnancy** (life threatening) – acute abdominal pain; positive beta-HCG, negative ultrasound for sac; can also have missed period, vaginal bleeding, hypotension
  - **Risk factors for ectopic pregnancy**: previous tubal manipulation, PID, previous ectopic pregnancy
  - Significant shock and hemorrhage can occur from an ectopic pregnancy

ENDOMETRIOSIS
- Symptoms: dysmenorrhea, infertility, dyspareunia
- Can involve the rectum and cause bleeding during menses → endoscopy shows **blue mass**
- **Ovaries** – most common site
- Tx: OCPs

PELVIC INFLAMMATORY DISEASE
- Has ↑ risk of infertility and ectopic pregnancy
- Symptoms: pain, nausea, vomiting, fever, vaginal discharge
  - Most commonly occurs in the first ½ of the menstrual cycle
- Risk factors: multiple sexual partners
- Dx: cervical motion tenderness, cervical cultures, positive Gram stain
- Tx: ceftriaxone, doxycycline
- **Complications**: persistent pain, infertility, ectopic pregnancy
- **HSV** – vesicles; **HPV** – condylomata
- **Syphilis** – positive dark-field microscopy, chancre
- **Gonococcus** – diplococci

MITTELSCHMERZ
- Rupture of graafian follicle
- Causes pain that can be confused with appendicitis
- Occurs 14 days after the 1st day of menses

VAGINAL CANCER
- #1 primary – squamous cell CA
- **DES** (diethylstilbestrol) – can cause clear cell CA of vagina
- **Botryoides** – rhabdosarcoma that occurs in young girls
- **XRT** – used for most cancers of vagina

VULVAR CANCER
- Elderly, nulliparous, obese; usually unilateral
- Tx: **< 2 cm** (stage I) – **WLE** and <u>ipsilateral</u> **inguinal node dissection**
  - **> 2 cm** (stage II or greater) – **radical vulvectomy** (bilateral labia) with <u>bilateral inguinal dissection</u>, postop **XRT** if close margins (< 1 cm)
  - Paget's VIN III or higher – **premalignant**
  - VIN – vulvar intra-epithelial neoplasia

OVARIAN CANCER
- **Leading cause of gynecologic death**
- Abdominal or pelvic pain; change in stool or urinary habits; vaginal bleeding
- ↓ **risk** – OCPs, bilateral tubal ligation
- ↑ **risk** – nulliparity, late menopause, early menarche
- **Types** – teratoma, granulosa-theca (estrogen secreting, precocious puberty); Sertoli–Leydig (androgens, masculinization); struma ovarii (thyroid tissues); choriocarcinoma (beta-HCG); mucinous; serous; and papillary
- **Clear cell type** – worst prognosis

Staging of Ovarian Cancer	
Stage	Location
I	One or both ovaries only
II	Limited to pelvis
III	Spread throughout abdomen
IV	Distant metastases

Modified from AJCC. *Cancer Staging Handbook*. 6th ed. New York, NY: Springer-Verlag; 2002:309–310.

- **Bilateral ovary** involvement still **stage I**
- **MC initial site of regional spread** – other ovary
- **Debulking tumor** – can be effective; including omentectomy (helps chemo and XRT)
- Tx: **total abdominal hysterectomy** and **bilateral oophorectomy** for all stages; *plus*:
  - Pelvic and para-aortic LN dissection
  - Omentectomy
  - 4 quadrant washes
  - Chemotherapy: cisplatin and paclitaxel (Taxol)
- **Krukenberg tumor** – stomach CA that has metastasized to ovary
  - Pathology classically shows **signet ring cells**
- **Meige's syndrome** – pelvic ovarian fibroma that causes **ascites** and **hydrothorax**
  - Excision of tumor cures syndrome

ENDOMETRIAL CANCER
- **Most common malignant tumor in female genital tract**
- **Risk factors** – nulliparity, late 1st pregnancy, obesity, tamoxifen, unopposed estrogen
- Vaginal bleeding in postmenopausal patient is endometrial CA until proved otherwise
- Uterine polyps have very low chance of malignancy (0.1%)
- **Serous** and **papillary** subtypes – worst prognosis

Staging and Treatment

Stage	Location	Treatment
I	Endometrium	Total abdominal hysterectomy and BSO or XRT
II	Cervix	Total abdominal hysterectomy and BSO or XRT
III	Vagina, peritoneum, and ovary	Total abdominal hysterectomy and BSO and XRT
IV	Bladder and rectum	Total abdominal hysterectomy and BSO and XRT

BSO, bilateral salpingo-oophorectomy; XRT, radiotherapy. Modified from AJCC. *Cancer Staging Handbook*. 6th ed. New York, NY: Springer-Verlag; 2002:301–302.

CERVICAL CANCER
- Goes to **obturator nodes 1st**
- Associated with **HPV 16** and **18**
- Squamous cell CA – most common

Staging of Cervical Cancer

Stage	Location
I	Cervix
II	Upper ⅔ of vagina
III	Pelvis, side wall, and lower ⅓ of vagina; hydronephrosis
IV	Bladder and rectum

Modified from AJCC. *Cancer Staging Handbook*. 6th ed. New York, NY: Springer-Verlag; 2002:294–296.

- Tx: **microscopic disease** without basement membrane invasion → **cone biopsy** (conization sufficient to remove disease)
  - **Stages I and IIa** – total abdominal hysterectomy (TAH)
  - **Stages IIb to IV** – XRT

OVARIAN CYSTS
- **Postmenopausal patient**
  - If **septated**, has ↑ **vascular flow** on Doppler, has **solid components**, or has **papillary projections** → oophorectomy with intraoperative frozen sections; TAH if ovarian CA
  - If none of the above are present, follow with ultrasound for 1 year → if persists or gets larger → oophorectomy with intraoperative frozen sections; TAH if ovarian CA
- **Premenopausal patient**
  - If **septated**, has ↑ **vascular flow** on Doppler, has **solid components**, or has **papillary projections** → oophorectomy with intraoperative frozen sections usual
    - Algorithm becomes very complicated after this, weighing how aggressive the cancer is (based on histology and stage at the time of operation) compared with whether the patient desires future pregnancy
  - If none of the above are present → can follow with ultrasound; surgery if suspicious findings appear

INCIDENTAL OVARIAN MASS AT THE TIME OF LAPAROTOMY FOR ANOTHER PROCEDURE
- Biopsy mass, 4 quadrant wash, biopsy omentum, look for metastases and biopsy
- If original procedure elective (eg gastric bypass), may need to abort procedure depending on findings
- **Do not perform oophorectomy**

ABNORMAL UTERINE BLEEDING

- < **40** years old – if **anovulation**. Tx: **clomiphene citrate**
  - If **leiomyomas** → Tx: **GnRH agonists** (leuprolide)
- > **40** years old – **cancer or menopause** → need biopsy

OTHER GYNECOLOGIC CONSIDERATIONS

- **Contraindications to estrogen therapy** – endometrial CA, thromboembolic disease, undiagnosed vaginal bleeding, breast CA
- **Uterine endometrial polyp** – can present as progressively heavier menses
- **Uterine fibroids** (leiomyomas) – under hormonal influence; recurrent abortions, infertility, bleeding
- **Most common vaginal tumor** – invasion from surrounding or distant structure
- **Hydatidiform mole** – malignancy risk with <u>partial mole</u>; complete mole is of paternal origin; Tx: chemo (methotrexate)
- **Toxic shock syndrome** – fever, erythema, diffuse desquamation, nausea, vomiting; associated with highly absorbent tampons
- **Ovarian torsion** – Tx: remove torsion and check for viability
- **Adnexal torsion with vascular necrosis** – Tx: adnexectomy
- **Ruptured tuboovarian abscess** – Tx: percutaneous drainage
- **Ovarian vein thrombosis** – Dx: CT scan; Tx: heparin
- **Postpartum pelvic thrombophlebitis** – can lead to ovarian vein, IVC, and hepatic vein thrombosis; get liver failure with ascites after pregnancy; Tx: **heparin** and **antibiotics**

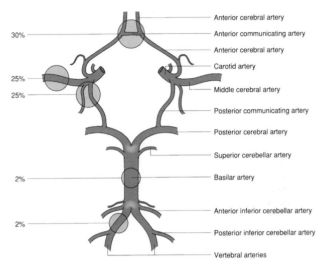

Locations of aneurysms of the circle of Willis and their relative occurrence.

CIRCLE OF WILLIS
- **Vertebral arteries** – come together to form a single **basilar artery**, which branches into 2 **posterior cerebral arteries**
- **Posterior communicating arteries** – connect **middle cerebral arteries** to **posterior cerebral arteries**
- **Anterior cerebral arteries** – branches off **middle cerebral arteries** and are connected to each other through the 1 **anterior communicating artery**

NERVE INJURY
- **Neurapraxia** – no axonal injury (temporary loss of function, foot falls asleep)
- **Axonotmesis** – disruption of **axon** with preservation of axon sheath, will improve
- **Neurotmesis** – disruption of **axon** and **axon sheath** (whole nerve is disrupted), may need surgery for recovery
- Regeneration of nerves occurs at a rate of **1 mm/day**
- **Nodes of Ranvier** – bare sections; allow salutatory conduction

ANTIDIURETIC HORMONE (ADH)
- Release controlled by **supraoptic nucleus of hypothalamus**, which descends into the posterior pituitary gland
- Released in response to high plasma osmolarity; ADH increases water absorption in collecting ducts
- **Diabetes insipidus** ($\downarrow$ ADH) – $\uparrow$ urine output, $\downarrow$ urine specific gravity, $\uparrow$ serum Na, and $\uparrow$ serum osmolarity
  - Can occur with ETOH, head injury
  - Tx: DDAVP, free water

- **SIADH** (↑ ADH) – ↓ urine output, concentrated urine, ↓ serum Na, and ↓ serum osmolarity
    - Can occur with head injury
    - Tx: fluid restriction, then diuresis

HEMORRHAGE

- **Arteriovenous malformations** – 50% present with hemorrhage; are congenital
    - Usually in patients < 30; sudden headache and loss of consciousness
    - Tx: resection if symptomatic
    - Can coil embolize these prior to resection
- **Cerebral aneurysms** – usually occur in patients > 40; most are congenital
    - Can present with bleeding, mass effect, seizures, or infarcts
    - Occur at branch points in artery, most off middle cerebral artery
    - Tx: often place coils before clipping and resecting aneurysm
- **Subdural hematoma** – caused by **torn bridging veins**
    - Has crescent shape on head CT and conforms to brain
    - Higher mortality than epidural hematoma
    - Tx: operate for significant neurologic degeneration or mass effect (shift > 1 cm)

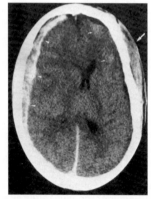

Acute subdural hematoma imaged by noncontrast computed tomography.

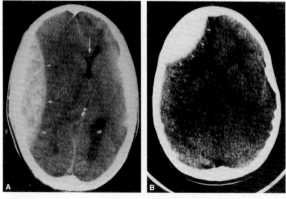

Two examples of acute epidural hematoma imaged by noncontrast computed tomography.

■ **Epidural hematoma** – caused by injury to **middle meningeal artery**
  • Has lens shape on head CT and pushes brain away
  • Patients classically lose consciousness, have a lucid interval, and then lose consciousness again
  • Tx: operate for significant neurologic degeneration or mass effect (shift > 0.5 cm)
■ **Subarachnoid hemorrhage** (nontraumatic)
  • Caused by cerebral aneurysms (50% middle cerebral artery) and AVMs
  • Symptoms: stiff neck (nuchal rigidity), severe headache, photophobia, neurologic defects
  • Tx: goal is to isolate the aneurysm from systemic circulation (clipping vascular supply), maximize cerebral perfusion to overcome vasospasm, and prevent rebleeding; use hypervolemia and calcium channel blockers to overcome vasospasm
  • Go to OR **only if neurologically intact**
  • Can get subarachnoid hemorrhages with trauma as well
■ **Intracerebral hematomas** – temporal lobe most often affected
  • Those that are large and cause focal deficits should be drained
■ **Symptoms** of ↑ ICP – stupor, headache, nausea and vomiting, stiff neck
■ **Signs** of ↑ ICP – hypertension, HR lability, slow respirations
  • **Intermittent bradycardia** is a sign of severely elevated ICP and impending herniation
  • **Cushing's triad** – hypertension, bradycardia, slow respiratory rate

SPINAL CORD INJURY
■ **Cord injury with deficit** → give **high-dose steroids (↓ swelling)**
■ **Complete cord transection** – areflexia, flaccidity, anesthesia, and autonomic paralysis below the level of the lesion
■ **Spinal shock** – hypotension, **normal or slow heart rate**, and **warm extremities** (vasodilated)
  • Occurs with spinal cord injuries above T5 (loss of sympathetic tone)
  • Tx: fluids initially, may need phenylephrine drip (alpha agonist)
■ **Anterior spinal artery syndrome** – most commonly occurs with acutely ruptured cervical disc
  • **Bilateral loss of motor, pain,** and **temperature** sensation below the level of lesion
  • **Preservation of position–vibratory sensation and light touch**
  • About 10% recover to ambulation
■ **Brown-Sequard syndrome** – incomplete cord transection (hemisection of cord); most commonly due to penetrating injury
  • **Loss of ipsilateral motor** and **contralateral pain/temperature** below level of lesion
  • About 90% recover to ambulation
■ **Central cord syndrome** – most commonly occurs with hyperflexion of the cervical spine
  • **Bilateral loss motor, pain,** and **temperature** sensation in **upper extremities**; lower extremities spared
■ **Cauda equina syndrome** – pain and weakness in lower extremities due to compression of lumbar nerve roots
■ **Spinothalamic tract** – carries pain and temperature sensory neurons
■ **Corticospinal tract** – carries motor neurons
■ **Rubrospinal tract** – carries motor neurons
■ **Dorsal nerve roots** – are generally afferent; carry sensory fibers
■ **Ventral nerve roots** – are generally efferent; carry motor neuron fibers

BRAIN TUMORS
■ Symptoms: **headache**, seizures, progressive neurologic deficit, and persistent vomiting
■ Adults – ⅔ supratentorial
■ Children – ⅔ infratentorial

- **Gliomas** – most common primary brain tumor in adults and overall
  - **Glioma multiforme** – most common subtype, uniformly fatal
- **Lung** – #1 metastasis to brain
- Most common brain tumor in children – **medulloblastoma**
- Most common metastatic brain tumor in children – **neuroblastoma**
- **Acoustic neuroma** – arises from the **8th cranial nerve** at **cerebellopontine angle**
  - Symptoms – hearing loss, unsteadiness, vertigo, nausea, and vomiting
  - Tx: surgery usual

SPINE TUMORS
- Overall, most are benign; #1 tumor overall **neurofibroma**
- **Intradural tumors** are more likely benign, and **extradural tumors** are more likely malignant
- **Paraganglionoma** – check for metanephrines in urine

PEDIATRIC NEUROSURGERY
- **Intraventricular hemorrhage** (subependymal hemorrhage)
  - Seen in premature infants secondary to rupture of the fragile vessels in germinal matrix
  - Patients go on to get intraventricular hemorrhage
  - Risk factors: ECMO, cyanotic congenital heart disease
  - Symptoms: bulging fontanelle, neurologic deficits, ↓ BP, and ↓ Hct
  - Tx: ventricular catheter for drainage and prevention of hydrocephalus
- **Myelomeningocele**
  - Neural cord defect – herniation of spinal cord and nerve roots through defect in vertebra
  - Most commonly occurs in the lumbar region

MISCELLANEOUS
- **Wernicke's area** – speech comprehension, temporal lobe
- **Broca's area** – speech motor, posterior part of anterior lobe
- **Pituitary adenoma**, **undergoing XRT**, **patient now in shock**
  - Dx: pituitary apoplexy
  - Tx: steroids
- **Cervical nerves roots 3–5** innervate diaphragm
- **Microglial cells** – act as brain macrophages

Cranial Nerves

Nerve	Name	Function	Muscle
I	Olfactory	Smell	
II	Optic	Sight	
III	Oculomotor		Motor to eye
IV	Trochlear		Superior oblique (eye)
V	Trigeminal: ophthalmic, maxillary, and mandibular branches	Sensory to face	Muscles of mastication
VI	Abducens		Lateral rectus (eye)
VII	Facial	Taste to anterior ⅔ of tongue	Motor to face
VIII	Vestibulocochlear	Hearing	
IX	Glossopharyngeal	Taste to posterior ⅓ of tongue	Swallowing muscles
X	Vagus	Many functions	
XI	Accessory		Trapezius Sternocleidomastoid
XII	Hypoglossal		Tongue

BACKGROUND
- **Osteoblasts** – synthesize nonmineralized bone cortex
- **Osteoclasts** – reabsorb bone
  - Stages of bone healing – 1) inflammation, 2) soft callus formation, 3) mineralization of the callus, 4) remodeling of the callus
- Cartilage receives nutrients from synovial fluid (osmotic)
- **Salter-Harris** fractures **III**, **IV**, and **V** – cross the epiphyseal plate and can affect the growth plate of the bone; need open reduction and internal fixation (**ORIF**)
- **Salter-Harris** fractures **I** and **II** – **closed reduction**

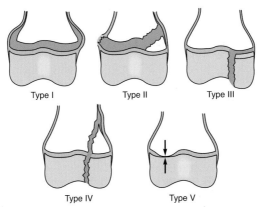

Type I   Type II   Type III

Type IV   Type V

Salter-Harris classification of epiphyseal injuries. Type I injury is an epiphysiolysis of the involved growth plate without associated fracture. Type II has an additional metaphyseal fracture fragment; type I and II injuries have a good prognosis and are usually treated with closed reduction and casting. Type III injury results in a fracture through the growth plate and epiphysis. Type IV fracture crosses the epiphysis, growth plate (physis), and metaphysis. Type III and IV injuries require careful open reduction and internal fixation if displaced. Type V injury involves a crush of the growth plate without a fracture and is usually detected late by asymmetric or premature closure of the growth plate.

- Fractures associated with **avascular necrosis** (AVN) – scaphoid, femoral neck, talus
- Fractures associated with **nonunion** – clavicle, 5th metatarsal fracture (Jones' fracture)
- Fractures associated with **compartment syndrome** – supracondylar humerus, tibia
- **Biggest risk factor for nonunion** – smoking

LOWER EXTREMITY NERVES
- **Obturator nerve** – hip adduction
- **Superior gluteal nerve** – hip abduction
- **Inferior gluteal nerve** – hip extension
- **Femoral nerve** – knee extension

LUMBAR DISC HERNIATION
- Presents with back pain, sciatica
- Herniated **nucleus pulposus**

- Nerve root compression affects 1 nerve root below disc:
  - **L3 nerve** compression (L2–3 disc) – weak hip flexion
  - **L4 nerve** compression (L3–4 disc) – weak knee extension (quadriceps), weak patellar reflex
  - **L5 nerve** compression (L4–5 disc) – weak dorsiflexion (foot drop)
    - ↓ sensation in big toe web space
  - **S1 nerve** compression (L5–S1 disc) – weak plantar flexion, weak Achilles reflex
    - ↓ sensation in lateral foot
- Dx: patients with neurologic findings need **MRI**
- Tx: NSAIDs, heat, and rest; surgery for substantial/progressive neurologic deficit, refractory cases, severe sciatica, or disc fragments that have herniated into the cord

TERMINAL BRANCHES OF BRACHIAL PLEXUS
- **Ulnar nerve**
  - **Motor** – <u>intrinsic musculature of hand</u> (palmar interossei, palmaris brevis, adductor pollicis, and hypothenar eminence); finger abduction (spread fingers); wrist flexion
  - **Sensory** – all of 5th and ½ 4th fingers, back of hand
  - Injury results in **claw hand**
- **Median nerve**
  - **Motor** – thumb apposition (anterior interosseous muscle, OK sign); finger flexors
  - **Sensory** – most of palm and 1st 3 and ½ 4th fingers on palmar side
  - Nerve is involved in **carpal tunnel syndrome**
- **Radial nerve**
  - **Motor** – wrist extension, finger extension, thumb extension, and triceps; <u>no</u> hand muscles
  - **Sensory** – 1st 3 and ½ 4th fingers on dorsal side
- **Axillary nerve** – motor to deltoid (abduction)
- **Musculocutaneous nerve** – motor to biceps, brachialis, and coracobrachialis

CERVICAL RADICULOPATHY
- **C1**, **C2**, **C3**, and **C4 nerve compression** (C1–2, C2–3, C3–4 discs) – neck and scalp pain
- **C5 nerve compression** (C4–5 disc) – weak deltoid and biceps
  - Weak biceps reflex
- **C6 nerve compression** (C5–6 disc) – weak deltoid and biceps, weak wrist extensors
  - Weak biceps reflex and brachioradialis reflex
- **C7 nerve compression** (most common, C6–7 disc) – weak triceps
  - Weak triceps reflex
- **C8 nerve compression** (C7–T1 disc) – weak triceps, weak intrinsic muscles of hand and wrist flexion
  - Weak triceps reflex
- **Radial nerve** – C5–C8
- **Median nerve** – C6–T1
- **Ulnar nerve** – C8–T1
- **Musculocutaneous nerve** – C5–C7
- **Axillary nerve** – C5–C6
- **Radial nerve roots** – on the superior portion of the brachial plexus
- **Ulnar nerve roots** – on the inferior portion of the brachial plexus

UPPER EXTREMITY
- **Clavicle fracture** – usually just treated with sling (risk of vascular impingement)
- **Shoulder dislocation**
  - **Anterior** (90%) risk of **axillary <u>nerve</u> injury**. Tx: closed reduction
  - **Posterior** (seizures, electrocution) risk of **axillary <u>artery</u> injury**. Tx: closed reduction

- **Acromioclavicular separation** – Tx: sling (risk of brachial plexus and subclavian vessel injury)
- **Scapula fracture** – sling unless glenoid fossa involved, then need internal fixation
- **Midshaft humeral fracture** – Tx: sling for almost all
- **Supracondylar humeral fracture** – adults → <u>ORIF</u>
  - **children: nondisplaced** → <u>closed reduction</u>; **displaced** → <u>ORIF</u>
- **Monteggia fracture** – proximal ulnar fracture and radial head dislocation
  - Tx: ORIF
- **Colles fracture** – fall on outstretched hand, distal radius. Tx: closed reduction
- **Nursemaid's elbow** – subluxation of the radius at the elbow caused by pulling on an extended, pronated arm. Tx: closed reduction
- **Combined radial and ulnar fracture**
  - **Adults** – ORIF
  - **Children** – closed reduction
- **Scaphoid fracture** – snuffbox tenderness; can have negative x-ray
  - Tx: all patients require cast to elbow, may need fixation; risk of **avascular necrosis**
- **Volkmann's contracture**: supracondylar humerus fracture → occluded **anterior interosseous artery** → closed reduction of humerus → artery opens up → reperfusion injury, edema, and **forearm compartment syndrome** (flexor compartment most affected)
  - Symptoms: forearm pain with passive extension; weakness, tense forearm, hypesthesia
  - **Median nerve** most affected by swelling
  - Tx: **forearm fasciotomies**
- **Forearm fasciotomies** – need to open volar and dorsal compartments
- **Dupuytren's contracture** – associated with diabetes, ETOH
  - Progressive proliferation of the **palmar fascia of hand** results in contractures that usually affect the **4th** and **5th digits** (cannot extend fingers)
  - Tx: NSAIDs, steroid injections; excision of involved fascia for significant contraction
- **Carpal tunnel syndrome** – median nerve compression by transverse carpal ligament
  - Tx: splint, NSAIDs, and steroid injections; **transverse carpal ligament** release if that fails
- **Trigger finger** – tenosynovitis of the flexor tendon that catches at the MCP joint when trying to extend finger
  - Tx: splint, tendon sheath steroid injections (not the tendon itself); if that fails, can release the pulley system at the MCP joint
- **Suppurative tenosynovitis**
  - Infection that spreads along flexor tendon sheaths of digits (can destroy sheath)
  - **4 classic signs**: tendon sheath tenderness, pain with passive motion, swelling along sheath, and semi-flexed posture of the involved digit
  - Tx: *midaxial longitudinal incision and drainage*
- **Rotator cuff tears** – supraspinatus, infraspinatus, teres minor, and subscapularis
  - Acutely → sling and conservative treatment
  - Surgical repair if the patient needs to retain a high level of activity or if ADL affected
- **Paronychia** – infection under nail bed; painful. Tx: antibiotics; remove nail if purulent
- **Felon** – infection in the terminal joint space of the finger
  - Tx: incision over the tip of the finger and along the medial and lateral aspects to prevent necrosis of tip of finger

LOWER EXTREMITY
- **Hip dislocation**
  - **Posterior** (90%) – patients have internal rotation and adduction of leg; risk of **sciatic nerve injury**. Tx: closed reduction
  - **Anterior** – patients have external rotation and abduction of leg; risk of injury to **femoral artery**. Tx: closed reduction

- **Isolated anterior ring with minimal ischial displacement** – Tx: weight-bearing as tolerated
- **Femoral shaft fracture** – ORIF with intramedullary rod
- **Femoral neck fracture** – ORIF → risk of avascular necrosis if open reduction delayed
- **Lateral knee trauma** – can result in injury to **anterior cruciate ligament, posterior cruciate ligament, and medial meniscus**
- **Anterior cruciate ligament injury** – positive anterior drawer test
  - Present with **knee effusion** and **pain with pivoting action**; MRI confirms diagnosis
  - Tx: surgery with knee instability (reconstruction with patellar tendon or hamstring tendon); otherwise physical therapy with leg-strengthening exercise
- **Posterior cruciate ligament injury** – positive posterior drawer test
  - Much less common than ACL injury; present with knee pain and joint effusion
  - Tx: conservative therapy initially; surgery for failure of medical management
- **Collateral ligaments**
  - **Medial collateral ligament injury** – lateral blow to knee
  - **Lateral collateral ligament injury** – medial blow to knee
  - Tx: **small tear** – brace; **large tear** – surgery
  - These injuries are associated with injuries to the corresponding **meniscus**
- **Meniscus tears** – joint line tenderness; can treat with arthroscopic repair or debridement
- **Posterior knee dislocation** – all patients need angiogram to rule out popliteal artery injury
- **Patellar fracture** – long leg cast unless comminuted, then need internal fixation
- **Tibial plateau fracture** and **tibia–fibula fracture** – ORIF fixation unless open, then need external fixator until tissue heals
- **Plantaris muscle rupture** – pain and mass below popliteal fossa (contracted plantaris) and ankle ecchymosis
- **Ankle fracture** – most treated with cast and immobilization; bimalleolar or trimalleolar fractures need ORIF
- **Metatarsal fracture** – cast immobilization or brace for 6 weeks
- **Calcaneus fracture** – cast and immobilization if nondisplaced; ORIF for displacement
- **Talus fracture** – closed reduction for most; ORIF for severe displacement
- **Nerve most commonly injured with lower extremity fasciotomy** – superficial peroneal nerve (foot eversion)
- **Footdrop** after **lithotomy position** or after **crossing legs for long periods** or **fibula head fracture** – common peroneal nerve (foot-drop)

LEG COMPARTMENTS
- **Anterior** – anterior tibial artery, deep peroneal nerve
  - **Muscles** – anterior tibialis, extensor hallucis longus, extensor digitorum longus, and communis
- **Lateral** – superficial peroneal nerve
  - **Muscles** – peroneal muscles
- **Deep posterior** – posterior tibial artery, peroneal artery, and tibial nerve
  - **Muscles** – flexor hallucis longus, flexor digitorum longus, and posterior tibialis
- **Superficial posterior** – sural nerve
  - **Muscles** – gastrocnemius, soleus, and plantaris

COMPARTMENT SYNDROME
- Most likely to occur in the **anterior compartment of leg** (get footdrop) after **vascular compromise, restoration of blood flow**, and subsequent **reperfusion injury** with **swelling of the leg compartment**
- Can also occur from crush injuries
- Symptoms: pain with passive motion; swollen extremity

■ **Distal pulses can be present** with compartment syndrome → last thing to go
■ Pressure > 20–30 mm Hg abnormal
■ Dx: based on clinical suspicion
■ Tx: **fasciotomy**

PEDIATRIC ORTHOPEDICS
■ **Osteomyelitis** – can occur in metaphysis of long bones in children; most commonly staph
  • Symptoms: pain, ↓ use of extremity
  • Dx: MRI, bone biopsy
  • Tx: incision and drainage; antibiotics
■ **Idiopathic adolescent scoliosis** – prepubertal females, right thoracic curve most common, usually asymptomatic
  • Curves 20–45 degrees need bracing to slow progression, which can occur with growth spurt
  • Curves > 45 degrees or those likely to progress → spinal fusion
■ **Osgood–Schlatter disease** – tibial tubercle apophysitis; caused by traction injury from the quadriceps in adolescents aged 13–15; most commonly have pain in front of the knee
  • X-ray: irregular shape or fragmenting of the tibial tubercle
  • Tx: mild symptoms → activity limitation; severe symptoms → cast 6 weeks followed by activity limitation
■ **Legg–Calvé–Perthes disease** – AVN of the femoral head; children 2 years and older
  • Can result from a hypercoagulable state; bilateral in 10%
  • Symptoms: painful gait limp
  • X-ray: flattening of the femoral head
  • Tx: maintain range of motion with limited exercise; **femoral head will remodel without sequelae**
  • Surgery if femoral head is not covered by the acetabulum
■ **Slipped capital femoral epiphysis**
  • Males aged 10–13; ↑ risk of AVN of the femoral head; painful gait
  • X-ray: widening and irregularity of the epiphyseal plate
  • Tx: surgical pinning
■ **Congenital dislocation of the hip**
  • More common in females
  • Tx: Pavlik harness, which keeps the legs abducted and the femoral head reduced in the acetabulum
■ **Clubfoot** – Tx: serial casting

BONE TUMORS
■ Most common is metastatic disease (#1 breast, #2 prostate)
  • Tx: internal fixation with impending fracture (> 50% cortical involvement); followed by XRT
■ **Multiple myeloma** – most common primary malignant tumor of bone
  • Tx: chemotherapy for systemic disease; internal fixation for impending fractures
■ **Pathologic fractures** – treat with internal fixation
  • XRT can be used for pain relief in patients with painful bony metastases
■ **Osteogenic sarcoma** – most common primary bone sarcoma, usually around the knee
  • 80% in patients < 20 years old
  • X-ray: **Codman's triangle** → periosteal reaction
  • Tx: limb-sparing resection; XRT and **doxorubicin-based** chemotherapy can be used preoperatively to increase chance of limb-sparing resection

■ **Benign bone tumors treated with curettage ± bone graft** – osteoid osteoma, endo-chondroma (may be able to observe), osteochondroma (resection only if cosmetic defect or causing symptoms), chondroblastoma, nonossifying fibroma (may be observed), and fibrodysplasia

■ **Giant cell** tumor of bone – total resection ± XRT (benign but 30% risk of recurrence; also has malignant degeneration risk)

OTHER ORTHOPEDIC CONDITIONS

■ **Spondylolisthesis** – formed by subluxation or slip of one vertebral body over another
  • Most commonly occurs in lumbar region
  • Most common cause of lumbar pain in adolescents (gymnasts)
  • Tx: depends on degree of subluxation and symptoms – ranges from conservative treatment to surgical fusion

■ **Cervical stenosis** – surgical decompression if significant myelopathy present

■ **Lumbar stenosis** – surgical decompression for cases refractory to medical treatment

■ **Torus fracture** – buckling of the metaphyseal cortex seen in children (ie distal radius)

■ **Open fractures** – need incision and drainage, antibiotics, fracture stabilization, and soft tissue coverage

- **Foregut** – lungs, esophagus, stomach, pancreas, liver, gallbladder, bile duct, and duodenum proximal to ampulla
- **Midgut** – duodenum distal to ampulla, small bowel, and large bowel to distal ⅓ of transverse colon
- **Hindgut** – distal ⅓ of transverse colon to anal canal
- Midgut rotates 270 degrees counterclockwise normally
- Low birth weight < 2,500 g; premature < 37 weeks
- **Immunity at birth** – **IgA** from mother's milk; **IgG** crosses the placenta
- **#1 cause of childhood death** – <u>trauma</u>
  - Trauma bolus – 20 cc/kg × 2, then give blood 10 cc/kg
  - **Tachycardia** – best indicator of shock (neonate > 150; < 1 year > 120; rest > 100)
  - Want urine output > 2–4 cc/kg/hr
  - Children (< 6 months) only have **25% the GFR capacity of adults** – poor concentrating ability
- ↑ alkaline phosphatase in children compared with adults → **bone growth**
- **Umbilical vessels** – 2 arteries and 1 vein

MAINTENANCE INTRAVENOUS FLUIDS
- 4 cc/kg/hr for 1st 10 kg
- 2 cc/kg/hr for 2nd 10 kg
- 1 cc/kg/hr for everything after that

CONGENITAL CYSTIC DISEASE OF THE LUNG
- **Pulmonary sequestration**
  - Lung tissue has **anomalous systemic arterial supply** (thoracic aorta or abdominal aorta through inferior pulmonary ligament)
  - Have either systemic venous or pulmonary vein drainage
  - **Extra-lobar** – more likely to have <u>systemic</u> venous drainage (azygous system)
  - **Intra-lobar** – more likely to have <u>pulmonary vein</u> drainage
  - Do <u>not</u> communicate with tracheobronchial tree
  - Most commonly presents with infection; can also have respiratory compromise or an abnormal CXR
  - Tx: **lobectomy**
- **Congenital lobar overinflation** (emphysema)
  - Cartilage fails to develop in bronchus, leading to air trapping with expiration
  - Vascular supply and other lobes are normal (except compressed by hyperinflated lobe)
  - Can develop hemodynamic instability (same mechanism as tension PTX) or respiratory compromise
  - LUL most commonly affected
  - Tx: **lobectomy**
- **Congenital cystic adenoid malformation**
  - Communicates with airway
  - Alveolar structure is poorly developed, although lung tissue is present
  - Symptoms: respiratory compromise or recurrent infection
  - Tx: lobectomy
- **Bronchiogenic cyst**
  - Most common cysts of the mediastinum; usually posterior to the carina
  - Are **extra-pulmonary cysts** formed from bronchial tissue and cartilage wall

- Usually present with a mediastinal mass filled with milky liquid
- Can compress adjacent structures or become infected; have malignant potential
- Occasionally are intra-pulmonary
- Tx: resect cyst

MEDIASTINAL MASSES IN CHILDREN

- **Neurogenic tumors** (neurofibroma, neuroganglioma, neuroblastoma) – <u>most common</u> mediastinal tumor in children; usually located posteriorly
- **Respiratory symptoms**, **dysphagia** – common to all mediastinal masses regardless of location
- **Anterior** – T cell lymphoma, **teratoma**, and other germ cell tumors (most common type of anterior mediastinal mass in children), thyroid CA
- **Middle** – T cell lymphoma, teratoma, cyst (cardiogenic or bronchiogenic)
- **Posterior** – T cell lymphoma, neuroblastoma, neurogenic tumor
- *Thymoma is <u>rare</u> in children*

CHOLEDOCHAL CYST

- Need to resect – risk of cholangiocarcinoma, pancreatitis, cholangitis, and obstructive jaundice; caused by **reflux of pancreatic enzymes** into the biliary system **in utero**

Choledochal Cysts

Type	%	Description	Treatment
I	85%	Fusiform dilation of entire common bile duct, mildly dilated common hepatic duct, normal intrahepatic ducts	Resection, hepaticojejunostomy
II	3%	A true diverticulum that hangs off the common bile duct	Resection off common bile duct; may be able to preserve common bile duct and avoid hepaticojejunostomy
III	1%	Dilation of distal intramural common bile duct; involves sphincter of Oddi	Resection, choledochojejunostomy
IV	10%	Multiple cysts, both intrahepatic and extrahepatic	Resection; may need liver lobectomy; possible TXP
V	1%	Caroli's disease: intrahepatic cysts; get hepatic fibrosis; may be associated with congenital hepatic fibrosis and medullary sponge kidney	Resection; may need lobectomy; possible liver TXP

LYMPHADENOPATHY

- Usually acute suppurative adenitis associated with URI or pharyngitis
- **If fluctuant** → FNA, culture and sensitivity, and antibiotics; may need incision and drainage if it fails to resolve
  - **Chronic causes** – cat scratch fever, atypical mycoplasma
- **Asymptomatic** – antibiotics for 10 days → excisional biopsy if no improvement
  - This is lymphoma until proved otherwise
- **Cystic hygroma** (lymphangioma) – usually found in lateral cervical regions in neck; gets infected; is usually **lateral** to the sternocleidomastoid (SCM) muscle
  - Tx: resection

DIAPHRAGMATIC HERNIAS AND CHEST WALL
- Overall survival 50%
- Increased on **left side** (80%); can have severe **pulmonary HTN**
- 80% have associated anomalies (cardiac and neural tube defects mostly; malrotation)
- Diagnosis can be made with prenatal ultrasound
- Symptoms: respiratory distress
- CXR – bowel in chest
- Tx: high-frequency ventilation; inhaled nitric oxide; may need ECMO
  - Stabilize these patients before operating on them
  - Need to reduce bowel and repair defect ± mesh (abdominal approach)
  - Look for visceral anomalies (run the bowel)
- **Bochdalek's hernia** – most common, located posteriorly
- **Morgagni's hernia** – rare, located anteriorly

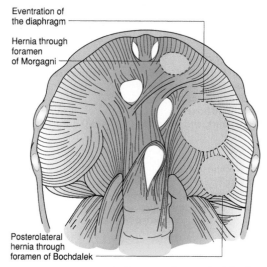

Eventration of the diaphragm

Hernia through foramen of Morgagni

Posterolateral hernia through foramen of Bochdalek

Anatomy of the diaphragm showing the location of congenital diaphragmatic defects.

- **Pectus excavatum** (sinks in) – sternal osteotomy, need strut; performed if causing respiratory symptoms or emotional stress
- **Pectus carinatum** (pigeon chest) – strut not necessary; repair for emotional stress

BRANCHIAL CLEFT CYST
- Leads to cysts, sinuses, and fistulas
- **1st branchial cleft cyst** – angle of mandible; may connect with **external auditory canal**
  - Often associated with **facial nerve**
- **2nd branchial cleft cyst** (<u>most common</u>) – on anterior border of mid-SCM muscle
  - Goes through **carotid bifurcation** into **tonsillar pillar**
- **3rd branchial cleft cyst** – lower neck, **medial** to or through the lower SCM
- Tx for all branchial cysts: resection

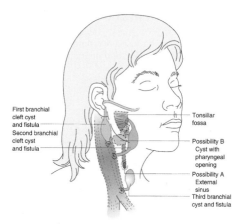

Types of first, second, and third branchial cleft remnants. Sinuses and fistulas are seen most often in infants and young children, whereas cysts usually appear at a later age.

THYROGLOSSAL DUCT CYST
- From the descent of the thyroid gland from the **foramen cecum**
- May be only thyroid tissue patient has
- Presents as a **midline** cervical mass
- Goes through the **hyoid bone**
- Tx: excision of **cyst**, **tract**, and **hyoid bone** (at least the central portion)

HEMANGIOMA
- Appears at birth or shortly after
- Rapid growth during first 6–12 months of life, then begins to involute
- Tx: **observation** – most resolve by age 7–8
- If lesion has **uncontrollable growth**, **impairs function** (eyelid or ear canal), or is **persistent after age 8** → can treat with **oral steroids** → laser or resection if steroids are not successful

NEUROBLASTOMA
- **#1 solid abdominal malignancy in children**
- Usually presents as asymptomatic mass
- Can have secretory diarrhea, raccoon eyes (orbital metastases), **HTN**, and opsomyoclonus syndrome (unsteady gait)
- Most often on **adrenals**; can occur anywhere along the sympathetic chain
- Most common in **1st 2 years of life**
  • Children < 1 year have best prognosis
- Most have ↑ **catecholamines**, **VMA**, **HVA**, and **metanephrines** (HTN)
- Derived from **neural crest cells**
- Encases vasculature rather than invades
- **Rare metastases** – go to lung and bone
- **Abdominal x-ray**: may show stippled calcifications in the tumor
- NSE, LDH, HVA, **diploid tumors**, and **N-myc amplification** (> 3 copies) – have _worse_ prognosis
- NSE is ↑ in all patients with **metastases**
- Tx: resection (**adrenal gland** and **kidney** taken; 40% cured)
- Initially unresectable tumors may be resectable after **doxorubicin**-based chemo

Staging of Neuroblastoma	
Stage	Description
I	Localized, complete excision
II	Incomplete excision but does not cross midline
III	Crosses midline ± regional nodes
IV	Distant metastases (nodes or solid organ)
IV-S	Localized tumor with distant metastases

WILMS TUMOR (NEPHROBLASTOMA)

- Usually presents as asymptomatic mass; can have hematuria or HTN; 10% bilateral
- Mean age at diagnosis – **3 years**
- Prognosis based on **tumor grade** (anaplastic and sarcomatous variations have worse prognosis)
- Frequent metastases to **bone** and **lung**
- Can resect pulmonary metastases if resectable
- Abdominal CT – replacement of renal parenchyma and <u>not</u> displacement (differentiates it from neuroblastoma)
- Tx: **nephrectomy** (90% cured)
  - If venous extension occurs in the renal vein, the tumor can be extracted from the vein
  - Need to examine the contralateral kidney and look for peritoneal implants
  - Avoid rupture of tumor with resection, which will ↑ stage
  - **Actinomycin** and **vincristine** based chemo in all unless Stage I and < 500 g tumor

Staging of Wilms Tumor	
Stage	Description
I	Limited to kidney, completely excised
II	Beyond kidney but completely excised
III	Residual nonhematogenous tumor
IV	Hematogenous metastases
V	Bilateral renal involvement

HEPATOBLASTOMA

- Most common malignant liver tumor in children; ↑ **AFP** in 90%
- Fractures, precocious puberty (from beta-HCG release)
- Better prognosis than hepatocellular CA
- Can be pedunculated; vascular invasion common
- Tx: resection optimal; otherwise **doxorubicin**- and **cisplatin**-based chemotherapy → may downstage tumors and make them resectable
- Survival is primarily related to resectability
- **Fetal histology** has best prognosis

MOST COMMONS

#1 children's malignancy overall – **leukemia** (ALL)
#1 solid tumor class – **CNS tumors**
#1 general surgery tumor – **neuroblastoma**
    #1 in child < 2 years → **neuroblastoma**
    #1 in child > 2 years → **Wilms tumor**

#1 cause of duodenal obstruction in newborns (< 1 week) – **duodenal atresia**
#1 cause of duodenal obstruction after newborn period (> 1 week) and overall –
    malrotation
#1 cause of colon obstruction – **Hirschsprung's disease**
#1 liver tumor in children – **hepatoblastoma**; ⅔ of liver tumors in children are malignant
#1 lung tumor in children – **carcinoid**
Painful lower GI bleeding – **#1 benign anorectal lesions** (fissures, etc.)
Painless lower GI bleeding – **#1 Meckel's diverticulum**
Upper GI bleeding – 0–1 year → **gastritis, esophagitis**
    1 year to adult → **esophageal varices, esophagitis**

MECKEL'S DIVERTICULUM
- Found on **antimesenteric border** of small bowel
- Embryology – **persistent vitelline duct**
- Rule of 2s – 2 feet from ileocecal valve, 2% population, 2% symptomatic, 2 tissue types (**pancreatic** – <u>most common</u>; **gastric** – most likely to be <u>symptomatic</u>), and 2 presentations (diverticulitis and bleeding)
- **#1 cause of painless lower GI bleeding in children**
- Can get Meckel's diverticulum scan with pertechnetate if suspicious of Meckel's diverticulum and having trouble locating
- Tx: resection with symptoms, suspicion of gastric mucosa, or narrow neck
  - Diverticulitis involving the base or if the base is > ⅓ the size of the bowel, need to perform segmental resection

PYLORIC STENOSIS
- 3–12 weeks, firstborn males
- **Projectile vomiting**
- Can feel **olive mass** in stomach
- Get **hypochloremic, hypokalemic metabolic alkalosis**
- Ultrasound – pylorus ≥ 4-mm thick, ≥ 14-mm long
- For severe dehydration, resuscitate with **normal saline boluses** until making urine, then switch to D5 normal saline with 10 mEq K maintenance
  - *Avoid fluid resuscitation with K-containing fluids in children with severe dehydration as hyperkalemia can quickly develop*
  - *Avoid non–salt-containing solutions in infants as hyponatremia can quickly develop*
  - *Infants should always have a maintenance fluid with **glucose** because of their limited reserves for gluconeogenesis and vulnerability for hypoglycemia*
- Tx: **pyloromyotomy** (RUQ incision; proximal extent should be the circular muscles of stomach)

INTUSSUSCEPTION
- Usually 3 months to 3 years
- **Currant jelly stools** (from vascular congestion, <u>not</u> an indication for resection), sausage mass, abdominal distention, RUQ pain, and vomiting
- Invagination of one loop of intestine into another
- Lead points in children – enlarged **Peyer's patches** (#1), lymphoma, and Meckel's diverticulum
- 15% recurrence after reduction
- Tx: reduce with **air-contrast enema** → 80% successful; <u>no</u> surgery required if reduced
  - Max pressure with air-contrast enema – **120 mm Hg**
  - Max column height with barium enema – **1 meter (3 feet)**
  - High perforation risk beyond these values → need to proceed to OR if you have reached these values

- Need to go to OR with peritonitis or free air, or if unable to reduce
  - When reducing in OR, do <u>not</u> place traction on proximal limb of bowel; need to apply pressure to the distal limb
  - Usually do <u>not</u> require resection unless associated with lead point (Meckel's, etc.)
- **Adults presenting with intussusception** – patient most likely has **malignant lead point** (ie colon CA in cecum) → OR for resection

INTESTINAL ATRESIAS
- Develop as a result of **intrauterine vascular accidents**
- Symptoms: bilious emesis, distention; most do not pass meconium
- More common in jejunum; can be <u>multiple</u>
- Get rectal biopsy to R/O Hirschsprung's before surgery
- Tx: resection

DUODENAL ATRESIA
- #1 cause of duodenal obstruction in newborns (< 1 week)
- Usually distal to ampulla of Vater and causes **bilious vomiting**, feeding intolerance
- Associated with polyhydramnios in mother
- Associated with cardiac, renal, and other GI anomalies
- 20% of these patients have **Down's syndrome** (check chromosomal studies)
- Abdominal x-ray – shows **double-bubble sign**
- Tx: resuscitation; duodenoduodenostomy or duodenojejunostomy

TRACHEOESOPHAGEAL FISTULAS (TEF)
- **Type C** – most common type (85%)
  - **Proximal esophageal atresia** (blind pouch) and **distal TE fistula**
  - Symptoms: newborn spits up feeds, has excessive drooling, and respiratory symptoms with feeding; cannot place NG tube in stomach
  - Abdominal x-ray – distended, gas-filled stomach
- **Type A** – second most common type (5%)
  - Esophageal atresia and no fistula
  - Symptoms: similar to type C
  - Abdominal x-ray – patients have gasless abdomen
- **VACTERL syndrome** – **v**ertebral, **a**norectal (imperforate anus), **c**ardiac, **TE** fistula, **r**adius/renal, and **l**imb anomalies
- Tx: **right extrapleural thoracotomy** for most; perform primary repair; and place G-tube
  - Azygous vein often needs to be divided
- **Infants that are premature**, **< 2,500 g**, or **sick** → Replogle tube, treat respiratory symptoms; place G-tube; <u>delay</u> repair
- **Complications of repair** – GERD, leak, empyema, stricture, and fistula
- Survival related to birth weight and associated anomalies

MALROTATION
- Sudden onset of **bilious vomiting** (Ladd's bands cause duodenal obstruction, coming out from the right retroperitoneum)
- Volvulus associated with compromise of the SMA, leading to infarction of the intestine
- Failure of normal counterclockwise rotation (270 degrees)
- 75% in the 1st month; 90% present by 1 year of age
- *Any child with bilious vomiting needs a UGI to rule out malrotation*
- Dx: **UGI** – duodenum does not cross midline; duodenal-jejunal junction displaced to the right
- Tx: resect Ladd's bands, counterclockwise rotation (may require multiple turns), place cecum in LLQ (cecopexy), place duodenum in RUQ, and appendectomy

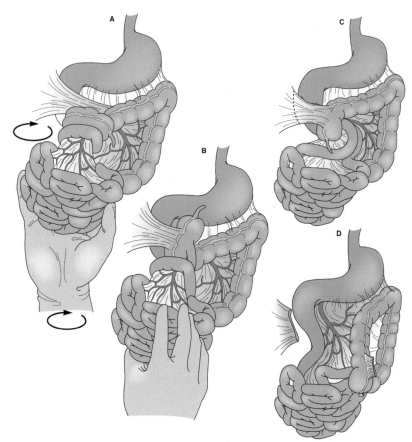

Correction of malrotation. *(A and B)* Detorsion of midgut. *(C and D)* Division of peritoneal attachments (Ladd's bands) of cecum to abdominal cavity.

MECONIUM ILEUS

- Causes **distal ileal obstruction**, abdominal distention, bilious vomiting, and distended loops of bowel
- Need sweat chloride test or PCR for Cl channel defect
- Occurs in 10% of children with **cystic fibrosis**
- Abdominal x-ray: dilated loops of small bowel without air-fluid levels (because the meconium is too thick to separate from the bowel wall); can have ground glass or soapsuds appearance
- Can cause perforation, leading to meconium pseudocyst or free perforation → requires laparotomy
- Tx: **Gastrografin enema** (effective in 80%); can also make the diagnosis and potentially treat the patient
- Can also use *N*-acetylcysteine enema
  - If surgery required, manual decompression and create a vent for ***N*-acetylcysteine antegrade enemas**

NECROTIZING ENTEROCOLITIS (NEC)
■ Classically presents with **bloody stools after 1st feeding** in **premature neonate**
■ Risk factors: prematurity, hypoxia, sepsis
■ Symptoms: lethargy, respiratory decompensation, abdominal distention, vomiting, blood per rectum
■ Abdominal x-ray: may show pneumatosis intestinalis, free air, or portal vein air
■ Need serial lateral decubitus films to look for perforation
■ Initial Tx: resuscitation, NPO, antibiotics, TPN, and orogastric tube
■ Indications for operation: free air, peritonitis, clinical deterioration → resect dead bowel and bring up ostomies
■ Need barium contrast enema before taking down ostomies to rule out distal obstruction from stenosis
■ Mortality 10%

CONGENITAL VASCULAR MALFORMATION
■ Surgery for hemorrhage, ischemia, CHF, nonbleeding ulcers, functional impairment, or limb-length discrepancy
■ Tx: **embolization** (may be sufficient on its own) and/or resection

IMPERFORATE ANUS
■ More common in males
■ Check for associated renal, cardiac, and vertebral (VACTERL) anomalies
■ **High** (above levators) – meconium in **urine** or **vagina** (fistula to bladder/vagina/prostatic urethra)
   • Tx: **colostomy**, later anal reconstruction with **posterior sagittal anoplasty**
■ **Low** (below levators) – meconium to perineal skin; perform **posterior sagittal anoplasty** (pull anus down into sphincter mechanism); **no colostomy needed**
■ Need postop anal dilatation to avoid stricture; these patients are prone to constipation

GASTROSCHISIS
■ **Intrauterine rupture of umbilical vein**; does <u>not</u> have a peritoneal sac
■ ↓ congenital anomalies (only 10%) except malrotation
■ To the right of midline, no peritoneal sac, stiff bowel from exposure to amniotic fluid
■ Tx: initially place saline-soaked gauzes and resuscitate the patient; can lose a lot of fluid from the exposed bowel; TPN, NPO
   • Repair when patient is stable
   • At operation, try to place bowel back in abdomen, may need Vicryl mesh silo
   • Primary closure at a later date if silo used

OMPHALOCELE
■ **Failure of embryonal development**; <u>has peritoneal sac</u> with cord attached
■ ↑ congenital anomalies (50%); midline defect
■ Sac can contain intra-abdominal structures other than bowel (liver, spleen, etc.)
■ **Cantrell pentalogy**
   • **Cardiac** defects
   • **Pericardium** defects (usually at diaphragmatic pericardium)
   • **Sternal** cleft or absence of lower sternum
   • **Diaphragmatic** septum transversum absence
   • **Omphalocele**

- Tx: initially place saline-soaked gauzes and resuscitate the patient; can lose a lot of fluid from the exposed bowel; TPN, NPO
  - Repair when patient is stable
  - At operation, try to place bowel back in abdomen; may need Vicryl mesh silo
  - Primary closure at a later date of mesh used
- Worse overall prognosis compared with gastroschisis secondary to congenital anomalies
- **Malrotation** can occur with both gastroschisis and omphalocele

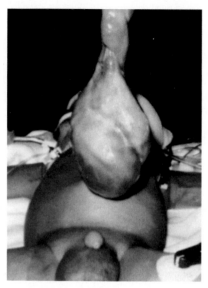

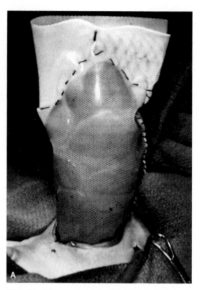

Omphalocele. The herniated intestines and liver are visible inside the sac. The umbilical cord attaches to the sac.

Silastic chimney or silo for temporary coverage of giant omphalocele.

HIRSCHSPRUNG'S DISEASE
- #1 cause of colonic obstruction in infants; more common in males
- **Most common sign** → infants fail to pass meconium in 1st 24 hours
  - Can also present in older age groups as chronic constipation (age 2–3)
- Get **distention**; occasionally get colitis
- Can get explosive release of watery stool with anorectal exam
- **Rectal biopsy** diagnostic (**absence of ganglion cells in myenteric plexus**)
- Is due to failure of the neural crest cells (ganglion cells) to progress in caudad direction
- Need to resect colon until proximal to where ganglion cells appear
- Tx: may need to bring up a colostomy initially, eventually connect the colon to the anus (Soave or Duhamel procedure)
- **Hirschsprung's colitis** – may be rapidly progressive; manifested by abdominal distention and foul-smelling diarrhea
  - Lethargy and signs of sepsis may be present
  - Tx: rectal irrigation to try and empty colon; may need emergency colectomy

UMBILICAL HERNIA
- Failure of closure of linea alba; most close by age 3, rare incarceration
- Increased in African Americans and premature infants
- Tx: surgery if not closed by age 5, incarceration, or if patient has a VP shunt

INGUINAL HERNIA

- Due to **persistent processus vaginalis**; 3% of infants, M > F
- Right in 60%, left in 30%, bilateral in 10%
- Extension of the hernia into the internal ring differentiates hernia from hydrocele
- Tx: emergent operation if not able to reduce; otherwise, elective repair with high ligation
- Consider exploring the contralateral side if left sided, female, or child < 1 year
- Need operation within 24 hours after reduction

HYDROCELE

- Most disappear by 1 year; noncommunicating will resolve; should transilluminate
- Tx: surgery at 1 year if not resolved or if thought to be communicating (waxing and waning size); **resect hydrocele** and **ligate processus vaginalis**

CYSTIC DUPLICATION

- Most common in ileum; often on mesenteric border
- Tx: resect cyst

BILIARY ATRESIA

- Most common cause of neonatal jaundice requiring surgery
- Progressive jaundice persisting > 2 weeks after birth suggests atresia
- Can involve either the extrahepatic or intrahepatic biliary tree or both
- Dx: liver biopsy → periportal fibrosis, bile plugging, eventual cirrhosis
  - Ultrasound and cholangiography can reveal atretic biliary tree
- Get cholangitis, continued cirrhosis, and eventual hepatic failure
- Try Kasai procedure (hepaticoportojejunostomy) – ⅓ get better, ⅓ go on to liver transplant, and ⅓ die
  - Involves resecting the atretic extrahepatic bile duct segment

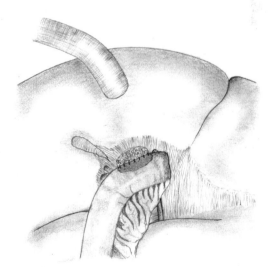

Anastomosis of Roux-en-Y hepatoportoenterostomy to liver. (From Qureshi FG, Ergun O, Ford HR. Biliary atresia. In: Fischer JE, Bland KI, et al, eds. *Mastery of Surgery*. 5th ed. Philadelphia, PA: Lippincott Williams & Wilkins; 2007, with permission.)

- Need to perform Kasai procedure **before age 3 months**, o/w get irreversible liver damage

TERATOMA
- ↑ AFP and **beta-HCG**
- **Neonates** – sacrococcygeal; **adolescents** – ovarian
- Tx: excision
- **Sacrococcygeal teratomas**
  - 90% benign at birth (almost all have exophytic component)
  - Great potential for malignancy
  - AFP – good marker
  - 2-month mark is a huge transition – **< 2 months** → usually benign; **> 2 months** → usually malignant
  - Tx: **coccygectomy** and long-term follow-up

UNDESCENDED TESTICLES
- Wait until 2 years old to treat
- Higher risk of testicular CA in these children
- Cancer risk stays the same even if testicles brought into scrotum
- Get **seminoma**
- If undescended bilaterally, get chromosomal studies
- If you cannot feel the testes in the inguinal canal, you need to get an MRI to confirm their presence
- Tx: orchiopexy through inguinal incision; if not able to get testicles down → close and wait 6 months and try again; if will not come down, perform division of spermatic vessels

TRACHEOMALACIA
- Elliptical, fragmented tracheal rings instead of C-shaped
- Wheezing, usually get better after 1–2 years
- **Surgical indications** – dying spell, failure to wean from ventilator, recurrent infections
- Surgery – **aortopexy** (aorta sutured to the back of the sternum, opens up trachea)

LARYNGOMALACIA
- Most common cause of airway obstruction in infants
- Symptoms: intermittent respiratory distress and stridor exacerbation in the supine position
- Caused by immature epiglottis cartilage with intermittent collapse of the epiglottis airway
- Most children outgrow this by 12 months
- Surgical tracheostomy reserved for a very small number of patients

CHOANAL ATRESIA
- Obstruction of choanal opening (nasal passage) by either bone or mucous membrane, usually unilateral
- Symptoms: intermittent respiratory distress, poor suckling
- Tx: surgical correction

LARYNGEAL PAPILLOMATOSIS
- Most common tumor of the pediatric larynx
- Frequently **involutes after puberty**
- Can treat with endoscopic removal or laser but frequently comes back
- Thought to be caused from HPV in the mother during passage through the birth canal

CEREBRAL PALSY
- Many develop **GERD**

Neonatal Intestinal Obstruction

Diagnosis	History	Physical Examination	Diagnostic Studies
Intestinal atresia or stenosis	Bilious emesis	Abdominal distention	Plain abdominal film
Duodenal atresia or stenosis	Failure to pass meconium	Acholic meconium Gastric distention	Contrast enema Plain abdominal film
	Bilious emesis	Trisomy 21	Upper GI contrast study
Imperforate anus	Failure to pass meconium	Absent anus or visible fistula	Plain chest, abdominal film
	Bilious emesis (late)	Abdominal distention	Ultrasound kidneys, sacrum, rectum
		VACTERL association	Echocardiogram
Necrotizing enterocolitis	High-risk, premature infant	Abdominal distention	Plain abdominal film
	Bilious emesis	Hematochezia, guaiac-positive stool	
Meconium ileus	Cystic fibrosis (10%)	Acholic meconium	Plain abdominal film
	Bilious emesis	Abdominal distention	Contrast enema
Malrotation	Bilious emesis	No abdominal distention	Plain abdominal film
	Term, healthy infant		Upper GI contrast study
Hirschsprung's disease	Delayed passage of meconium	Abdominal distention	Plain abdominal film
	Bilious emesis	Trisomy 21	Contrast enema

GI, gastrointestinal; VACTERL, vertebral, anal, cardiac, tracheal, esophageal, renal, and limb anomalies.

- **Type I error** – rejects null hypothesis incorrectly → falsely assumed there was a difference when no difference exists
- **Type II error** – accepts null hypothesis incorrectly because of **small sample size** → the treatments are interpreted as equal when there is actually a difference
- **Null hypothesis** – hypothesis that no difference exists between groups
- **$p < 0.05$ rejects the null hypothesis**
  - **$p < 0.05$** = > 95% likelihood that the difference between the populations is true
  - < 5% likelihood that the difference is not true and occurred by chance alone
- **Variance** – spread of data around a mean
- **Parameter** – population
- **Numeric terms** – example: 2, 7, 7, 8, 9, 11, 15
  - **Mode** – most frequently occurring value = 7
  - **Mean** – average = 9
  - **Median** – middle value of a set of data (50th percentile) = 8

TRIALS AND STUDIES
- **Randomized controlled trial** – prospective study with random assignment to treatment and nontreatment groups
  - **Avoids treatment biases**
- **Double-blind controlled trial** – prospective study in which patient and doctor are blind to the treatment
  - **Avoids observational biases**
- **Cohort study** – prospective study → compares disease rate between exposed and unexposed groups (nonrandom assignment)
- **Case-control study** – retrospective study in which those who have the disease are compared with a similar population who do not have the disease; the frequency of the suspected risk factor is then compared between the 2 groups
- **Meta-analysis** – combining data from <u>different studies</u>

QUANTITATIVE VARIABLES
- **Student's t test** – 2 independent groups and variable is **quantitative** → compares means (mean weight between 2 groups)
- **Paired t tests** – variable is **quantitative**; before and after studies (eg weight before and after, drug versus placebo)
- **ANOVA** – compares **quantitative** variables (means) for more than 2 groups

QUALITATIVE VARIABLES
- **Nonparametric statistics** – compare categorical (qualitative) variables **(race, sex, medical problems and diseases, medications)**
- **Chi-squared test** – compares 2 groups with **categorical (qualitative) variables** (number of obese patients with and without diabetes versus number of nonobese patients with and without diabetes)
- **Kaplan-Meyer** – small groups → estimates survival
- **Relative risk** = incidence in exposed/incidence in unexposed
- **Power of test** = probability of making the correct conclusion = 1 − probability of type II error
  - Likelihood that the conclusion of the test is true
  - Larger sample size increases power of a test

- **Prevalence** – number of people with disease in a population (eg number of patients in United States with colon CA)
  - Long-standing disease increases prevalence
- **Incidence** – number of new cases diagnosed over a certain time frame in a population (eg number of patients in United States newly diagnosed with colon CA in 2003)
- **Sensitivity** – ability to detect disease = true-positives/(true-positives + false-negatives)
  - Indicates the number of people who have the disease who test positive
  - **With high sensitivity**, a <u>negative test result means patient is very unlikely to have disease</u>

	Positive Test	Negative Test
Have disease	True-positive (TP)	False-negative (FN)
No disease	False-positive (FP)	True-negative (TN)

- **Specificity** – ability to state no disease is present = true-negatives/(true-negatives + false-positives)
  - Indicates the number of people who do not have the disease who test negative
  - **With high specificity**, a <u>positive test result means patient is very likely to have disease</u>
- **Positive predictive value** = true-positives/(true-positives + false-positives)
  - Likelihood that with a positive result, the patient actually has the disease
- **Negative predictive value** = true-negatives/(true-negatives + false-negatives)
  - Likelihood that with a negative result, the patient does not have the disease
- **Accuracy** = true-positives + true-negatives/true-positives + true-negatives + false-positives + false-negatives
- **Predictive value** – depends on disease prevalence
- **Sensitivity** and **specificity** – are independent of prevalence

PATIENT SAFETY
- **National Surgical Quality Improvement Program** (NSQIP) – seeks to collect outcome data to measure and improve surgical quality in the United States. Outcomes are reported as observed vs. expected ratios.
- **JCAHO prevention of wrong site/procedure/patient protocol**:
  - Pre-op verification of **patient** and **procedure**
  - **Operative site** and **side** (marking if left or right or multiple levels; must be visible after the patient is prepped)
  - **Time out** before incision made (verifying <u>patient</u>, <u>procedure</u>, <u>position site + side</u>, and availability of <u>implants</u> or <u>special requirements</u>)
- **Promoting culture of safety**
  - Confidential system of reporting errors
  - Emphasis on learning over accountability
  - Flexibility in adapting to new situations or problems
- **RFs for retained object after surgery** (MC sponge) – emergency procedure, unplanned change in procedure, obesity, towel used for closure
- **Sentinel Event** (JCAHO) – unexpected occurrence involving death or serious injury, or the risk thereof; hospital undergoes **root cause analysis** to prevent and minimize future occurrences (eg **wrong site surgery**)
- **GAP protection technique** – gaps in care (eg change in caregiver, divisions of labor, shift changes, transfers) can lead to loss of information and error; **prevention** – **structured handoffs** and **checklists** (face to face if possible); standardizing orders; reading back orders if verbal

↑	increased *or* high
↓	decreased *or* low
2,3-DPG	2,3-diphosphoglycerate
5FU	5-fluorouracil
AAA	abdominal aortic aneurysm
Ab	antibody
Abd	abdominal
abx	antibiotic
AC	doxorubicin (Adriamycin) and cyclophosphamide (Cytoxan)
ACE	angiotensin-converting enzyme
Ach	acetylcholine
ACT	activated clotting time
ACTH	adrenocorticotropic hormone
AD	autosomal dominant
ADH	antidiuretic hormone
ADL	activities of daily living
AFP	alpha-fetoprotein
Ag	antigen
AIDS	acquired immunodeficiency syndrome
AKA	above-knee amputation
ALL	acute lymphoblastic leukemia
ALND	axillary lymph node dissection
ALT	alanine aminotransferase
angio	angiography
ANOVA	analysis of variance
AP	aortopulmonary
APACHE	acute physiology and chronic health evaluation
APR	abdominoperineal resection
APUD	amine precursor uptake and decarboxylation
ARDS	acute respiratory distress syndrome
ASA	acetylsalicylic acid
ASD	atrial septal defect
AST	aspartate aminotransferase
ATGAM	antithymocyte gamma globulin
AT-III	antithrombin III
ATN	acute tubular necrosis
ATP	adenosine triphosphate
ATPase	adenosine triphosphatase
A-V	arteriovenous
AV	atrioventricular
AVM	arteriovenous malformation
AVN	avascular necrosis
AXR	abdominal radiograph
BCG	bacille Calmette-Guérin
BKA	below-knee amputation
BM	bowel movement
BPH	benign prostatic hypertrophy
BSA	body surface area
BT shunt	Blalock-Taussig shunt
BUN	blood urea nitrogen
Bx	biopsy
Ca	calcium
CA	cancer, carcinoma
CABG	coronary artery bypass graft
cAMP	cyclic adenosine monophosphate
CaO_2	arterial oxygen content
CBD	common bile duct
CCK	cholecystokinin
cCMP	3,5-cyclic monophosphate (cytidine)
CD	cluster of differentiation (eg CD4, CD8)
CEA	carcinoembryonic antigen
CEA	carotid endarterectomy
cGMP	cyclic guanosine-3, 5-monophosphate
chemo	chemotherapy
CHF	chronic heart failure
CI	cardiac index
CLL	chronic lymphocytic leukemia
CMF	cyclophosphamide (Cytoxan), methotrexate, and 5-fluorouracil
CML	chronic myelogenous leukemia
CMV	cytomegalovirus
CN	cranial nerve
CNS	central nervous system
CO	cardiac output
COPD	chronic obstructive pulmonary disease
CPAP	continuous positive airway pressure
CPP	cerebral perfusion pressure
CPR	cardiopulmonary resuscitation
Cr	creatinine
CRH	corticotropin-releasing hormone
CSA	cyclosporin
CSF	cerebrospinal fluid
CT	computed tomography
CVA	cerebrovascular accident (stroke)
CVHD	continuous venovenous hemodialysis
CvO_2	venous oxygen content

CVP	central venous pressure
Cx	complication
CXR	chest radiograph
D/C	discontinue
DAG	diacylglycerol
DBP	diastolic blood pressure
DCIS	ductal carcinoma in situ
DDAVP	desmopressin acetate, 1-desamino-8-d-arginine-vasopressin
DES	diethylstilbestrol
DIC	disseminated intravascular coagulation
DIT	diiodotyrosine
DKA	diabetic ketoacidosis
DLCO	diffusing capacity of the lung for carbon monoxide
DM	diabetes mellitus
DPL	diagnostic peritoneal lavage
DVT	deep venous thrombosis
Dx	diagnosis
DZ	disease
EBV	Epstein-Barr virus
ECA	external carotid artery
ECHO	echocardiogram
ECMO	extracorporeal membrane oxygenation
EDRF	endothelium-derived relaxing factor
EDV	end-diastolic volume
EEG	electroencephalogram
EF	ejection fraction
EGD	esophagogastroduodenoscopy
EGF	epidermal growth factor
EKG	electrocardiogram
ELAM	endothelial leukocyte adhesion molecule
EPI	epinephrine
ER	emergency room *or* endoplasmic reticulum
ERCP	endoscopic retrograde cholangiopancreatography
ERV	expiratory reserve volume
ESR	erythrocyte sedimentation rate
ESWL	extracorporeal shock wave lithotripsy
ET	endotracheal
ETCO$_2$	end-tidal CO$_2$
ETOH	ethanol, alcohol
F/U	follow-up
FAP	familial adenomatous polyposis
FAST	focused abdominal sonography for trauma

Fc	antibody fragment, crystallizable
FEV$_1$	forced expiratory volume in 1 second
FFP	fresh frozen plasma
FGF	fibroblastic growth factor
FiO$_2$	fraction of inspired oxygen
FNA	fine needle aspiration
FRC	functional residual capacity
FSH	follicle-stimulating hormone
FTSG	full-thickness skin graft
FTT	failure to thrive
Fx	fracture
G6PD	glucose-6-phosphate dehydrogenase
GCS	Glasgow Coma Scale
GCSF	granulocyte colony–stimulating factor
GDA	gastroduodenal artery
GERD	gastroesophageal reflux disease
GFR	glomerular filtration rate
GH	growth hormone
GHRH	growth hormone–releasing hormone
GI	gastrointestinal
GIP	gastric inhibitory peptide
GIST	gastrointestinal stromal tumor
GNR	gram-negative rod
GnRH	gonadotropin-releasing hormone
GPC	gram-positive cocci
GPR	gram-positive rod
GRP	gastrin-releasing peptide
GSH	glutathione
GU	genitourinary
H and P	history and physical
HA	headache
HBIG	hepatitis B immunoglobulin
HBV	hepatitis B virus
HCG	human chorionic gonadotropin
HCl	hydrochloric acid; hydrochloride
Hct	hematocrit
HCT	hematocrit
HCV	hepatitis C virus
HETE	hydroxyeicosatetraenoic acid
HGB/Hgb	hemoglobin
HIDA	hepatic iminodiacetic acid
HIT	heparin-induced thrombocytopenia
HIV	human immunodeficiency virus
HLA	human leukocyte antigen
HMG CoA	_-hydroxy-_-methylglutaryl-CoA

HMW	high molecular weight	LTC$_4$	leukotriene C$_4$
HPETE	hydroperoxyeicosatetraenoic acid	LTD$_4$	leukotriene D$_4$
		LTE$_4$	leukotriene E$_4$
HPF	high-power field	LV	left ventricle *or* left ventricular
HPV	human papillomavirus	LVEDV	left ventricular end-diastolic volume
HR	heart rate		
HSV	herpes simplex virus	LVEF	left ventricular ejection fraction
HTLV-1	human T-cell leukemia virus 1	LVESV	left ventricular end-systolic volume
HTN	hypertension		
HUS	hemolytic uremic syndrome	LVOT	left ventricular outflow tract
HVA	homovanillic acid	MAC	minimum alveolar concentration
IABP	intra-aortic balloon pump		
IBW	ideal body weight	MALT	mucosa-associated lymphoid tissue
ICA	internal carotid artery		
ICAM	intracellular adhesion molecule	MAO	monoamine oxidase
ICP	intracranial pressure	MAOI	monoamine oxidase inhibitor
ICU	intensive care unit	MAP	mean arterial pressure
Ig	immunoglobulin	MEN	multiple endocrine neoplasia
IJ	internal jugular	MHC	major histocompatibility complex
IL	interleukin		
IMA	inferior mesenteric artery *or* internal mammary artery	MI	myocardial infarction
		MIBG	radioactive iodine meta-idobenzoguanidine
IMF	intramaxillary fixation		
IMV	inferior mesenteric vein	MIT	monoiodotyrosine
INF	interferon	MRA	magnetic resonance angiogram
INH	isoniazid	MRCP	magnetic resonance cholangiopancreatography
INR	international normalized ratio		
ITP	idiopathic thrombocytopenic purpura	MRM	modified radical mastectomy
		MRND	modified radical neck dissection
IV	intravenous		
IVC	inferior vena cava	MRSA	methicillin-resistant *S. aureus*
IVF	intravenous fluid	MS	mental status
IVP	intravenous pyelogram	MSH	melanocyte-stimulating hormone
L	liter		
LA	left atrium	MTP	metatarsophalangeal
LAD	left anterior descending (coronary artery)	MTX	methotrexate
		N/V	nausea and vomiting
LAK	lymphokine-activated killer	NADH	nicotinamide adenine dinucleotide
LAR	low anterior resection		
LATS	long-acting thyroid stimulator	NADPH	nicotinamide adenine dinucleotide phosphate
LCIS	lobular carcinoma in situ		
LD$_{50}$	dose that will kill 50% of test subjects	NAPA	*N*-acetylprocainamide
		NE	norepinephrine
LDH	lactate dehydrogenase	NEC	necrotizing enterocolitis
LES	lower esophageal sphincter	NGT	nasogastric tube
LFT	liver function test	NHL	non-Hodgkin's lymphoma
LH	luteotropic hormone	NIF	negative inspiratory force
LHRH	luteinizing hormone–releasing hormone	NO	nitric oxide
		NPO	nil per os (nothing by mouth)
LLQ	left lower quadrant	NS	normal saline (solution)
LR	lactated Ringer's	NSAID	nonsteroidal anti-inflammatory drug
LS ratio	lecithin:sphingomyelin ratio		
LTA$_4$	leukotriene A$_4$	NSE	neuron-specific enolase
LTB$_4$	leukotriene B$_4$	NTG	nitroglycerine

OCP	oral contraceptive pills
OKT3	murine monoclonal anti-CD3 antibody therapy
Op-DDD	2,4-dichlorodiphenyl-dichloroethane (mitotane)
OR	operating room
ORIF	open reduction and internal fixation
PA	pulmonary artery
PABA	p-aminobenzoic acid
PADP	pulmonary artery diastolic pressure
PAF	platelet-activating factor
PAS	periodic acid–Schiff stain
PCN	penicillin
PCR	polymerase chain
PDA	patent ductus arteriosus
PDGF	platelet-derived growth factor
PE	pulmonary embolism
PECAM	platelet/endothelial cell adhesion molecule
PEEP	positive end-expiratory pressure
PEG	percutaneous endoscopic gastrostomy
PGD_2	prostaglandin D_2
PGE_1	prostaglandin E_1
PGE_2	prostaglandin E_2
PGF_2	prostaglandin F_2
PGG_2	prostaglandin G_2
PGH_2	prostaglandin H_2
PGI_2	prostaglandin I_2 (prostacyclin)
PMHx	past medical history
PMN	polymorphonuclear leukocytes
PNA	pneumonia
PNMT	phenylethanolamine-N-methyl-transferase
POD	postoperative day
PPN	peripheral line parenteral nutrition
PRBC	packed red blood cells
PSA	prostate-specific antigen
PSSS	postsplenectomy sepsis syndrome
PT	prothrombin time
PTA	percutaneous transluminal angioplasty
PTC	percutaneous transhepatic cholangiography
PTCA	percutaneous transluminal coronary angioplasty
PTFE	polytetrafluoroethylene
PTH	parathyroid hormone
PTHrP	parathyroid hormone–related peptide
PTT	partial thromboplastin time
PTU	propylthiouracil
PTX	pneumothorax
PUD	peptic ulcer disease
PVC	premature ventricular contraction
PVR	pulmonary vascular resistance
Qp/Qs	pulmonary-to-systemic flow ratio
R/O	rule out
RA	right atrium
RBC	red blood cell
RLL	right lower lobe
RLN	recurrent laryngeal nerve
RND	radical neck dissection
ROM	range of motion
RPR	rapid plasma reagin
RQ	respiratory quotient
RR	respiratory rate
RUG	retrograde urethrogram
RUL	right upper lobe
RUQ	right upper quadrant
RV	residual volume *or* right ventricle
S/E	side effect
S–B	Sengstaken–Blakemore (tube)
SBFT	small bowel follow-through
SBO	small bowel obstruction
SBP	spontaneous bacterial peritonitis
SBP	systolic blood pressure
SCC	squamous cell carcinoma
SCD	sequential compression device
SCM	sternocleidomastoid
SCV	subclavian
SFA	superficial femoral artery
SIRS	systemic inflammatory response syndrome
SLE	systemic lupus erythematosus
SMA	superior mesenteric artery
SMV	superior mesenteric vein
SOB	shortness of breath
STSG	split-thickness skin graft
SVC	superior vena cava
SvO_2	mixed venous oxygen saturation
SVR	systemic vascular resistance
SVRI	systemic vascular resistance index
SVT	supraventricular tachycardia
Sx	symptom

T bili	total bilirubin		TXA_2	thromboxane A_2
TAG	triacylglyceride		TXP	transplant
TAH	total abdominal hysterectomy		U/S	ultrasound
TB	tuberculosis		UC	ulcerative colitis
TBG	thyroid-binding globulin		UDCA	ursodeoxycholic acid
TCOM	transcutaneous oxygen measurement		UES	upper esophageal sphincter
			UGI	upper gastrointestinal
TCR	T-cell receptor		URI	upper respiratory tract infection
TE	tracheoesophageal			
TEN	toxic epidermal necrolysis		UTI	urinary tract infection
TFT	thyroid function test		UV	ultraviolet
TGF-β	transforming growth factor-beta		V/Q	ventilation/perfusion
			VC	vital capacity
TIA	transient ischemic attack		VCAM	vascular cell adhesion molecule
TIPS	transjugular intrahepatic portosystemic shunt			
			V-fib	ventricular fibrillation
TLC	total lung capacity		VIP	vasoactive intestinal peptide
TMJ	temporomandibular joint		VIPoma	vasoactive intestinal peptide–producing tumor
TNF	tumor necrosis factor			
TOS	thoracic outlet syndrome		VLDL	very-low-density lipids
tPA	tissue plasminogen activator		VMA	vanillylmandelic acid
TPN	total parenteral nutrition		VO_2	oxygen consumption
TRALI	transfusion-related acute lung injury		VP-16	etoposide
			VRE	vancomycin-resistant *Enterococcus*
TRAM	transverse rectus abdominis myocutaneous			
			VSD	ventricular septal defect
TRH	thyrotropin-releasing hormone		V-tach	ventricular tachycardia
			vWD	von Willebrand's disease
TSH	thyroid-stimulating hormone		vWF	von Willebrand factor
TSI	thyroid-stimulating immunoglobulin		W/U	workup
			WBC	white blood cell
TTP	thrombotic thrombocytopenic purpura		WDHA	watery diarrhea, hypokalemia, achlorhydria
TURP	transurethral resection of the prostate; transurethral prostatectomy		wedge	pulmonary artery wedge pressure
			WLE	wide local excision
TV	tidal volume		XRT	radiation therapy
Tx	treatment		Z–E/ZES	Zollinger–Ellison syndrome

INDEX

Note: Page numbers in *italics* denote figures; those followed by a "t" denote tables

A

Abdominal aorta, *152*
Abdominal aortic aneurysms, 151–154, 153t
Abdominal aortic disease. *See* Vascular
  disorders
Abdominal compartment syndrome, 57
Abdominoperineal resection (APR), 230, *231*
Abnormal bleeding, causes of. *See also under*
  Hematology
  ASA, 7
  coumadin, 8
  disseminated intravascular coagulation, 8
  epistaxis, 8
  factor VII deficiency, 6–7
  H and P, 8
  hemophilia A, 7
  hemophilia B, 7
  heparin-induced thrombocytopenia, 7
  incomplete hemostasis, 6
  menorrhagia, 8
  normal circumcision, 8
  platelet disorders, 7
  platelets, 8
  prostate surgery, 8
  tonsillectomy, 8
  tooth extraction, 8
  von Willebrand's disease, 6–7
Abnormal hypercoagulability, 8–9
Abnormal uterine bleeding, 258
Abnormal wound healing, 54
ABO blood-type antigens, 2
Abortions, 255
Abscesses
  anorectal, 241
  benign breast disease, 126
  head and neck (*See under* Head and neck)
  infection, 15
  liver (*See under* Liver)
Acalculous cholecystitis, 198
Accelerated rejection, 46
Access grafts, 163
Accessory breast tissue (polythelia), 126
Accessory nipples, 126
Accessory spleen, 213
Achalasia, 170

Acid–base balance, 34t
Acidosis, 82
Acoustic neuroma, 103, 262
Acquired A-V fistula, 163
Acquired hypercoagulability, 8
Acquired thrombocytopenia, 7
Acral lentiginous melanoma, 94
Acromegaly, 107
Acromioclavicular separation, 265
Actin, 4
Actinic keratosis, 97
Actinomyces, 17, 236
Acute arterial emboli, 158
Acute arterial thrombosis, 158
Acute hemolysis, 11
Acute pancreatitis, 206–207
Acute rejection
  heart transplantation, 48
  in kidney transplantation, 46
  in liver transplantation, 47
  lung transplantation, 48
Acute renal failure, 34, 35
Acute respiratory distress syndrome, 82, *82*, 82t
Acute septic arthritis, 18
Acute subdural hematoma, *260*
Acyclovir, 22
Addison's disease, 111
Adenocarcinoma, 172, 223, 243
Adenoid cystic adenoma, 139
Adenoid cystic CA, 101
Adenomas
  adenoid cystic, 139
  adrenal, 111
  bronchial, 139
  multiple, 121
  pituitary, 123
  single, 121
Adenomatous polyps, 182
Adenosine, 25
Adjuvant therapy, 133
Adrenal
  adenoma, 111
  cortex, 109–111
  hyperplasia, 111
  insufficiency, 78, 110
  medulla, 111–112